AF712647

Social Disparities in Health and Health Care

Series editors

Ronald J. Angel, Austin, TX, USA
William R. Avison, London, ON, Canada

More information about this series at http://www.springer.com/series/8142

Mandi M. Larsen

Health Inequities Related to Intimate Partner Violence Against Women

The Role of Social Policy in the United States, Germany, and Norway

Springer

Mandi M. Larsen
Jacobs University Bremen
Bremen
Germany

Social Disparities in Health and Health Care
ISBN 978-3-319-29563-3 ISBN 978-3-319-29565-7 (eBook)
DOI 10.1007/978-3-319-29565-7

Library of Congress Control Number: 2016930273

© Springer International Publishing Switzerland 2016
This work is subject to copyright. All rights are reserved by the Publisher, whether the whole or part of the material is concerned, specifically the rights of translation, reprinting, reuse of illustrations, recitation, broadcasting, reproduction on microfilms or in any other physical way, and transmission or information storage and retrieval, electronic adaptation, computer software, or by similar or dissimilar methodology now known or hereafter developed.
The use of general descriptive names, registered names, trademarks, service marks, etc. in this publication does not imply, even in the absence of a specific statement, that such names are exempt from the relevant protective laws and regulations and therefore free for general use.
The publisher, the authors and the editors are safe to assume that the advice and information in this book are believed to be true and accurate at the date of publication. Neither the publisher nor the authors or the editors give a warranty, express or implied, with respect to the material contained herein or for any errors or omissions that may have been made.

Printed on acid-free paper

This Springer imprint is published by SpringerNature
The registered company is Springer International Publishing AG Switzerland

Acknowledgements

This book is based on my doctoral dissertation at the University of Bremen and Jacobs University Bremen in Germany. First and foremost, I am very grateful for the financial and institutional support of the Bremen International Graduate School of Social Sciences (BIGSSS), without which I may never have embarked upon the path of doctoral study. My sincerest gratitude goes to Heinz Rothgang and Karin Gottschall for guiding my research and sharing their welfare state expertise with me. I owe Petra Brzank many thanks for her willingness many years ago to meet an American newcomer for coffee in Hamburg's *Hauptbahnhof*, and for her continuing mentorship in the field of violence against women. A research stay in Norway greatly enriched both my doctoral work and my ancestral connection to the country. *Tusen takk* to Lars Kristofersen and Jon Ivar Elstad of NOVA in Oslo, as well as to Terje Eikemo of the Norwegian University of Science and Technology in Trondheim, for their tremendous Norwegian hospitality.

I am deeply indebted to the many friends and colleagues who have provided commentary and feedback on my research. In particular, I extend my gratitude toward Nate Breznau, Alexi Gugushvili, Zsófia Ignácz, and Katja Möhring for making the time to share valuable comments on earlier versions of these chapters in their dissertation form. My research has also benefited greatly from the critique provided by Lorraine Frisina Doetter, Ralf Götze, Alexander Haarmann, Simone Haasler, Markus Kiesel, and Simone Scherger during the BIGSSS Colloquia. Any errors found in this work are solely my own.

My heartfelt thanks go to my dear friend Daniel Senkowski for always believing in me, even in the moments when I did not. Above all, I would never have made it this far without the unconditional love and encouragement of my family—my parents Terry and Sandra Larsen, my brother Chad Larsen, my sister and brother-in-law Kirsten and David Geyer, and my nephews Coen and Blake Geyer.

Words cannot express how much their support has meant to me in all of my adventures and endeavors thus far, even when it has meant being thousands of miles apart.

Bremen
November 2015

Mandi M. Larsen

Contents

Abbreviations

AFDC	Aid to Families with Dependent Children
BIC	Bayesian information criterion
BMFSFJ	*Bundesministerium für Familie, Senioren, Frauen und Jugend*
CAHRV	Coordination Action on Human Rights Violations
CDC	US Centers for Disease Control and Prevention
CTS	Conflict Tactics Scales
EU	European Union
FMLA	Family and Medical Leave Act
FRA	European Union Agency for Fundamental Rights
GDP	Gross domestic product
IPV	Intimate partner violence
IRR	Incident risk ratio
NAV	Norwegian Labor and Welfare Administration
NGO	Nongovernmental organizations
NIBR	Norwegian Institute of Urban and Regional Research
NIJ	US National Institute of Justice
NIS	Norwegian National Insurance Scheme
NOK	Norwegian Kroner
OECD	Organisation for Economic Co-operation and Development
OR	Odds ratio
PCP	Primary care provider
PMM	Predictive mean matching
PPACA	US Patient Protection and Affordable Care Act
PTSD	Post-traumatic stress disorder
RQ	Research question
RRR	Relative risk ratio
SAH	Self-assessed health
SHI	Statutory health insurance
SOEP	Socio-Economic Panel Study
SSB	Statistics Norway
TANF	Temporary Assistance for Needy Families

UK	United Kingdom
US	United States of America
VAWA	US Violence Against Women Act
WHO	World Health Organization
ZIF	*Zentrale Informationsstelle Autonomer Frauenhäuser*

Chapter 1
Introduction

Abstract Violence against women is a major source of health inequalities, necessitating the investigation of the relationships between violence and economic inequality, weak social safety nets, and poverty. While the health effects of intimate partner violence (IPV) have been well researched, there is a gap in knowledge regarding the factors contributing to women's individual risk of IPV, as well as those which contribute to the stratification of IPV within and across societies. This book aims to close this gap, and this chapter begins by defining key terminology, especially regarding IPV, the welfare state, and health inequities. In naming this book's research puzzle, the conceptual framework is briefly mentioned before describing the key contributions of this work. The chapter closes with a chapter-by-chapter overview of the book.

Violence against women is a phenomenon occurring worldwide. More than two decades ago, the 'Declaration on the Elimination of Violence Against Women' explicitly acknowledged it as an international human rights concern (United Nations General Assembly 1993). Since then, international prevalence surveys have established that violence within an intimate partnership is one of the most common forms of violence against women, occurring across social, economic, and cultural boundaries (Ellsberg et al. 2008). A recent survey has shown that 22 % of women in the European Union (EU) have experienced physical or sexual violence from a partner (European Union Agency for Fundamental Rights [FRA] 2014). Moreover, another survey found that 24 % of US women report having experienced severe physical violence from a partner in their lifetime (Black et al. 2011). Given its prevalence, there is a growing consensus that intimate partner violence (IPV) and its consequences represent a serious societal and political burden.

All forms of violence against women are known to lead to negative health consequences and worldwide it is a major source of health inequalities (Heise et al. 1999; Krug et al. 2002). Researchers have recently begun to demonstrate that poor self-perceived health and psychological distress may be more strongly associated with IPV than other forms of violence against women (Vives-Cases et al. 2011). An international spectrum of studies has shown that when compared to nonabused women, victims of IPV have poorer overall health, more symptoms, and are more than twice as likely to report a disability (Bonomi et al. 2006; Coker et al. 2005;

© Springer International Publishing Switzerland 2016
M.M. Larsen, *Health Inequities Related to Intimate Partner Violence Against Women*, Social Disparities in Health and Health Care,
DOI 10.1007/978-3-319-29565-7_1

Eberhard-Gran et al. 2007; Garcia-Moreno et al. 2005; Hagemann-White 2005; Wijma et al. 2003). Using national survey data, an Australian study concluded that IPV presents a larger population health risk than high blood pressure, tobacco use, and being overweight (Vos et al. 2006). The negative physical and mental health effects are even more pronounced for women who experience a greater severity of IPV (Dutton et al. 2005; Ford-Gilboe et al. 2009; Straus et al. 2009; Wuest et al. 2010). Likewise, more recent exposure and longer duration of IPV are associated with incrementally worse health outcomes (Bonomi et al. 2006). Another critical finding is that IPV continues to negatively impact women's health up to 5 years after leaving a violent relationship (Alsaker et al. 2007; Campbell and Lewandowski 1997; Ford-Gilboe et al. 2009). Taken together, these studies demonstrate the devastating and often sustained negative impact of IPV on women's health.

While the health effects of IPV have been well researched, there is a gap in knowledge regarding the factors contributing to women's individual risk of IPV, as well as those which contribute to the stratification of IPV within and across societies (Heise 2012). Thus, some researchers argue that the focus needs to shift away from the question of whether abuse affects health, and instead examine "*who* recovers from these problems, who is most at-risk of sustained poor health, and how the *conditions of women's lives* impact outcomes *over time* …" (Ford-Gilboe et al. 2009, p. 1021, emphasis in original). Essentially, if effective policies and services addressing IPV are to be evidence-based, then it is vital to examine who is most vulnerable to IPV and its health consequences, and whether these vulnerabilities are a result of systematic stratification. This focal shift serves as the launching point for this book.

Before continuing, however, it may be helpful to explain some of the key terminology used in this book. The term 'intimate partner violence' is used as opposed to a number of other common terms that have been applied to this phenomenon since the feminist movement of the 1970s first labeled it as a social problem. Originally, 'wife battering' and 'spouse abuse' were commonly used (see for example, Labell 1979; Martin 1976), and gradually the term 'domestic violence' came into favor as it became clear that violence also occurs in unmarried couples (Nicolaidis and Paranjape 2009). While the term 'domestic violence' is still commonly used, the term 'intimate partner violence' was recommended by the United States Centers for Disease Control and Prevention (CDC) and the World Health Organization (WHO) in order to distinguish violence between partners from other common forms of violence common in families (e.g., child or elder abuse) (Nicolaidis and Paranjape 2009; Saltzman et al. 1999). Thus, in order to be clear, this book refers to IPV against women. Relatedly, women who have experienced IPV are referred to interchangeably as both 'victims' and 'survivors,' acknowledging both the imbalance in power inherent in IPV and women's active resistance to the violence.

The definition of the welfare state applied in this book centers around the extent to which state interventions attempt to alter the structures of social inequality (Orloff 1993; Pfau-Effinger 1998). This is often operationalized in the form of pensions and financial protection (i.e., in cases of disability, unemployment, accidents, or sickness). In combining the work of Esping-Andersen (1990) with Korpi (1989), three key dimensions of the welfare state emerge: *state–market relations,* as well as to what extent the welfare state influences *social stratification* and *decommodification*. The first dimension looks at the balance of provision between the state and the market. In other words, whether these social protections are primarily provided by the state or left up to the market. Regarding the second mechanism of social stratification, Esping-Andersen (1990, p. 23) describes the welfare state as "an active force in the ordering of social relations." For example, offering pensions to retired workers can prevent poverty among the elderly, while other employment provisions protect workers against poverty during spells of unemployment or sickness. While resource redistribution and alleviation of poverty are traditionally understood by some as being the broad, overarching goals of welfare policy, others prefer to objectively examine whether social policies are indeed "aimed at, or actually produce, greater equality among citizens" (Orloff 1993, p. 304), arguing that social provision can also have the effect of stratifying based on economic or occupational class. This is closely related to the third dimension of decommodification, that is, whether social provisions from the welfare state enable an acceptable standard of living independent of the market. This is also related to whether provision is universally available to all as a right of social citizenship, based on employment and financial contributions, or rather means-tested and available only to the very poor (Korpi 1989).

Based on these dimensions, Esping-Andersen (1990) proposed a threefold typology of "worlds of welfare capitalism" (e.g., liberal, social democratic, and conservative) to aid in the comparative analysis of welfare states. For example, the market dominates the liberal regime, where benefits from the state are typically modest and means-tested, and little is done to reduce poverty or inequality (e.g., Australia, Canada, and the United States). In this type of regime, Esping-Andersen (1990, p. 28), claims that "concepts of gender matter less than the sanctity of the market," so although all adults (mothers included) are dependent on the labor market, there is little state intervention to enable women's participation. At the opposite end of the spectrum are the social democratic welfare regimes, seeking to dramatically alleviate poverty and inequalities by providing generous benefits based upon social citizenship and intervention by the state to ensure full employment and income protection (e.g., Denmark, Finland, Norway, and Sweden). This type of regime is founded on the idea that both men and women should be integrated into the labor market, and thus the welfare state must structure its policies to make this possible. Finally, the conservative regimes have relatively generous earnings-related assistance administered through employers, which typically reinforce existing patterns of social inequality, but minimize the role of the market (e.g., Austria, Belgium, France, and Germany). These regimes are predicated upon the idea that men are the primary breadwinners and thus policies are not oriented towards ensuring women's integration into the labor market. While there are many who criticize these regime types and their usefulness (as will be detailed in Chap. 3), Esping-Andersen's typology is frequently used in comparative welfare state literature in order to be able to make claims about the various impacts of social policy.

Overall, the empirical research tends to demonstrate that the welfare state is a predominant factor in shaping life chances and inequalities (Esping-Andersen 2002; Olafsdottir and Beckfield 2011) and that welfare state generosity (e.g., in unemployment, sickness, and pension benefits) decreases poverty and economic inequality (Brady 2005; Korpi and Palme 1998; Möller et al. 2012). For example, in a comparison of the US, Germany, and Sweden, the likelihood of falling into poverty (and staying there) was higher in the US given its limited state interventions (DiPrete 2002). Likewise, levels of income inequality are found to be the lowest among social democratic welfare regimes, slightly higher in the conservative regimes, and the highest among liberal welfare regimes (Olafsdottir and Beckfield 2011).

In addition, the term 'health inequities' is used throughout this book rather than 'health inequalities.' The latter refers to differences in health outcomes between groups. However, the former is based upon a "comparative principle, a judgment about how a person or a group of people is situated relative to others" (Peters and Evans 2001, p. 27). By identifying a health difference as inequitable, one appeals to ethical norms and a judgment of whether such differences are avoidable, unfair, socially produced, and systematic (Evans et al. 2001; Solar and Irwin 2010). Individual differences in health outcomes that concentrate themselves within certain social groups and are related to education, income, or health care access, are unfair by definition. Thus, insofar as the cause of health inequalities are related to "modifiable social arrangements … they may be considered unjust" (Diderichsen et al. 2001, p. 14). This implies the necessity of a systematic response to reduce health inequities not only from the health sector, but from the social, political, and economic sectors as well. Indeed, this book is founded on the idea that if certain groups of IPV victims are more vulnerable to poor health than others, then these differences are systematically and socially produced, and are therefore inequitable.

1.1 The Research Puzzle

At the individual level, research shows that socioeconomic factors, community characteristics, and societal characteristics influence health outcomes (e.g., Ansari et al. 2003). Social determinants such as education, housing, income, unemployment, chronic stress, and social exclusion, are sometimes better predictors of health status than behavioral variables like diet or exercise (Raphael 2006). Moreover, the distribution of resources which promote health is substantially skewed to favor those with higher socioeconomic statuses. Socioeconomic status serves as a 'fundamental cause' of poor health because those with access to resources (e.g., money, power) can make use of their status to avoid health risks and reduce the costs of poor health (Link and Phelan 1995). In other words, "no matter what the current profile of diseases and known risks happens to be, those who are best positioned with regard to important social and economic resources will be less afflicted by disease" (Link and Phelan 1995, p. 87). This is highly relevant for women in abusive relationships who may be more economically dependent on their partners, have more restricted access to employment and income, or may be more socially deprived (Davis et al. 1999; Ford-Gilboe et al. 2009; Moe and Bell 2004; Tolman and Rosen 2001). Thus, the combination of IPV exposure and limited socioeconomic resources may alter the pathway leading toward health outcomes.

While addressing the social determinants of health is the key to improving health and combating inequities, "the social factors promoting and undermining the health of individuals and populations should not be confused with the social processes underlying their unequal distribution" (Graham 2004, p. 101). Hence, attention should also be paid to the effect of broader factors on health. In particular, how a welfare state allocates resources among its citizens plays a significant role in the health opportunities accorded to different population groups (Burstrom et al. 2010; Evans et al. 2001). Given that social policies are meant to protect against income loss and redistribute resources, thereby affecting key social determinants of health, social policy at the macro-level should be a significant means of affecting population health (Lundberg et al. 2010).

Together, this raises the topic of health inequities for women who have experienced IPV as a research puzzle. Specifically, it is thus far not well understood what individual factors lead to IPV exposure and poor health, and which groups are most susceptible. Moreover, the contribution of the broader social structure in which women are embedded has not been systematically examined (Whitaker 2014). To address these gaps in knowledge, a conceptual framework is applied which was developed by Diderichsen et al. (2001), proposing that health inequities are shaped by the social and policy context through the interconnected mechanisms of *social stratification*, *differential exposure* to health risks, and *differential vulnerability* to ill health. By identifying these mechanisms, the framework also proposes a number of points where policy could intervene in order to reduce inequities. In adapting this conceptual framework to IPV, it is hypothesized that exposure to IPV varies systematically according to socioeconomic resources, and that IPV and limited socioeconomic resources mutually increase the vulnerability to the health consequences of IPV. Furthermore, it is expected that the extent to which the policy context provides a safety net for women shapes their exposure to IPV and their health outcomes.

1.2 Contributions to the Literature

This book addresses several key gaps in the literature on IPV exposure, health inequities, and social policy. Firstly, it directly investigates the intersections of social position and IPV exposure in their impact on health, which has often been neglected in the research from a gendered perspective. Much of the early feminist research on IPV controlled for effects of social position in order to emphasize that IPV cuts across all social divisions and is a problem of gender oppression, rather than a class, racial, or ethnic issue (Goodman et al. 2009; Meier 1997; Raphael 2003). Over time, however, feminist theorizing and empirical research has begun to expand beyond the one-factor explanation of patriarchal structure, incorporating socioeconomic explanations as well. However, even though a review of the research would seem to infer that violence and poverty may magnify one another in their impact on health (Goodman et al. 2009; Loya 2014), these bodies of literature tend not to intersect (Romito et al. 2005). Studies investigating the health consequences of IPV often do not account for variation in women's socioeconomic status and access to resources, and thus little is known about the role of social position (Briere and Jordan 2004; Ford-Gilboe et al. 2009). By specifically examining these intersections, my research sheds new light on the health outcomes of IPV survivors and where social position may play a systematic role.

Secondly, the research presented here uses nationally representative data covering a wider spectrum of socioeconomic, IPV, and health outcomes than is often available for research on IPV. For practical reasons, research from a feminist or gendered perspective on this topic tends to draw its sample from the population of women seeking services from domestic violence programs, women's shelters, criminal justice programs, or health care. While this certainly facilitates access to an otherwise hard-to-reach population, women who seek services are not necessarily representative of women who do not seek help, nor of women who do not identify their relationships as violent (Ruiz-Pérez et al. 2007). In order to understand the complexities of IPV, all of these groups of women must be included in research studies (Grauwiler 2008). Nationally representative surveys are, therefore, vital for detecting and measuring IPV among a broader cross-section of women. Thus, this book provides a wider, and presumably, more accurate lens for examining differentials in health for this population.[1]

Thirdly, while it is assumed that macro-level factors affect prevalence of IPV exposure (Kaya and Cook 2010; Whitaker 2014), little is known about the role of institutional welfare arrangements in affecting the health of IPV survivors. This book addresses this crucial gap in two ways. First, the conceptual framework guiding the analysis explicitly links individual level factors and policy context to health inequities. Second, a cross-national comparative approach using the diverse cases of the US, Germany, and Norway is applied. Examining the policy contexts in which IPV survivors experience health inequities allows for a broader discussion of the impact of macro-level societal structures. In doing so, this research has vital implications for policy makers. By shedding light on which groups are most susceptible to poorer health outcomes, and under which structural conditions, welfare state policy can then be targeted towards reducing IPV exposure and eliminating health inequities.

[1]Differences in IPV measurement methods, as well as how this influences the theoretical understanding of IPV, will be explored in detail in Chap. 2.

1.3 Structure of the Book

Figure 1.1 provides an outline of the 10 chapters contained in this book. This first chapter presented the research puzzle, namely, the question of individual and policy factors contributing to health inequities for IPV survivors. Chapter 2 provides an overview of how IPV is defined, its various sociological theoretical explanations, and the controversies which surround both the definition and the theories. Additionally, empirical evidence for both the economic and health factors related to abusive relationships, as well as their intersections, are explored.

Chapter 3 offers a theoretical review of the welfare state literature relevant to women's socioeconomic resources and their health, followed respectively by a review of the empirical literature related to family and health policy. In order to piece this literature together into a complete picture connecting the welfare state with women's health outcomes, a conceptual model highlighting mechanisms leading to health inequities is introduced. Moving towards the application of this model to IPV, the gaps in the literature regarding IPV, health, and the welfare state are reviewed. Finally, the conceptual framework is adapted to IPV and serves as the foundation for elucidating four specific research questions regarding individual and

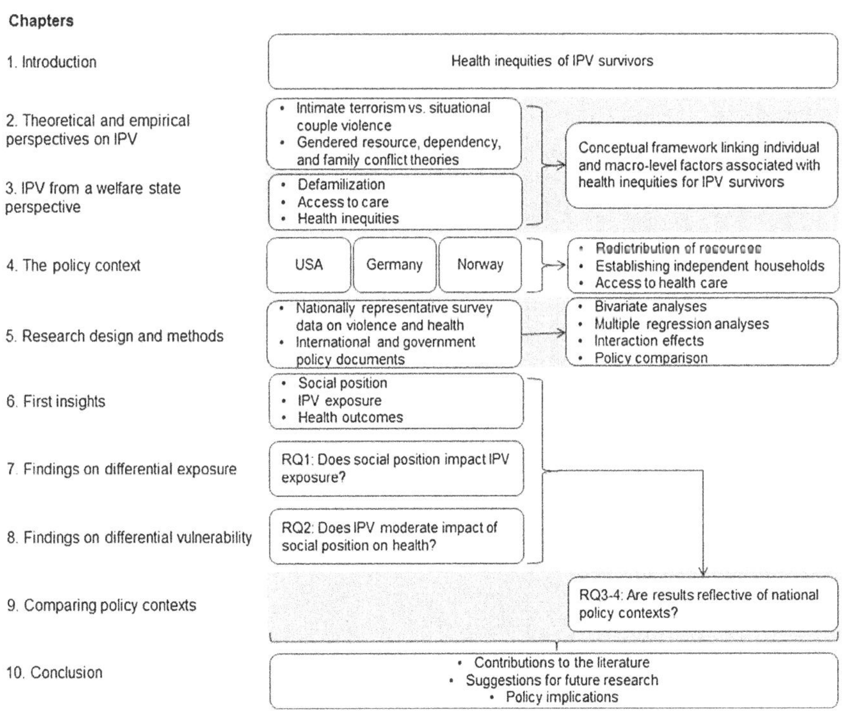

Fig. 1.1 Overview of the book

macro-level factors related to differential exposure to IPV and differential vulnerability to poor health.

Chapter 4 presents a justification of the selection of the US, Germany, and Norway as diverse cases, along with a detailed description of the relevant policy contexts. Country by country, each case description begins with background information on the prevalence of IPV, the history of policies on violence against women, and the available services. Next, the aspects of the welfare state influencing social stratification are highlighted, such as unemployment benefits, sickness benefits, and benefits directed at single, low-income mothers. This is followed by an exploration of family policies influencing defamilization and women's resources for establishing independent households. Finally, the situation for each country in terms of access to health care is described, specifically looking at entitlement to care, availability of health care providers, and affordability of out-of-pocket payments by patients. The chapter closes by comparing and contrasting the policy contexts of the US, Germany, and Norway.

The research design and methods applied in this book are introduced in Chap. 5. The chapter begins with a discussion of the three sets of national survey data used in the analyses: the 1995 *National Violence Against Women Survey* in the US, the 2003 *Health, Well-being, and Safety of Women in Germany* Survey, and the 2003–04 *Survey of Everyday Safety* in Norway. Next are a description of the sample selection, and the operationalization of the social position, IPV exposure, health, and control variables. Following this is an account of the univariate, bivariate, and multivariate statistical methods applied in the analysis, as well as a description of the exploratory cross-national policy comparison.

Chapter 6 is the first of three chapters presenting findings from the quantitative analyses used to test the hypotheses. It first offers a descriptive overview of the US, German, and Norwegian samples. Following this is a presentation of the bivariate analyses used to determine the initial relationships between the variables. These analyses offer a clear picture of the composition of each of the country samples and provide the first clues towards answering my research questions.

Findings regarding social position's impact on IPV exposure are presented in Chap 7. Based on the literature linking socioeconomic resources to the ability to end abusive relationships and establish independent households, it is examined whether women with lower social positions may be differentially exposed to IPV. To do this, a multinomial logit regression model was fit for each country using IPV exposure as the dependent variable, with household income, education, and employment as predictors. The results of the regression models are presented in terms of relative risk ratios, as well as in predicted probabilities of minor and severe IPV at each level of social position.

As the final quantitative empirical chapter, Chap. 8 presents the findings on whether women with IPV exposure are differentially vulnerable to social position's impact on health outcomes. From a statistical standpoint, the question posed is one of the moderating effects of IPV exposure on the relationship between social position and health. Findings from a series of nested models are presented, first establishing whether social position affects health, and then whether IPV contributes to health outcomes, before finally testing the interaction between social position and IPV exposure. Logit regression models are used for self-assessed health as the first dependent variable, presenting the results in terms of odds ratios. Negative binomial regression models are also fit for mental health complaints as the second dependent variable, presenting the results in terms of incident rate ratios. Furthermore, calculations of predicted probabilities of poor self-assessed health and predicted counts of mental health complaints, taking into account IPV exposure and social position, are also presented.

Chapter 9 explores the macro-level policy context related to my research questions. The comparison of the US, Germany, and Norway enables a discussion of whether patterns in differential exposure to IPV and differential vulnerability to poor health found in the quantitative analyses vary across institutional arrangements. This chapter brings together evidence from the detailed policy descriptions in Chap. 4 and the empirical findings from Chaps. 6, 7, and 8. This allows for an exploration of whether policy contexts may contribute to systematic differences in health outcomes for IPV survivors.

In closing, Chap. 10 discusses the main findings related to each of my four research questions and their theoretical implications. This is followed by a brief look at possible critical issues of the presented research, as well as some suggestions for future research that arise from my results. Finally, based on the conceptual framework, the implications for welfare policy and where it may intervene to improve health outcomes for IPV survivors are discussed.

References

Alsaker, K., Moen, B. E., & Kristoffersen, K. (2007). Health-related quality of life among abused women one year after leaving a violent partner. *Social Indicators Research, 86*(3), 497–509. doi:10.1007/s11205-007-9182-7

Ansari, Z., Carson, N. J., Ackland, M. J., Vaughan, L., & Serraglio, A. (2003). A public health model of the social determinants of health. *Sozial und Präventivmedizin, 48*(4), 242–251.

Black, M. C., Basile, K. C., Breiding, M. J., Smith, S. G., Walters, M. L., Merrick, M. T., et al. (2011). *The National Intimate Partner and Sexual Violence Survey (NISVS): 2010 summary report*. Atlanta, GA: CDC.

Bonomi, A. E., Thompson, R. S., Anderson, M., Reid, R. J., Carrell, D., Dimer, J. A., et al. (2006). Intimate partner violence and women's physical, mental, and social functioning. *American Journal of Preventive Medicine, 30*, 458–466. doi:10.1016/j.amepre.2006.01.015

Brady, D. (2005). The welfare state and relative poverty in rich western democracies, 1967–1997. *Social Forces, 83*(4), 1329–1364. doi:10.1353/sof.2005.0056

Briere, J., & Jordan, C. E. (2004). Violence against women: Outcome complexity and implications for assessment and treatment. *Journal of Interpersonal Violence, 19*(11), 1252–1276. doi:10.1177/0886260504269682

Burstrom, B., Whitehead, M., Clayton, S., Fritzell, S., Vannoni, F., & Costa, G. (2010). Health inequalities between lone and couple mothers and policy under different welfare regimes—The example of Italy, Sweden and Britain. *Social Science and Medicine, 70*, 912–920. doi:10.1016/j.socscimed.2009.11.014

Campbell, J. C., & Lewandowski, L. A. (1997). Mental and physical health effects of intimate partner violence on women and children. *The Psychiatric Clinics of North America, 20*(2), 353–374. doi:10.1016/S0193-953X(05)70317-8

Coker, A. L., Smith, P. H., & Fadden, M. K. (2005). Intimate partner violence and disabilities among women attending family practice clinics. *Journal of Women's Health, 14*, 829–838. doi:10.1089/jwh.2005.14.829

Davis, M. F., Renzetti, C. M., & Edelson, J. L. (1999). The economics of abuse: How violence perpetuates women's poverty. In R. Brandwein & J. L. Edelson (Eds.), *Battered women, children, and welfare reform: The ties that bind* (pp. 17–30). Thousand Oaks, CA: Sage.

Diderichsen, F., Evans, T., & Whitehead, M. (2001). The social basis of disparities in health. In T. Evans, M. Whitehead, F. Diderichsen, A. Bhuyia, & M. Wirth (Eds.), *Challenging inequities in health: From ethics to action* (pp. 12–23). New York, NY: Oxford University Press.

DiPrete, T. A. (2002). Life course risks, mobility regimes, and mobility sonsequences: A comparison of Sweden, Germany, and the United States. *American Journal of Sociology, 108* (2), 267–309. doi:10.1086/344811

Dutton, M., Kaltman, S., Goodman, L. A., Weinfurt, K., & Vankos, N. (2005). Patterns of intimate partner violence: Correlates and outcomes. *Violence and Victims, 20*, 483–497. doi:10.1891/0886-6708.2005.20.5.483

Eberhard-Gran, M., Schei, B., & Eskild, A. (2007). Somatic symptoms and diseases are more common in women exposed to violence. *Journal of General Internal Medicine, 22*(12), 1668–1673. doi:10.1007/s11606-007-0389-8

Ellsberg, M., Jansen, H. A. F. M., Heise, L., Watts, C. H., & García-Moreno, C. (2008). Intimate partner violence and women's physical and mental health in the WHO multi-country study on women's health and domestic violence: An observational study. *The Lancet, 371*, 1165–1172. doi:10.1016/S0140-6736(08)60522-X

Esping-Andersen, G. (1990). *The three worlds of welfare capitalism*. London: Polity.

Esping-Andersen, G. (2002). *Why we need a new welfare state*. Oxford, UK: Oxford University Press.

European Union Agency for Fundamental Rights (FRA). (2014). In *Violence against women: An EU-wide survey*. Luxembourg: Publications Office of the European Union. http://fra.europa.eu/sites/default/files/fra-2014-vaw-survey-main-results_en.pdf. Accessed November 01, 2014.

Evans, T., Whitehead, M., Diderichsen, F., Bhuiya, A., & Wirth, M. (2001). Introduction. In T. Evans, M. Whitehead, F. Diderichsen, A. Bhuiya, & M. Wirth (Eds.), *Challenging inequities in health: From ethics to action* (pp. 2–11). New York, NY: Oxford University Press.

Ford-Gilboe, M., Wuest, J., Varcoe, C., Davies, L., Merritt-Gray, M., Campbell, J. C., et al. (2009). Modelling the effects of intimate partner violence and access to resources on women's health in the early years after leaving an abusive partner. *Social Science and Medicine, 68*, 1021–1029. doi:10.1016/j.socscimed.2009.01.003

Garcia-Moreno, C., Heise, L., Jansen, H. A. F. M., Ellsberg, M., & Watts, C. (2005). Public health. Violence against women. *Science, 310*(5752), 1282–1283. doi:10.1126/science.1121400

Goodman, L. A., Smyth, K. F., Borges, A. M., & Singer, R. (2009). When crises collide: How intimate partner violence and poverty intersect to shape women's mental health and coping? *Trauma, Violence, and Abuse, 10*, 306–329. doi:10.1177/1524838009339754

Graham, H. (2004). Social determinants and their unequal distribution: Clarifying policy understandings. *The Milbank Quarterly, 82*(1), 101–124. doi: 10.1111/j.0887-378X.2004.00303.x

Grauwiler, P. (2008). Voices of women: Perspectives on decision-making and the management of partner violence. *Children and Youth Services Review, 30*, 311–322. doi:10.1016/j.childyouth.2007.10.008

Hagemann-White, C. (2005). Surveying prevalence of violence against women in the context of the German National Action Plan. *Statistical Journal of the United Nations, 22*, 301–309.

Heise, L. (2012). *Determinants of partner violence in low and middle-income countries: Exploring variation in individual and population level risk*. London, UK: London School of Hygiene Tropical Medicine. http://researchonline.lshtm.ac.uk/682451/1/560822.pdf. Accessed July 13, 2014.

Heise, L., Ellsberg, M., & Gottemoeller, M. (1999). *Ending violence against women. Population reports*. Baltimore, MD: Johns Hopkins University School of Public Health.

Kaya, Y., & Cook, K. J. (2010). A cross-national analysis of physical intimate partner violence against women. *International Journal of Comparative Sociology, 51*(6), 423–444. doi:10.1177/0020715210386155

Korpi, W. (1989). Power, politics, and state autonomy in the development of social citizenship: Social rights during sickness in eighteen OECD countries since 1930. *American Sociological Review, 54*(3), 309–328.

Korpi, W., & Palme, J. (1998). The paradox of redistribution and strategies of equality: Welfare state institutions, inequality, and poverty in the Western countries. *American Sociological Review, 63*(5), 661–687.

Krug, E. G., Dahlberg, L. L., Mercy, J. A., Zwi, A. B., & Lozano, R. (2002). *World report on violence and health*. Geneva: World Health Organization. http://apps.who.int/iris/bitstream/10665/42495/1/9241545615_eng.pdf. Accessed November 24, 2010.

Labell, L. S. (1979). Wife abuse—A sociological study of battered women and their mates. *Victimology, 4*(2), 258–267.

Link, B. G., & Phelan, J. (1995). Social conditions as fundamental causes of disease. *Journal of Health and Social Behavior, 35*(Extra Issue), 80–94.

Loya, R. M. (2014). The role of sexual violence in creating and maintaining economic insecurity among asset-poor women of color. *Violence Against Women, 20*(11), 1299–1320. doi:10.1177/1077801214552912

Lundberg, O., Fritzell, J., Åberg Yngwe, M., & Kölegård, M. L. (2010). The potential power of social policy programmes: Income redistribution, economic resources and health. *International Journal of Social Welfare, 19*, S2–S13. doi:10.1111/j.1468-2397.2010.00727.x

Martin, D. (1976). *Battered wives*. Volcano, CA: Volcano Press.

Meier, J. (1997). Domestic violence, character, and social change in the welfare reform debate. *Law & Policy, 19*(2), 205–263. doi:10.1111/1467-9930.00028

Moe, A. M., & Bell, M. P. (2004). Abject economics. *Violence Against Women, 10*(1), 29–55. doi:10.1177/1077801203256016

Möller, A. S., Backstrom, T., Sondergaard, H. P., & Helstrom, L. (2012). Patterns of injury and reported violence depending on relationship to assailant in female Swedish sexual assault victims. *Journal of Interpersonal Violence, 27*(16), 3131–3148. doi:10.1177/0886260512441261

Nicolaidis, C., & Paranjape, A. (2009). Defining intimate partner violence: Controversies and implications. In C. Mitchell & D. Anglin (Eds.), *Intimate partner violence: A health-based perspective* (pp. 19–30). New York, NY: Oxford University Press.

Olafsdottir, S., & Beckfield, J. (2011). Health and the social rights of citizenship: Integrating welfare-state theory and medical sociology. In B. A. Pescosolido, J. K. Martin, J. D. McLeod, & A. Rogers (Eds.), *Handbook of the sociology of health, illness, and healing* (pp. 101–115). New York, NY: Springer. doi:10.1007/978-1-4419-7261-3_6

Orloff, A. (1993). Gender and the social rights of citizenship: The comparative analysis of gender relations and welfare states. *American Sociological Review, 58*(3), 303–328.

Peters, F., & Evans, T. (2001). Ethical dimensions of health equity. In T. Evans, M. Whitehead, F. Diderichsen, A. Bhuiya, & M. Wirth (Eds.), *Challenging inequities in health: From ethics to action* (pp. 24–33). Oxford, UK: Oxford University Press.

Pfau-Effinger, B. (1998). Gender cultures and the gender arrangement—A theoretical framework for cross-national gender research. *Innovation: The European Journal of Social Science Research, 11*(2), 147–166. doi:10.1080/13511610.1998.9968559

Raphael, J. (2003). Battering through the lens of class. *Journal of Gender, Social Policy and the Law, 11*(2), 367–375.

Raphael, D. (2006). Social determinants of health: Present status, unanswered questions, and future directions. *International Journal of Health Services, 36*(4), 651–677. doi:10.2190/3MW4-1EK3-DGRQ-2CRF

Romito, P., Turan, J. M., & De Marchi, M. (2005). The impact of current and past interpersonal violence on women's mental health. *Social Science and Medicine, 60*, 1717–1727. doi:10.1016/j.socscimed.2004.08.026

Ruiz-Pérez, I., Plazaola-Castaño, J., & Vives-Cases, C. (2007). Methodological issues in the study of violence against women. *Journal of Epidemiology and Community Health, 61*(Supp II), ii26–ii31. doi:10.1136/jech.2007.059907

Saltzman, L. E., Fanslow, J. L., McMahon, P. M., & Shelley, G. A. (1999). *Intimate partner violence surveillance: Uniform definitions and recommended data elements, version 1.0.* Atlanta, GA: National Center for Injury Prevention and Control, Centers for Disease Control and Prevention. http://www.cdc.gov/ncipc/pub-res/ipv_surveillance/IntimatePartnerViolence.pdf. Accessed January 05, 2011.

Solar, O., & Irwin, A. (2010). *A conceptual framework for action on the social determinants of health*. Geneva: World Health Organization.

Straus, H., Cerulli, C., McNutt, L. A., Rhodes, K. V., Conner, K. R., Kemball, R. S., et al. (2009). Intimate partner violence and functional health status: Associations with severity, danger, and self-advocacy behaviors. *Journal of Women's Health, 18*(5), 625–631.

Tolman, R. M., & Rosen, D. (2001). Domestic violence in the lives of women receiving welfare: Mental health, substance dependence, and economic well-being. *Violence Against Women, 7* (2), 141–158. doi:10.1177/10778012201007002003

United Nations General Assembly. (1993). Declaration on the elimination of violence against women. Geneva. http://www.un.org/documents/ga/res/48/a48r104.htm. Accessed May 15, 2014.

Vives-Cases, C., Ruiz-Cantero, M. T., Escribà-Agüir, V., & Miralles, J. J. (2011). The effect of intimate partner violence and other forms of violence against women on health. *Journal of Public Health, 33*, 15–21. doi:10.1093/pubmed/fdq101

Vos, T., Astbury, J., Piers, L., Magnus, A., Heenan, M., Stanley, L., et al. (2006). Measuring the impact of intimate partner violence on the health of women in Victoria, Australia. *Bulletin of the World Health Organization, 84*(9), 739–744. doi:10.1590/S0042-96862006000900017

Whitaker, M. P. (2014). Linking community protective factors to intimate partner violence perpetration. *Violence Against Women, 20*(11), 1338–1359. doi:10.1177/1077801214552854

Wijma, B., Schei, B., Swahnberg, K., Hilden, M., Offerdal, K., Pikarinen, U., et al. (2003). Emotional, physical, and sexual abuse in patients visiting gynaecology clinics: A Nordic cross-sectional study. *The Lancet, 361*(9375), 2107–2113. doi:10.1016/S0140-6736(03)13719-1

Wuest, J., Ford-Gilboe, M., Merritt-Gray, M., Wilk, P., Campbell, J. C., Lent, B., et al. (2010). Pathways of chronic pain in survivors of intimate partner violence. *Journal of Women's Health, 19*(9), 1665–1674. doi:10.1089/jwh.2009.1856

Chapter 2
Theoretical and Empirical Perspectives on Intimate Partner Violence

Abstract The social production of health inequities for women who have experienced IPV spans a wide disciplinary spectrum, touching on aspects of sociology, public health, and gender studies. Therefore, the present chapter begins with a look at how IPV is defined and how it is theoretically explained and understood from a sociological perspective. Based on this background, empirical evidence for both the socioeconomic and health factors related to abusive relationships are explored, specifically highlighting the intersection between social position and health outcomes for survivors of IPV. This lays the foundation for the later theoretical and empirical review of the role of the welfare state in health inequities for female survivors of IPV.

The social production of health inequities for women who have experienced IPV spans a wide disciplinary spectrum, touching on aspects of sociology, public health, and gender studies. Therefore, the present chapter begins with a look at how IPV is defined and how it is theoretically explained and understood from a sociological perspective. Based on this background, empirical evidence for both the socioeconomic and health factors related to abusive relationships are explored, specifically highlighting the intersection between social position and health outcomes for survivors of IPV. This lays the foundation for Chap. 3's theoretical and empirical review of the role of the welfare state in health inequities for female survivors of IPV.

2.1 Definitions of IPV

The WHO understands IPV as "any behavior within a present or former intimate relationship that causes physical, psychological, or sexual harm" (Heise and García-Moreno 2012, p. 90). The types of behavior typically considered to constitute IPV include physical abuse (e.g., slapping, hitting, kicking, beating), psychological abuse (e.g., intimidation, humiliation), sexual abuse (e.g., sexual coercion, forced intercourse), or other controlling behaviors (e.g., isolating a partner from family and friends, restricting access to financial resources). These abusive

© Springer International Publishing Switzerland 2016

M.M. Larsen, *Health Inequities Related to Intimate Partner Violence Against Women*, Social Disparities in Health and Health Care,
DOI 10.1007/978-3-319-29565-7_2

behaviors tend to overlap in violent relationships, with physical violence being accompanied by psychological abuse and sexual violence in about half of violent relationships.

However, a more comprehensive definition in terms of IPV's gender symmetry is still hotly contested. A feminist definition views IPV as a continual pattern of behaviors used to assert control over an intimate partner (Nicolaidis and Paranjape 2009). Rather than being understood as isolated behaviors, importance is placed upon power dynamics, as well as the intent and consequences of the violence. From this point of view, IPV is commonly perceived of as male violence against a female partner. By and large, this definition of IPV was developed by clinicians and academics through the lens of feminist theory, based primarily on qualitative research with abused women accessing help services (e.g., Dobash and Dobash 1979; Walker 1979). The family conflict viewpoint, however, understands the majority of IPV to occur as a response to occasional conflict in the family, perpetrated equally by men and women. In this definition, the focus is specifically on behaviors. Such factors as relationship dynamics, intents, and consequences are purposely excluded from the definition. This viewpoint stems from some of the first attempts by sociologists to study IPV using community-based surveys (e.g., Straus et al. 1980). These different perspectives have generated much unresolved debate (Winstok 2011). The feminist perspective contends that defining IPV without addressing the context of violence neglects that behaviors have fundamentally different consequences and are inherently gendered (DeKeseredy 2011; Dobash et al. 1992; Johnson 2011). Researchers from the family conflict perspective, however, argue that making assumptions about gender ideologies overlooks the needs of male victims (Dutton 2012; Straus 1999) and denies that ending women's violence against men is also "morally, legally, and therapeutically necessary" (Straus 2011, p. 286).

Meanwhile, a number of researchers have attempted to reconcile these conflicting perspectives. For example, in a meta-analytic review of the literature, Archer (2000) found that when specifically examining more severe forms of violence, men are more likely to be the perpetrator against women. However, when examining more minor forms of violence, there is a greater degree of gender symmetry between victims and perpetrators. Another potential reconciliation comes from Johnson (1995),[1] who suggested that researchers may in fact be examining two different phenomena which vary by the occurrence of coercive control. In later research, he expanded upon this theory and proposed four discrete types of IPV based on both coercive control and aggression: intimate terrorism, violent resistance, situational couple violence, and mutual violent control (Johnson 2006, 2011).

[1]It is important to note that Johnson clearly identifies himself as coming from the feminist perspective (2011).

The former two are rather gender asymmetrical. *Intimate terrorism* is the exertion of control over one's partner using a range of violent and nonviolent tactics, usually perpetrated by men over women, typically escalating in severity. Johnson argues that intimate terrorism is most frequently seen among women seeking help services for an abusive relationship, fitting with the feminist understanding of IPV, but most likely only represents a small percentage of overall violence in partnerships. On the other hand, *violent resistance* is one partner's response to intimate terrorism, although it is clear that the violent resistor remains in the position of least power, and this is typically perpetrated by women against men. The latter two types of IPV, however, tend to be gender symmetrical. *Situational couple violence* is understood as violence that occurs during conflict, but which is not fixed in systematic domination and control of one partner over another. He asserts that this type of violence is less severe and is often revealed through population-based surveys, fitting with the family conflict perspective of IPV, and is the most common type of violence in partnerships. Finally, Johnson hypothesizes that *mutual violent control* occurs when both partners simultaneously seek to dominate the other, although this may occur only rarely.

Critics of Johnson's categorizations wonder if perhaps the question lies in clarifying the *degree* of violence rather than *types* of violence (Heise 2012). An attempt at empirically testing Johnson's concepts of intimate terrorism and situational couple violence using a US representative sample concluded that,

> there may not be as sharp a demarcation between the two hypothetical forms of IPV as has been proposed but rather a continuum where both controlling behaviors and injury and violence escalation are just three factors that characterize the various forms of IPV that may evolve over time in the course of a relationship (Frye et al. 2006, p. 1303).

Although the jury is still out on whether IPV is made up of distinct categories or rather a spectrum of severity, Johnson's work has at least opened the door to discussions that perhaps not all instances of IPV are equal (Heise 2012), even if it has not ended the debate between the feminist and family conflict perspectives (e.g., Dutton 2012; Straus 2011). This book focuses on the understandings of IPV as both intimate terrorism and situational couple violence perpetrated against women, and the next sections of this chapter explore their theoretical foundations and empirical support.[2]

---

[2]Although it is beyond the scope of this book, it is important to highlight an ever-increasing body of literature challenging heteronormative assumptions around IPV, asserting that imbalances in power and dependence also propagate patterns of abuse in homosexual relationships (e.g., Cruz 2000; Jeffries and Ball 2008; McClennen et al. 2002; Oliffe et al. 2014; Renzetti 1992). The complex intersections of gender, sexuality, and power in abusive relationships among lesbian, gay, bisexual, and transgender individuals necessitate even further research to understand the underpinnings of IPV in these communities.

2.2 Theoretical Explanations of IPV

In delving into the definitions of IPV, one cannot avoid also touching upon its theoretical underpinnings. There is a vast body of theoretical approaches from different disciplines attempting to explain the causes of IPV and its risk factors. The theoretical realm spans psychological (e.g., frustration–aggression theory, social learning theory, cognitive behavioral theory), biobehavioral (e.g., neurochemical mechanisms), criminological, economic, and sociological explanations (Heise 2012; Mitchell and Vanya 2009). For the purposes of this book, however, this section focuses specifically on the most relevant sociological theories endeavoring to explain IPV, including: feminist theory, family conflict theory, resource theory and its offshoots of relative resource theory and gendered resource theory, and dependency theory. Although there are significant differences between them, these theories share common ideas about the importance of structure (patriarchal or otherwise), socioeconomic resources, and status.

According to some of the earliest *feminist theorizing*, IPV is primarily the result of a patriarchal system which exerts men's domination and control over women (Dobash and Dobash 1979). This occurs either "directly, through cultural norms of deference and obedience backed if necessary by the use of force; or indirectly, by shaping women's opportunities and constraints in basic institutions such as the family and work that reinforce women's subordination" (Rodriguez-Menes and Safranoff 2012, p. 585). Simply put, a high level of gender inequality in laws, the social order, and institutions plays itself out in a high level of men's violence against women, but levels of IPV will decrease as a society's gender equity increases. Research which applies feminist theory emphasizes "power and control in relationships, social norms condoning wife beating, and structural and economic forces that keep women trapped in abusive relationships" (Heise 2012, p. 47). Arguably, one of the primary contributions of feminist theory is its argument that social context is vital to understanding IPV, whereas prior to the feminist movement, victims were often implicitly or explicitly blamed for the violence they experienced (e.g., ascribing them with deviant, masochistic personalities) (Mitchell and Vanya 2009).

Much of the early feminist-based research on IPV typically controlled for socioeconomic variables in empirical research instead of directly investigating them (Cunradi et al. 2002; Goodman et al. 2009; Raphael 2003). This had to do with the deeply ingrained belief among early feminist activists that IPV cuts across all social divisions and therefore is a societal problem of gender oppression, not a class or ethnic problem (Meier 1997). While it has been shown that violence affects all levels of society, some feminist scholars have argued that a purely universalist strategy may have the unintended negative consequence of minimizing the significance of the differentials in vulnerabilities experienced by those in lower social positions (Humphreys 2007; Purvin 2007; Raphael 2003). Rather than reducing victims' vulnerability, this may instead compound it through uninformed services and policies which ignore the specific needs and difficulties facing poor women who are abused by their partners (Josephson 2002). In this sense, feminist theorizing has expanded beyond the one-factor explanation of patriarchal structure (Dekeseredy and Dragiewicz 2007; DeKeseredy 2011), and has begun to examine socioeconomic explanations as well.

Even so, this remains a central point of critics of feminist theory, arguing that societal gender inequality is only one of many factors involved in the occurrence of partner violence (Dutton 2006). Researchers from this standpoint instead propose a theory of *family conflict*, arguing that factors such as age, income, and employment status of couples play a more important role (Anderson 1997; Gelles 1993). Essentially, not every man is violent even in societies with high levels of gender inequality, and thus explanations must also take into account the difficulties of everyday family life. This theory of family conflict makes use of social structuralism in explaining violence in relationships. Basically, violence occurs as a reaction to "socially structured stress" (e.g., low income, unemployment, poor health) and the institutionalized inequalities among socioeconomic, gender, and racial divides (Gelles 1985, p. 361). In essence, IPV from this perspective is understood as, "the outcome of a pileup of stressors associated with a perceived excess of demands over resources" (Fox et al. 2002, p. 794). Thus, violence in the family is inherently related to a family's position in the social structure.

Even before feminist and family conflict theory, however, one of the first researchers to apply sociological theories to IPV was Goode (1971) with *resource theory*. He proposed that the power balance between partners is often dependent upon the resources individuals contribute to the relationship. Moreover, he hypothesized that "force and its threat can be used when other resources are unavailable or have proved ineffective" (Goode 1971, p. 628). In other words, men with fewer resources outside the relationship (e.g., when facing unemployment or financial hardship) are more likely to make use of violence in order to reestablish their control within the relationship. In contrast, men with sufficient external resources have little need to reassert their power through violence. An extension of resource theory known as *relative resource theory* focuses not on men's absolute resources, but rather on the (im)balance in economic and social resources between men and women in a relationship (Macmillan and Gartner 1999; McCloskey 1996). According to this theory, men who have fewer resources (e.g., education or income) as compared to their female partners are more likely to use violence to regain their power if they have no other means to do so. The flip side of this theory can also be used to hypothesize that women with comparatively lower education and status than their partners are also at increased risk if "violence is construed as a privilege of his greater resource contribution and simultaneously as a reflection of his partner's relative economic vulnerability" (Fox et al. 2002, p. 794). Developing these ideas even further, *gendered resource theory* proposes that IPV is rather an interaction between status inconsistencies in relationships and the male partner's gender ideology (Atkinson et al. 2005). Basically, if male partners view the relationship through the lens of egalitarianism and do not perceive the need to be the primary breadwinner, then they do not have any need to use violence to reassert their superiority over female partners with higher statuses.

Dependency theory takes a different approach and builds both on the ideas around the patriarchal structure of society, while also acknowledging the role of socioeconomic factors. It contends that women's absolute socioeconomic resources are the critical relevant factors in IPV rather than family resources, men's resources, or men's resources relative to women's (as in family conflict theory, resource theory, and relative resource theory, respectively). This line of argumentation states that the patriarchal structure of society can manifest itself in socioeconomic vulnerabilities among women. These "low opportunities and multiple constraints stemming from women's positions in the socioeconomic structure affect women's control over their lives, making them dependent on their male partners, and raising the probability of experiencing violence" (Rodriguez-Menes and Safranoff 2012, p. 586). In this sense, dependency theory is framed around women's resources and their ability to exercise agency given the patriarchal structure in which they are embedded. According to this theory, it is necessary to consider both individual and macro-level factors affecting women's standing in society and their exposure to IPV.

In sum, even though the theories mentioned above may lean toward explaining either intimate terrorism or situational couple violence (or perhaps both), there is a great deal of overlap amongst them. It is quite likely that these various theories all contain elements of truth. Therefore, many researchers have come to the conclusion that IPV is an intricate phenomenon that requires a multifaceted approach (Rodriguez-Menes and Safranoff 2012), and should be understood as occurring due to an interaction of multiple factors at the individual, household, community, and societal levels (Heise 1998). This, along with the differences between intimate terrorism and situational couple violence, is vital to keep in mind when examining the empirical research on IPV, socioeconomic resources, and health.

2.3 The Evidence on IPV and Economic Vulnerability

As predicted by many of the sociological theories of IPV, there is an unmistakable empirical link between IPV and socioeconomic resources, although the relationship may look slightly different according to structural and cultural context. This section begins with an exploration of empirical literature connecting IPV and socioeconomic status at the household level, followed by evidence related specifically to women's own socioeconomic resources, and the role of economic (in)dependence in women's abilities to exit abusive relationships. The conclusion of this section includes a brief discussion of what can be said in terms of directionality.

In the US, one of the primary correlates of IPV is *household income level*, with economic hardship and lower levels of income increasing the likelihood of violence (Bachman and Saltzman 1995; Tjaden and Thoennes 2000; Tolman and Rosen 2001; Vest et al. 2002). In fact, a US study found that household income has the greatest influence on the probability of experiencing IPV as compared to other risk factors (Cunradi et al. 2002). Likewise, an EU-wide representative survey found that on average, women who found it difficult to live on their household income were nearly twice as likely to have experienced physical and/or sexual violence from a current or former partner than women who found their level of household income to be comfortable (FRA 2014). In Germany specifically, there is a higher likelihood of experiencing physical or sexual violence from a current partner in households with lower incomes, but the differences between income levels are not quite as strong as those found in the US or EU-wide studies (Schröttle and Ansorge 2008).[3] A national Norwegian survey found that women who considered themselves as being financially worse off than others had increased exposure to IPV (Nerøien and Schei 2008). Depending on whether household income is related to IPV from a current or former partner, there are two different theoretical mechanisms for this association. For women in lower income households who have higher rates of IPV exposure from a *current* partner, it is supposed that financial burdens place undue stress on the relationship and men may express their frustration by resorting to violence, as suggested by the branch of resource theories or family conflict theory. For women in lower income households who report higher rates of IPV exposure from a *former* partner, this may reflect the economically vulnerable situation women find themselves in after ending an abusive relationship, perhaps related to dependency theory.

Focusing specifically on *women's socioeconomic resources* and IPV, there is a large degree of variation depending on the country context and men's relative resources. In Norway, women's lower educational levels and unemployment are strongly associated with IPV (Nerøien and Schei 2008). In contrast, an EU-wide survey demonstrated that women's level of education does not seem to impact IPV exposure from current or former partners (FRA 2014). A nationally representative survey of Germany found that women with incomes greater than their partners' income have the highest likelihood of IPV (Schröttle and Ansorge 2008). This was also found to be the case in the US, where women who have higher incomes than their partners (Anderson 1997; McCloskey 1996), or whose income increases over time relative to their partners (Fox et al. 2002), have a higher risk of IPV. Macmillan and Gartner's (1999) findings suggest that it may be even more nuanced: perhaps women's employment only increases the risk of IPV when her partner is unemployed, and risk of IPV decreases considerably when the abusive partner is also employed. The explanation for such findings goes back to relative resource theory: women's higher level of resources as compared to their partner's resources disrupts cultural norms and expectations of men as breadwinners, leading to greater levels of violence among men attempting to reassert their control in the relationship. However, it is also important to keep in mind that at least one study has found that women's share of relative resources increases the likelihood of violence only when their partners hold a traditional male breadwinner gender ideology (Atkinson et al. 2005).

---

[3]This may also be related to the German analysis focusing on IPV from a current partner, rather than current and former partners.

There is yet another body of literature around women's resources, but its focus is rather on women's *ability to end an abusive relationship* as opposed to their risk of IPV. It is clear that separation from an abusive partner requires women to have access to adequate financial resources and support. Due to this, women without their own resources who are economically dependent on their abusive partner find it difficult to end the abusive relationship, and instead are more likely to tolerate abuse for longer (Basu and Famoye 2004; Kalmuss and Straus 1982; Kim and Gray 2008). A review of US studies around women's decisions to leave or stay in an abusive relationship found that women's higher personal income levels and employment status were the strongest predictors of leaving (Anderson and Saunders 2003), and this was also found in a study of women leaving domestic violence shelters in Norway (Alsaker et al. 2007). Women also report lack of financial resources as a central barrier to leaving an abusive partner (Anderson et al. 2003; Schröttle and Ansorge 2008). It is, therefore, not surprising that a number of studies have demonstrated that access to economic opportunities (Farmer and Tiefenthaler 1997; Golden et al. 2013; Shobe and Dienemann 2008) and maintaining employment is of utmost importance for women seeking to establish independence from their abusive partners (Moe and Bell 2004).

While the association of IPV and socioeconomic status is clear, less so is the causal directionality of this relationship. The small number of longitudinal studies that do exist tend to provide evidence that abuse can occur as the result of poverty. The US National Survey of Family and Households found that employment instability and financial hardship increased the likelihood of abuse at later time points, even when IPV history was controlled for at baseline (Fox and Benson 2006). Likewise, Byrne et al. (1999) discovered that women living in poverty at baseline were almost twice as likely to report episodes of abuse in the subsequent waves of the study. On the other hand, there is considerable evidence in the other causal direction, demonstrating the disruptive effects of IPV on women's social position (Davies et al. 2015). For example, IPV decreases women's ability to both obtain and maintain employment, and it has a negative influence on income and housing stability (Goodman et al. 2009). Low-income victims of IPV have been found to be one-third less likely to be able to maintain employment (at least 30 h per week) in the 6 months following abuse than low-income women who have not been abused (Browne et al. 1999). A 3-year longitudinal study also found that unemployment at follow-up was more than twice as likely for women who experienced a new episode of violence over the course of the study than for women who did not (Byrne et al. 1999). Moreover, women with prior histories of IPV at baseline were more likely to have deteriorating income levels over subsequent observations if they had experienced a new episode of IPV. Even with these longitudinal studies, however, the causal directionality of social position and IPV is difficult to disentangle. This instead seems to indicate a rather cyclical relationship where women with lower social positions are at greater risk of IPV, and women who experience IPV are at greater risk of being in lower social positions (Byrne et al. 1999).

In sum, there seems to be strong evidence for theories of IPV considering both household resources and women's individual resources in analyses of IPV. Likewise, the cross-national differences found across various studies appear to lend support to dependency theory, emphasizing the importance of also taking macro-level structures into account.

2.4 The Evidence on IPV and Health

This second section on empirical evidence focuses on the health outcomes related to IPV which were alluded to in Chap. 1. The acute, intermediate, and long-term health consequences associated with IPV are reviewed, including: physical, (psycho-)somatic, reproductive, and psychological impairments. Physical injuries from IPV are the most visible and obvious health consequences of partner violence. In the US, IPV is one of the most common causes of injury for women seeking care for violence-related injuries in hospital emergency rooms (Rand 1997). Common injuries include bruises, scratches, burns, broken bones, head injuries, lacerations, miscarriages, and knife and gunshot wounds (Dutton et al. 2006; Tjaden and Thoennes 2000). In Germany, 64 % of those who have experienced IPV report having been injured (Müller and Schröttle 2004), while in Norway, this is true for 33 % of women who have experienced IPV (Nerøien and Schei 2008).

It is also important to consider the intermediate and long-term physical health effects which continue even after the abuse has ended (Garcia-Moreno et al. 2005). Among abused women, chronic pain (e.g., abdominal pain, pelvic pain, headaches, neck and back pain) is the most commonly reported symptom (Bonomi et al. 2007; Campbell et al. 2002; Coker et al. 2005; Sutherland et al. 2002), and greater severity of pain is related to longer duration of IPV exposure (Humphreys et al. 2011). A Canadian study of women who had left their abusive partners (an average of 20 months previously) found that 35 % reported high levels of debilitating pain, which is significantly higher than the national average of 18 % (Wuest et al. 2008). Associated with increased levels of chronic stress from abuse are also a loss of appetite, eating disorders, and gastrointestinal disorders like irritable bowel syndrome (Coker et al. 2000; Lindgren and Renck 2008). Moreover, often due to forced sex from the partner, gynecological disorders (e.g., chronic pelvic pain, vaginal bleeding or infection, sexually transmitted infections, and cervical cancer) are the "most consistent, longest lasting, and largest physical health difference" (Campbell 2002, p. 1332) between abused and nonabused women (Coker et al. 2000; Eby et al. 1995; Plichta and Abraham 1996; Schei and Bakketeig 1989; Schei 1991).

In addition to the myriad of physical health consequences, IPV also adversely affects mental health. International research has shown that women who have experienced IPV are three to five times more likely to report depression, suicidality, posttraumatic stress disorder (PTSD), and substance use than women without histories of IPV (Bonomi et al. 2006; Dillon et al. 2013; Golding 1999; Nerøien and

Schei 2008; O'Campo et al. 2006; Romito et al. 2005). Among these, depression and PTSD are the most frequent mental health outcomes for survivors of IPV (Cascardi et al. 1999; Dutton et al. 2006). In Australia, researchers have demonstrated that nearly 35 % of the disease burden presented by IPV can be attributed to depression (Vos et al. 2006), and US researchers have shown that PTSD and depression may act as mediators between IPV and women's physical health (Sutherland et al. 2002). Furthermore, cross-national studies have demonstrated a significant association between IPV and suicide in many different contexts. The likelihood of suicidal ideation is three times as likely and attempted suicide is four times as likely as among women who have experienced IPV than among women who have never experienced IPV (Devries et al. 2011; Ellsberg et al. 2008). As with physical health consequences, greater severity and a longer duration of IPV results in higher probability and more severe symptoms of depression and PTSD, as does experiencing more than one type (e.g., physical, sexual, psychological) of IPV (Ansara and Hindin 2011; Dillon et al. 2013; Dutton et al. 2005; Lindhorst and Beadnell 2011; Straus et al. 2009).

As evidenced by this wealth of literature, it is clear that IPV has negative health consequences for women.[4] However, the mechanisms by which IPV leads to poor health are less clearly understood (Ford-Gilboe et al. 2009; Scott-Storey 2011). The obvious exceptions to this, of course, are the acute and direct effects of physical injury, which may result in long-term disability. An indirect effect of IPV on health appears to occur through the presence of chronic stress, which accumulates over the course of abusive relationships, leading to long-term negative physical and mental health consequences (Dillon et al. 2013; Kendall-Tackett 2005; Plichta 2004; Sutherland et al. 2002). The presence of chronic stress can potentially lead to physiological changes in the body which create vulnerabilities to chronic illnesses and diseases (Kendall-Tackett 2005). Research also suggests that women who have experienced IPV tend to engage in more health risk behaviors (e.g., smoking, alcohol and drug use, unprotected sex) (Eby 2004; Golding 1999) and fewer healthy behaviors (Tomasulo and McNamara 2007) than women who have no exposure to IPV. These health behaviors potentially serve as a partial mediator between IPV and poor physical health. However, little is known about how the conditions of women's lives influence the health effects of IPV, which is detailed in Sect. 2.5 on the intersections of IPV, socioeconomic status, and health.

[4]It is worth noting that the studies cited in this section have utilized a variety of research methodologies, including surveys, clinical records, and qualitative interviews. Furthermore, they made use of population, community, shelter, and clinical samples for their research across a number of different cultural contexts. Despite these substantial differences, however, the health consequences appear to be relatively consistent across settings, thereby erasing doubt that IPV presents itself as a significant health concern (Dillon et al. 2013).

2.5 The Intersections: IPV, Economic Vulnerability, and Health

Due in part to early feminist theorizing which emphasized the universality of IPV (see Sect. 2.2), there are very few empirical studies attempting to clarify whether women's health outcomes ascribed to IPV may also be related to socioeconomic circumstances or vice versa. A notable exception is a US study that surveyed nearly 400 women of all income levels, including women with and without histories of IPV (Sutherland et al. 2001). The researchers found that IPV contributed to the variance in physical health outcomes above and beyond what could be explained by household income levels alone. Furthermore, while a similar negative trend in the relationship between IPV and health was found for all income levels, IPV was more strongly associated with poorer health among low-income women. Taken together, these findings suggest that abuse is especially harmful to the health of low-income women and that perhaps more economic resources could improve women's health.

The literature on women's access to resources in abusive relationships is also important to consider in its effect on health outcomes. A study by Ford-Gilboe et al. (2009) found that the combined total of women's personal, social, and economic resources mediated the relationship between IPV and health. Access to financial resources is often key to successfully ending an abusive relationship, and it follows that the more economically dependent a woman is on her abuser, the longer she stays with her partner. It is therefore plausible that this increases her risk for serious injury and illness through extended exposure to violence. Moreover, the long-term health effects (e.g., disability or chronic illness) resulting from IPV can present barriers to employment or result in poverty, further increasing her dependency on the abusive partner (Davis et al. 1999). Abused women reporting chronic pain, for example, were found in one study to be significantly more likely to be unemployed, to remain longer in a violent relationship, and to report more injuries (Humphreys et al. 2011). Women in the US taking part in focus groups described this as a dynamic interplay between the adverse health impact of IPV, the devastating effects of IPV on already-compromised health, and increasing dependency on the abuser due to illness or disability (Thomas et al. 2008). Likewise, a qualitative study with survivors in Germany confirms this finding, describing awareness that dependence on their partner exposed them to ongoing violence and had a continual detrimental impact on their health (Larsen et al. 2014).

2.6 Summary

This chapter has briefly described the theoretical assumptions and empirical evidence useful for understanding the occurrence of IPV and its outcomes. The great debates over IPV's definition highlight how crucial a nuanced understanding of the phenomenon is for research. Likewise, the overlap among sociological theories endeavoring to explain IPV hint at the necessity of taking a multifaceted approach in the investigation of partner violence. This includes taking into account both the individual-level factors of women's socioeconomic resources (e.g., income, education, employment) as well as societal-level factors (e.g., patriarchal structures, social policy) shaping the structure of women's lives. Empirical evidence suggests that the intersection between social position and IPV plays a role in women's health, potentially creating even greater vulnerabilities to poor health. However, these interactions are poorly understood and research on this topic only inconsistently addresses the structure of women's lives. This highlights the need for research on the health effects of IPV from a broader societal context. This sets the stage for Chap. 3, which provides the theoretical and empirical foundations of the welfare state's impact on health for women who have experienced IPV.

References

Alsaker, K., Moen, B. E., & Kristoffersen, K. (2007). Health-related quality of life among abused women one year after leaving a violent partner. *Social Indicators Research, 86*(3), 497–509. doi:10.1007/s11205-007-9182-7

Anderson, K. L. (1997). Gender, status, and domestic violence: An integration of feminist and family violence approaches. *Journal of Marriage and Family, 59*(3), 655–669.

Anderson, D. K., & Saunders, D. G. (2003). Leaving an abusive partner: An empirical review of predictors, the process of leaving, and psychological well-being. *Trauma, Violence, and Abuse, 4*(2), 163–191. doi:10.1177/1524838002250769

Anderson, M. A., Gillig, P. M., Sitaker, M., McCloskey, K., Malloy, K., & Grigsby, N. (2003). "Why doesn't she just leave?": A descriptive study of victim reported impediments to her safety. *Journal of Family Violence, 18*(3), 151–155. doi:10.1023/A:1023564404773

Ansara, D. L., & Hindin, M. J. (2011). Psychosocial consequences of intimate partner violence for women and men in Canada. *Journal of Interpersonal Violence, 26*(8), 1628–1645. doi:10.1177/0886260510370600

Archer, J. (2000). Sex differences in aggression between heterosexual partners: A meta-analytic review. *Psychological Bulletin, 126*(5), 651–680.

Atkinson, M. P., Greenstein, T. N., & Lang, M. M. (2005). For women, breadwinning can be dangerous: Gendered resource theory and wife abuse. *Journal of Marriage and Family, 67*(5), 1137–1148. doi:10.1111/j.1741-3737.2005.00206.x

Bachman, R., & Saltzman, L. E. (1995). *Violence against women: Estimates from the redesigned survey*. Washington, DC: U.S. Department of Justice.

Basu, B., & Famoye, F. (2004). Domestic violence against women, and their economic dependence: A count data analysis. *Review of Political Economy, 16*(4), 457–472. doi:10.1080/0953825042000256685

Bonomi, A. E., Thompson, R. S., Anderson, M., Reid, R. J., Carrell, D., Dimer, J. A., et al. (2006). Intimate partner violence and women's physical, mental, and social functioning. *American Journal of Preventive Medicine, 30*, 458–466. doi:10.1016/j.amepre.2006.01.015

Bonomi, A. E., Anderson, M. L., Rivara, F. P., & Thompson, R. S. (2007). Health outcomes in women with physical and sexual intimate partner violence exposure. *Journal of Women's Health, 16*(7), 987–997. doi:10.1089/jwh.2006.0239

Browne, A., Salomon, A., & Bassuk, S. S. (1999). The impact of recent partner violence on poor women's capacity to maintain work. *Violence Against Women, 5*(4), 393–426. doi:10.1177/10778019922181284

Byrne, C. A., Resnick, H. S., Kilpatrick, D. G., Best, C. L., & Saunders, B. E. (1999). The socioeconomic impact of interpersonal violence on women. *Journal of Consulting and Clinical Psychology, 67*(3), 362–366.

Campbell, J. C. (2002). Health consequences of intimate partner violence. *Lancet, 359*, 1331–1336. doi:10.1016/S0140-6736(02)08336-8

Campbell, J. C., Jones, A. S., Dienemann, J., Kub, J., Schollenberger, J., O'Campo, P., et al. (2002). Intimate partner violence and physical health consequences. *Archives of Internal Medicine, 162*, 1157–1163.

Cascardi, K., O'Leary, D., & Schlee, K. A. (1999). Co-occurrence and correlates of posttraumatic stress disorder and major depression in physically abused women. *Journal of Family Violence, 14*(3), 227–249. doi:10.1023/A:1022827915757

Coker, A. L., Smith, P. H., Bethea, L., King, M. R., & McKeown, R. E. (2000). Physical health consequences of physical and psychological intimate partner violence. *Archives of Family Medicine, 9*, 451–457.

Coker, A. L., Smith, P. H., & Fadden, M. K. (2005). Intimate partner violence and disabilities among women attending family practice clinics. *Journal of Women's Health, 14*, 829–838. doi:10.1089/jwh.2005.14.829

Cruz, M. J. (2000). Gay male domestic violence and the pursuit of masculinity. In P. Nardi (Ed.), *Gay masculinities: Research on men and masculinities*. Thousand Oaks, CA: Sage Publications.

Cunradi, C. B., Caetano, R., & Schafer, J. (2002). Socioeconomic predictors of intimate partner violence among White, Black, and Hispanic couples in the United States. *Journal of Family Violence, 17*(4), 377–389. doi:0885-7482/02/1200-0377/0

Davies, L., Ford-Gilboe, M., Willson, A., Varcoe, C., Wuest, J., Campbell, J., & Scott-Storey, K. (2015). Patterns of cumulative abuse among female survivors of intimate partner violence: Links to women's health and socioeconomic status. *Violence Against Women, 21*(1), 30–48. doi:10.1177/1077801214564076

Davis, M. F., Renzetti, C. M., & Edelson, J. L. (1999). The economics of abuse: How violence perpetuates women's poverty. In R. Brandwein & J. L. Edelson (Eds.), *Battered women, children, and welfare reform: The ties that bind* (pp. 17–30). Thousand Oaks, CA: Sage.

DeKeseredy, W. S. (2011). Feminist contributions to understanding woman abuse: Myths, controversies, and realities. *Aggression and Violent Behavior, 16*(4), 297–302. doi:10.1016/j.avb.2011.04.002

Dekeseredy, W. S., & Dragiewicz, M. (2007). Understanding the complexities of feminist perspectives on woman abuse: A commentary on Donald G. Dutton's Rethinking Domestic Violence. *Violence Against Women, 13*(8), 874–884. doi:10.1177/1077801207304806

Devries, K., Watts, C., Yoshihama, M., Kiss, L., Schraiber, L. B., Deyessa, N., et al. (2011). Violence against women is strongly associated with suicide attempts: Evidence from the WHO multi-country study on women's health and domestic violence against women. *Social Science and Medicine, 73*(1), 79–86. doi:10.1016/j.socscimed.2011.05.006

Dillon, G., Hussain, R., Loxton, D., & Rahman, S. (2013). Mental and physical health and intimate partner violence against women: A review of the literature. *International Journal of Family Medicine*, 1–15. doi:10.1155/2013/313909

Dobash, R. P., & Dobash, R. E. (1979). *Violence against wives: A case against the patriarchy*. New York, NY: Free Press.

Dobash, R. P., Dobash, R. E., Wilson, M., & Daly, M. C. (1992). The myth of sexual symmetry in marital violence. *Social Problems, 29*(1), 71–91. doi:10.2307/3096914

Dutton, D. G. (2006). *Rethinking domestic violence*. Vancouver, Canada: University of British Columbia Press.

Dutton, D. G. (2012). The case against the role of gender in intimate partner violence. *Aggression and Violent Behavior, 17*(1), 99–104. doi:10.1016/j.avb.2011.09.002

Dutton, M., Kaltman, S., Goodman, L. A., Weinfurt, K., & Vankos, N. (2005). Patterns of intimate partner violence: Correlates and outcomes. *Violence and Victims, 20*, 483–497. doi:10.1891/0886-6708.2005.20.5.483

Dutton, M., Green, B. L., Kaltman, S. I., Roesch, D. M., Zeffiro, T. A., & Krause, E. D. (2006). Intimate partner violence, PTSD, and adverse health outcomes. *Journal of Interpersonal Violence, 21*(7), 955–968. doi:10.1177/0886260506289178

Eby, K. (2004). Exploring the stressors of low-income women with abusive partners: Understanding their needs and developing effective community responses. *Journal of Family Violence, 19*(4), 221–232. doi:10.1023/B:JOFV.0000032632.59865.8e

Eby, K., Campbell, J. C., Sullivan, C. M., & Davidson, W. S. (1995). Health effects of experiences of sexual violence for women with abusive partners. *Health Care for Women International, 16* (6), 563–576.

Ellsberg, M., Jansen, H. A. F. M., Heise, L., Watts, C. H., & García-Moreno, C. (2008). Intimate partner violence and women's physical and mental health in the WHO multi-country study on women's health and domestic violence: An observational study. *The Lancet, 371*, 1165–1172. doi:10.1016/S0140-6736(08)60522-X

European Union Agency for Fundamental Rights [FRA]. (2014). *Violence against women: An EU-wide survey*. Luxembourg: Publications Office of the European Union. http://fra.europa.eu/sites/default/files/fra-2014-vaw-survey-main-results_en.pdf. Accessed November 01, 2014.

Farmer, A., & Tiefenthaler, J. (1997). An economic analysis of domestic violence. *Review of Social Economy, 55*(3), 337–358. doi:10.1080/00346769700000004

Ford-Gilboe, M., Wuest, J., Varcoe, C., Davies, L., Merritt-Gray, M., Campbell, J. C., et al. (2009). Modelling the effects of intimate partner violence and access to resources on women's health in the early years after leaving an abusive partner. *Social Science and Medicine, 68*, 1021–1029. doi:10.1016/j.socscimed.2009.01.003

Fox, G. L., & Benson, M. L. (2006). Household and neighborhood contexts of intimate partner violence. *Public Health Reports, 121*(4), 419–427.

Fox, G. L., Benson, M. L., DeMaris, A. A., & Wyk, J. (2002). Economic distress and intimate violence: Testing family stress and resources theories. *Journal of Marriage and Family, 64*(3), 793–807. doi:10.1111/j.1741-3737.2002.00793.x

Frye, V., Manganello, J., Campbell, J. C., Walton-Moss, B., & Wilt, S. (2006). The distribution of and factors associated with intimate terrorism and situational couple violence among a population-based sample of urban women in the United States. *Journal of Interpersonal Violence, 21*(10), 1286–1313. doi:10.1177/0886260506291658

Garcia-Moreno, C., Heise, L., Jansen, H. A. F. M., Ellsberg, M., & Watts, C. (2005). Public health. Violence against women. *Science, 310*(5752), 1282–1283. doi:10.1126/science.1121400

Gelles, R. J. (1985). Family violence. *Annual Review of Sociology, 11*(1), 347–367. doi:10.1146/annurev.so.11.080185.002023

Gelles, R. J. (1993). Through a sociological lens: Social structure and family violence. In R. J. Gelles & D. R. Loseke (Eds.), *Current controversies on family violence* (pp. 31–46). Newbury Park, CA: Sage Publications.

Golden, S. D., Perreira, K. M., & Durrance, C. P. (2013). Troubled times, troubled relationships: How economic resources, gender beliefs, and neighborhood disadvantage influence intimate partner violence. *Journal of Interpersonal Violence, 28*, 2134–2155. doi:10.1177/0886260512471083

Golding, J. M. (1999). Intimate partner violence as a risk factor for mental disorders: A meta-analysis. *Journal of Family Violence, 14*(2), 99–132.

Goode, W. J. (1971). Force and violence in the family. *Journal of Marriage and the Family, 33*(4), 624–636. doi:10.2307/349435

Goodman, L. A., Smyth, K. F., Borges, A. M., & Singer, R. (2009). When crises collide: How intimate partner violence and poverty intersect to shape women's mental health and coping? *Trauma, Violence, and Abuse, 10*, 306–329. doi:10.1177/1524838009339754

Heise, L. (1998). Violence against women: An integrated, ecological framework. *Violence Against Women, 4*(3), 262–290.

Heise, L. (2012). *Determinants of partner violence in low and middle-income countries: Exploring variation in individual and population level risk*. London, UK: London School of Hygiene Tropical Medicine. http://researchonline.lshtm.ac.uk/682451/1/560822.pdf. Accessed July 13, 2014.

Heise, L., & García-Moreno, C. (2012). Violence by intimate partners. In E. G. Krug, L. L. Dahlberg, J. A. Mercy, A. B. Zwi, & R. Lozano (Eds.), *World report on violence and health* (pp. 87–121). Geneva: World Health Organization.

Humphreys, C. (2007). A health inequalities perspective on violence against women. *Health and Social Care in the Community, 15*(2), 120–127. doi:10.1111/j.1365-2524.2006.00685.x

Humphreys, J., Cooper, B. A., & Miaskowski, C. (2011). Occurrence, characteristics, and impact of chronic pain in formerly abused women. *Violence Against Women, 17*(10), 1327–1343. doi:10.1177/1077801211425216

Jeffries, S., & Ball, M. J. (2008). Male same-sex intimate partner violence: A descriptive review and call for further research. *Murdoch e-Law Review, 15*(1), 134–179. http://eprints.qut.edu.au/17536/1/c17536.pdf. Accessed May 12, 2014.

Johnson, M. P. (1995). Patriarchal terrorism and common couple violence: Two forms of violence against women. *Journal of Marriage and Family, 57*(2), 283–294.

Johnson, M. P. (2006). Conflict and control: Gender symmetry and asymmetry in domestic violence. *Violence Against Women, 12*(11), 1003–1018. doi:10.1177/1077801206293328

Johnson, M. P. (2011). Gender and types of intimate partner violence: A response to an anti-feminist literature review. *Aggression and Violent Behavior, 16*(4), 289–296. doi:10.1016/j.avb.2011.04.006

Josephson, J. (2002). The intersectionality of domestic violence and welfare in the lives of poor women. *Journal of Poverty, 6*(1), 1–20. doi:10.1300/J134v06n01_01

Kalmuss, D. S., & Straus, M. A. (1982). Wife's marital dependency and wife abuse. *Journal of Marriage and Family, 44*(2), 277–286.

Kendall-Tackett, K. (2005). Exciting discoveries on the health effects of family violence: Where we are, where we need to go. *Journal of Interpersonal Violence, 20*(2), 251–257. doi:10.1177/0886260504267747

Kim, J., & Gray, K. A. (2008). Leave or stay? Battered women's decision after intimate partner violence. *Journal of Interpersonal Violence, 23*(10), 1465–1482. doi:10.1177/0886260508314307

Larsen, M., Krohn, J., Püschel, K., & Seifert, D. (2014). Experiences of health and health care among women exposed to intimate partner violence: Qualitative findings from Germany. *Health Care for Women International, 35*(4), 359–379. doi:10.1080/07399332.2012.738264

Lindgren, M. S., & Renck, B. (2008). "It is still so deep-seated, the fear": Psychological stress reactions as consequences of intimate partner violence. *Journal of Psychiatric and Mental Health Nursing, 15*, 219–228. doi:10.1111/j.1365-2850.2007.01215.x

Lindhorst, T., & Beadnell, B. (2011). The long arc of recovery: Characterizing intimate partner violence and its psychosocial effects across 17 years. *Violence Against Women, 17*(4), 480–499. doi:10.1177/1077801211404548

Macmillan, R., & Gartner, R. (1999). When she brings home the bacon: Labor-force participation and the risk of spousal violence against women. *Journal of Marriage and Family, 61*(4), 947–958.

McClennen, J. C., Summers, A. B., & Vaughan, C. (2002). Gay men's domestic violence. *Journal of Gay and Lesbian Social Services, 14*(1), 23–49. doi:10.1300/J041v14n01_02

McCloskey, L. A. (1996). Socioeconomic and coercive power with the family. *Gender and Society, 10*(4), 449–463. doi:10.1177/089124396010004006

Meier, J. (1997). Domestic violence, character, and social change in the welfare reform debate. *Law and Policy, 19*(2), 205–263. doi:10.1111/1467-9930.00028

Mitchell, C., & Vanya, M. (2009). Explanatory frameworks of intimate partner violence. In C. Mitchell & D. Anglin (Eds.), *Intimate partner violence: A health-based perspective* (pp. 39–52). New York, NY: Oxford University Press.

Moe, A. M., & Bell, M. P. (2004). Abject economics. *Violence Against Women, 10*(1), 29–55. doi:10.1177/1077801203256016

Müller, U., & Schröttle, M. (2004). *Lebenssituation, Sicherheit und Gesundheit von Frauen in Deutschland: Eine repräsentative Untersuchung zu Gewalt gegen Frauen in Deutschland [Health, well-being and personal safety of women in Germany: A representative study of violence against women in Germany]*. Berlin: Bundesministerium für Familie, Senioren, Frauen und Jugend.

Nerøien, A. I., & Schei, B. (2008). Partner violence and health: Results from the first national study on violence against women in Norway. *Scandinavian Journal of Public Health, 36*(2), 161–168. doi:10.1177/1403494807085188

Nicolaidis, C., & Paranjape, A. (2009). Defining intimate partner violence: Controversies and implications. In C. Mitchell & D. Anglin (Eds.), *Intimate partner violence: A health-based perspective* (pp. 19–30). New York, NY: Oxford University Press.

O'Campo, P., Kub, J., Woods, A., Garza, M., Jones, A. S., Gielen, A. C., et al. (2006). Depression, PTSD, and comorbidity related to intimate partner violence in civilian and military women. *Brief Treatment and Crisis Intervention, 6*(2), 99–110. doi:10.1093/brief-treatment/mhj010

Oliffe, J. L., Han, C., Maria, E. S., Lohan, M., Howard, T., Stewart, D. E., et al. (2014). Gay men and intimate partner violence: A gender analysis. *Sociology of Health and Illness, 36*(4), 564–579. doi:10.1111/1467-9566.12099

Plichta, S. B. (2004). Intimate partner violence and physical health consequences: Policy and practice implications. *Journal of Interpersonal Violence, 19*(11), 1296–1323. doi:10.1177/0886260504269685

Plichta, S. B., & Abraham, C. (1996). Violence and gynecologic health in women <50 years old. *American Journal of Obstetrics and Gynecology, 174*(3), 903–907. doi:10.1016/S0002-9378(96)70323-X

Purvin, D. M. (2007). At the crossroads and in the crosshairs: Social welfare policy and low-income women's vulnerability to domestic violence. *Social Problems, 54*(2), 188–210. doi:10.1525/sp.2007.54.2.188

Rand, M. (1997). *Violence-related injuries treated in hospital emergency departments*. Washington, DC: U.S. Department of Justice.

Raphael, J. (2003). Battering through the lens of class. *Journal of Gender, Social Policy and the Law, 11*(2), 367–375.

Renzetti, C. (1992). *Violent betrayal: Partner abuse in lesbian relationships*. Thousand Oaks, CA: Sage Publications.

Rodriguez-Menes, J., & Safranoff, A. (2012). Violence against women in intimate relations: A contrast of five theories. *European Journal of Criminology, 9*(6), 584–602. doi:10.1177/1477370812453410

Romito, P., Turan, J. M., & De Marchi, M. (2005). The impact of current and past interpersonal violence on women's mental health. *Social Science and Medicine, 60*, 1717–1727. doi:10.1016/j.socscimed.2004.08.026

Schei, B. (1991). Physically abusive spouse—A risk factor of pelvic inflammatory disease? *Scandinavian Journal of Primary Health Care, 9*(1), 41–45.

Schei, B., & Bakketeig, L. S. (1989). Gynaecological impact of sexual and physical abuse by spouse. A study of a random sample of Norwegian women. *British Journal of Obstetrics and Gynaecology, 96*(12), 1379–1383.

Schröttle, M., & Ansorge, N. (2008). *Gewalt gegen Frauen in Paarbeziehungen: Eine sekundäranalytische Auswertung zur Differenzierung von Schweregraden, Mustern, Risikofaktoren und Unterstützung nach erlebter Gewalt [Violence against women in relationships: A secondary analysis of the differentiation between severity, types, risk factors, and support after violent incidents]*. Berlin: Bundesministerium für Familie, Senioren, Frauen und Jugend.

Scott-Storey, K. (2011). Cumulative abuse: Do things add up? An evaluation of the conceptualization, operationalization, and methodological approaches in the study of the phenomenon of cumulative abuse. *Trauma, Violence, and Abuse, 12*(3), 135–150. doi:10.1177/1524838011404253

Shobe, M. A., & Dienemann, J. (2008). Intimate partner violence in the United States: An ecological approach to prevention and treatment. *Social Policy and Society, 7*(02), 185–195.

Straus, M. A. (1999). The controversy over domestic violence by women: A methodological, theoretical, and sociology of science analysis. In X. B. Arriaga & S. Oskamp (Eds.), *Violence in intimate relationships* (pp. 17–44). Thousand Oaks, CA: Sage Publications.

Straus, M. A. (2011). Gender symmetry and mutuality in perpetration of clinical-level partner violence: Empirical evidence and implications for prevention and treatment. *Aggression and Violent Behavior, 16*(4), 279–288. doi:10.1016/j.avb.2011.04.010

Straus, M. A., Gelles, R. J., & Steinmetz, S. K. (1980). *Behind closed doors: Violence in the American family*. Garden City, NJ: Anchor Books.

Straus, H., Cerulli, C., McNutt, L. A., Rhodes, K. V, Conner, K. R., Kemball, R. S., et al. (2009). Intimate partner violence and functional health status: Associations with severity, danger, and self-advocacy behaviors. *Journal of Women's Health, 18*(5), 625–631. doi:10.1089/jwh.2007.0521

Sutherland, C. A., Sullivan, C. M., & Bybee, D. I. (2001). Effects of intimate partner violence versus poverty on women's health. *Violence Against Women, 7*, 1122–1143. doi:10.1177/10778010122183775

Sutherland, C. A., Bybee, D. I., & Sullivan, C. M. (2002). Beyond bruises and broken bones: The joint effects of stress and injuries on battered women's health. *American Journal of Community Psychology, 30*(5), 609–636. doi:10.1023/a:1016317130710

Thomas, K. A., Joshi, M., Wittenberg, E., & McCloskey, L. A. (2008). Intersections of harm and health: A qualitative study of intimate partner violence in women's lives. *Violence Against Women, 14*, 1252–1273. doi:10.1177/1077801208324529

Tjaden, P., & Thoennes, N. (2000). *Extent, nature, and consequences of intimate partner violence: Findings from the National Violence Against Women Survey*. Washington, DC: U.S. Department of Justice.

Tolman, R. M., & Rosen, D. (2001). Domestic violence in the lives of women receiving welfare: Mental health, substance dependence, and economic well-being. *Violence Against Women, 7* (2), 141–158. doi:10.1177/1077801201007002003

Tomasulo, G. C., & McNamara, J. R. (2007). The relationship of abuse to women's health status and health habits. *Journal of Family Violence, 22*(4), 231–235. doi:10.1007/s10896-007-9076-0

Vest, J. R., Catlin, T. K., Chen, J. J., & Brownson, R. C. (2002). Multistate analysis of factors associated with intimate partner violence. *American Journal of Preventive Medicine, 22*(3), 156–164

Vos, T., Astbury, J., Piers, L., Magnus, A., Heenan, M., Stanley, L., et al. (2006). Measuring the impact of intimate partner violence on the health of women in Victoria, Australia. *Bulletin of the World Health Organization, 84*(9), 739–744. doi:10.1590/S0042-96862006000900017

Walker, L. E. (1979). *The battered woman*. New York, NY: Harper and Row Publishers.

Winstok, Z. (2011). The paradigmatic cleavage on gender differences in partner violence perpetration and victimization. *Aggression and Violent Behavior, 16*(4), 303–311. doi:10.1016/j.avb.2011.04.004

Wuest, J., Merritt-Gray, M., Ford-Gilboe, M., Lent, B., Varcoe, C., & Campbell, J. C. (2008). Chronic pain in women survivors of intimate partner violence. *The Journal of Pain, 9*(11), 1049–1057. doi:10.1016/j.jpain.2008.06.009

Chapter 3
IPV from a Welfare State Perspective

Abstract This chapter offers a review of the theoretical welfare state literature relevant to women's socioeconomic resources and their health, followed respectively by an examination of empirical research related to family and health policy. In order to piece this literature together into a complete picture connecting the welfare state with women's health outcomes, a conceptual model highlighting mechanisms leading to health inequities is introduced. Moving toward the application of this model to IPV, the gaps in the literature regarding IPV, health, and the welfare state are examined. Finally, the conceptual framework is adapted to IPV and serves as the foundation for elucidating four specific research questions regarding individual- and macro-level factors related to differential exposure to IPV and differential vulnerability to poor health.

This chapter offers a review of the theoretical welfare state literature relevant to women's socioeconomic resources and their health, followed respectively by an examination of empirical research related to family and health policy. In order to piece this literature together into a complete picture connecting the welfare state with women's health outcomes, a conceptual model highlighting mechanisms leading to health inequities is introduced. Moving toward the application of this model to IPV, the gaps in the literature regarding IPV, health, and the welfare state are examined. Finally, the conceptual framework is adapted to IPV and serves as the foundation for elucidating four specific research questions regarding individual- and macro-level factors related to differential exposure to IPV and differential vulnerability to poor health.

3.1 The Gendered Welfare State

Feminist scholarship has long critiqued the mainstream comparative welfare state research as offering little in the way of understanding that stratification and decommodification may differ for men and women (e.g., Orloff 1993, 2009a; Sainsbury 1994a; Sorensen and McLanahan 1987). While Esping-Andersen does not entirely ignore gender in his typologies, his early focus was primarily on the

© Springer International Publishing Switzerland 2016
M.M. Larsen, *Health Inequities Related to Intimate Partner Violence Against Women*, Social Disparities in Health and Health Care,
DOI 10.1007/978-3-319-29565-7_3

labor market and did not thoroughly consider the role of family and women's care work (Pfau-Effinger 1998). Therefore, it became necessary to also examine welfare state issues in the context of gender relations—for example, including the role of the family and caregiving in the analysis of the balance between market and state in social provision. One of the seminal works of this kind is Hobson's (1990) *No Exit, No Voice* article, where she makes the case that when social benefits are offered only to those participating in the labor market, and pension systems are based on status and wage contributions, this creates long-term negative consequences for women's economic well-being:

> We can no longer assume that redistributive policies based on family incomes necessarily improve the position of women in the family and society. Social and labor market policies that are designed for the family as a unit– where the man is the major breadwinner and a gendered division of labor exists in the household– may in fact deepen the gap between men's and women's power in the family and in society, and thus institutionalize gender inequality (Hobson 1990, p. 239).

Building upon Hirschman's (1970) work *Exit, Voice, and Loyalty*, Hobson contends that when women are economically dependent on their male partners, they have less of a 'voice' in decision-making within a relationship and are also not economically able to 'exit' the relationship if necessary.

There is some empirical evidence in this direction. At least at the national level, comparative cross-national studies have shown that increases in women's employment income results in a gendered shift in the allocation of household duties (Hook 2006; Stier and Lewin-Epstein 2007). Likewise, when men and women in the US contribute equally to income in a household, the chances of divorce or separation are higher if the relationship is unhappy (Rogers 2004; Sayer and Bianchi 2000). In other words, women's economic contribution to the family increases their decision-making power and also allows them to end unhappy partnerships. However, the data are not always so straightforward. In *Geld und Liebe [Money and love]*, Wimbauer (2003) argues that while the symbolic meaning of income can indeed create power and status inequalities in relationships, the situation is more complex than simply examining who earns more or less. Research in Germany has shown than even when women earn more than their partners, it does not necessarily mean that women hold the power in the relationship or that women's earnings are considered to be the primary household income (Lott 2009). Data from the US and Australia imply that once women provide the majority of the household income, couples appear to compensate for this deviation from gendered norms by returning to more traditional divisions of household duties (Bittman et al. 2003). This suggests that it is also necessary to consider societal gender cultures when analyzing women's voice and ability to exit a relationship.

Orloff (1993) builds upon Hobson's argument by claiming that the unbalanced power relationships resulting from women's economic dependency must be equalized by the welfare state through the promotion of independence for women from both markets and marriage. If those who carry out the caregiving within a family (usually women), "do not enter the labor market, or enter it only as secondary workers, the resulting distribution of income within the family and the availability of other income sources affects their own and their children's well-being" (Orloff 1993, p. 319). To address this imbalance through social policy involves strategies that provide women with incomes that allow them to support themselves and their children without making claims on the breadwinner's income. This is often referred to as the concept of *defamilization*: "the degree to which individual adults can uphold a socially acceptable standard of living, independently of family relationships, either through paid work or through social security provisions" (Lister 1997, p. 173). This acknowledges that women's economic dependency within the family is equivalent to dependency on the market (Esping-Andersen 1999, p. 45).

As an operationalization for the concept of defamilization, Orloff (1993) suggests two dimensions for comparatively investigating the effects of the welfare state: *women's access to paid work* and women's ability to *establish and maintain an independent household*. In terms of access to paid work, it is important to assess to what extent social policy is supporting women's ties to the labor market. Of course, employment is only one piece of the puzzle for having a 'voice' and choosing to 'exit' if needed, since women often earn lower wages due to gender pay gaps, work in lower paying sectors, and often work only part-time (Jaehrling et al. 2014; Misra et al. 2007a; Orloff 2009a). It is, therefore, vital to also consider whether women have sufficient resources to establish an independent household and to what extent the welfare state helps relieve (e.g., through social transfers) this "compulsion to enter or stay in a marriage because of economic vulnerability" (Orloff 1993, p. 321).

When seeking to examine women's economic dependency, Pfau-Effinger (1998, 2012) makes the claim that social policy has been afforded too much explanatory power and is too deterministic in its supposed impact on individual behavior. Instead, she calls for more complex theorizing around the relationship between structure and culture. She argues that the constant interchange between gender culture, gender order, and gender arrangements is central to welfare state comparisons. *Gender culture* is comprised of the values, models, and belief systems related to the 'proper' form of gender relations and the gendered division of labor. This gender culture serves as a reference point for the behavior of individuals and of social policy institutions, and can impact the gender order. The *gender order* is the gendered structure of the division of labor, as well as the gendered structure of the institutions of the welfare state, the family, and the market. Together, the gender culture and the gender order create the *gender arrangement*, which is essentially the social practice within households of the division of labor. Pfau-Effinger emphasizes that women's employment behavior and their economic (in)dependence are influenced by the interaction of gender culture, gender order, and social practices under the gender arrangement. The theory offers no clear causal chain linking these dimensions together (Kremer 2007). It does, however, propose ideal types of cultural family models which "connect cultural values in relation to the family-employment relationship of the adult family members, the gender division of labour within the family, and the most suitable form of care for children"

(Pfau-Effinger 2012, p. 533). She suggests the following ideal types for empirical cross-national comparisons of women's employment behavior: the *male breadwinner/female carer* model; the *male breadwinner/female part-time carer* model; the *dual breadwinner/external carer* (either the state or the market) model; and the *dual breadwinner/extended family care* model. Empirical studies from this standpoint have found that family policies encouraging women's employment are more successful in cultures which value a dual-earner family model, and less successful in cultures which place higher priority on women's roles as caregivers (Budig et al. 2012).

Despite approaching this issue from a different perspective, there are similarities to be found between Pfau-Effinger's cultural family models and some gendered welfare state classifications based on the ideas of defamilization (Lewis 1992; O'Connor 1993; Sainsbury 1994b). For example, Misra et al. (2007a) make use of Fraser's (1994) theoretical approach to welfare state support for caregiving. They developed four key welfare state strategies for women's roles: the *carer strategy*, with women viewed primarily as carers and secondarily as earners (e.g., Austria, Germany); *the earner strategy*, with women viewed primarily as earners and secondarily as carers (e.g., Canada, the US); the *choice strategy*, with women perceived as having a choice in being primarily earners or caregivers (e.g., France, Belgium); and the *earner–carer strategy*, with women (and men) seen as involved in both earning and caring equally (e.g., Sweden). Similarly, Ferrarini (2006) proposed three categories of family policy: the *general family policy* model is based on the traditional understanding of the male as breadwinner with a dependent female partner; the *dual-earner* model is based on both partners equally participating in the labor market; and the *market-oriented* model, which leaves families to address issues of caregiving privately.

The following paragraphs contain a review of the empirical literature which takes either a regime approach (i.e., comparing countries according to typologies like those previously mentioned) or an institutional approach (i.e., comparisons based rather on specific welfare institutions and policies) (Dahl and van der Wel 2013). Studies of family policy often investigate three related outcomes for women: (1) labor market participation, (2) economic dependency within relationships, and (3) poverty.

Starting with women's *labor market participation*, there is general agreement that publicly funded childcare has a positive effect on the employment of women with small children, in that it frees women of some of their care responsibilities (Gornick et al. 1997; Orloff 2009a; Pettit and Hook 2005). For women with school-aged children, public school schedules affect their employment since the length of the school day, whether students are sent home for lunch, length and frequency of vacations, and number of school weeks per year can conflict with typical employment schedules (Cook 2010; Gornick et al. 1997; Graves 2013). Moreover, generous parental leave typically has a positive impact on women's employment levels by allowing them to care for small children and return to their jobs afterward, but leaves which are too long can have the opposite effect. According to Pettit and Hook (2005), extensive parental leave has a negative effect on the levels of employment for women with small children, actually serving to disconnect them from the labor force. For women seeking a solution to combining work and family, policies mandating equal wages and working conditions for part-time employment can indeed support women's employment levels overall (Bleijenbergh et al. 2004; Gornick and Meyers 2009). Finally, joint-income tax systems (e.g., as in Germany) tend to penalize dual-earner couples by taxing the secondary income on top of the primary income, while systems of individual taxation (e.g., as in Sweden) encourage couples to be dual earners by adding lowly taxed secondary income to the primary income (Cook 2010; Gustafsson and Bruyn-Hundt 1991; Sainsbury 1999).

Second, based on the impact of these policies on women's labor market participation, inferences are also made regarding the impact of the social policy context on women's *economic dependence* in relationships. Data from the Luxembourg Income Study reveals that in Sweden, for example, higher levels of women's labor market participation are associated with lower levels of economic dependence, suggesting that policies which enable women's employment (e.g., paid parental leave, flexible working hours, individualized taxes, and state-subsidized childcare) help reduce economic dependency (Hobson 1990).[1] Other studies have also found a strong connection between women's labor force participation and their economic dependency. In their cross-national examination of these factors, Bianchi et al. (1999, p. 29) found their results fit "very neatly" into Esping-Andersen's welfare regime typology. Specifically, the lowest levels of labor force participation and the greatest levels of economic dependency were found among women in the conservative welfare states which promoted the traditional division of labor in the household (e.g., Germany, Belgium, and the Netherlands), while the exact opposite was found in the social democratic welfare states which supported women's employment (e.g., Finland, Sweden, Norway).

In research attempting to disentangle the effect of actual policies from the effect of welfare regime types on women's economic independence, greater availability of public childcare appears to increase women's relative contribution to household income and thereby increase their economic independence (Stier and Mandel 2009). On the other hand, policies supporting extensive maternity leave and part-time employment have the opposite effect for dual-earner couples (Huber et al. 2009; Stier and Mandel 2009). While these policies may allow women to maintain a nominal connection to the labor force, they incentivize extended separation from employment and decrease their relative contributions to the household. Part-time employment, for example, is associated with lower wages, limited access to social insurance, fewer opportunities for career advancement, and reduced retirement pensions (Bardasi and Gornick 2008). Thus, while it may prove to be a solution for solving immediate work–family conflicts, it prioritizes women's roles as carers and increases their economic dependence on their partners.

---

[1]Hobson is careful to note, however, that while the level of women's economic dependence in Sweden is the lowest among the nine Western countries compared, a considerable percentage of women are still economically dependent on their partners.

Finally, beyond labor market participation and economic dependency is also the question of whether the welfare state supports women in being able to establish an independent household without falling into *poverty*. The term 'feminization of poverty' was coined by Pearce (1978) to describe the situation of higher rates of poverty among women than men, which has been found to be the case in nearly all affluent democracies (Brady and Kall 2008). In this question, the research often focuses specifically on single mothers as a litmus test for how well social policy addresses women's economic vulnerabilities (Hobson 1994), because families led by single mothers tend to have higher poverty rates than other types of families (Christopher et al. 2002). It has been found that family allowances (i.e., cash transfers to families with children) and state provision of childcare for children under the age of two significantly reduced poverty levels for single mothers (Misra et al. 2007b). These family allowances raise single mothers' chances at increasing the household income above the poverty level, especially if earned income is not sufficient (Huber et al. 2009; Jaehrling et al. 2014). Regarding childcare, it is probable that poverty rates are reduced by easing women's care burden and minimizing their separation from the labor market. Likewise, while parental leave initially reduces poverty rates, very long parental leave *increases* them (Misra et al. 2007b). Extended absence from the workplace reduces women's attachment to the labor force and their employment opportunities upon returning to work, thereby contributing to poverty levels. Basically, "where welfare is not generous and employment support is left to market sources, solo mothers' relative poverty remains high" (Orloff 2009b, p. 327).

In sum, there is considerable evidence that the social policy context contributes in both positive and negative ways to women's labor market participation, economic independence, and poverty rates. For the most part, the strongest attachment to the labor force and ability to establish an independent household exist in welfare states which approach family policy from a dual-earner perspective.[2] On the other hand, the weakest connection to paid work and the resources for establishing an independent household tend to be found in the welfare states with policies viewing women as primarily caregivers and men primarily as breadwinners. Liberal welfare states which view women as primarily earners and leave caretaking up to the market, however, generally provide very little state intervention and thus fall somewhere in between.

[2]This book takes a rather institutional arrangement approach to its analysis and therefore does not specifically apply any of the regime typologies referred to in this section in its analyses. However, for purposes of simplification in the text, these regime labels are sometimes used to refer to specific groupings of family policies.

3.2 Welfare States and Health Care Systems

Above and beyond the welfare state and family policies already described in this chapter, health care is unquestionably considered to be one of the primary functions of the welfare state, with health care expenditures consuming one of the largest shares of resources across modern welfare states (Bambra 2005a; Beckfield et al. 2013; Moran 2000). In the words of Freeman and Moran, "Health care matters. Not often, but sometimes, it is a matter of life and death. More usually, it represents a powerful means of alleviating the anxiety, discomfort and incapacity that come from sickness and ill health" (Freeman and Moran 2000, p. 35). Systems of health care are made up of

> organizations that both deliver care and medical services (hospitals, physicians' practices, clinics) and that arrange for the financing of care (governments, agencies, states, local communities, and private insurance companies). These organizations are embedded within welfare states, which are based on particular institutional logics and distributional principles that restructure class relations in specific ways (Quadagno 2010, p. 126).

Although health policy is intertwined with other social policy, health care is rarely directly addressed in comparative welfare state literature or the general welfare regimes discussion (Bambra 2005a, b; Olafsdottir and Beckfield 2011). Whereas the feminist critique of mainstream welfare state research tends to add gendered dimensions to welfare regime theory, the internal debate and comparison in the health policy literature remains relatively disconnected from the broader welfare state discussion (Freeman and Moran 2000; Moran 1999, 2000). Some contend that this is due to the focus of Esping-Andersen's regime classification on social transfers while ignoring the provision of social services (e.g., health care, education, social care) (Bambra 2005b, 2007). This assumes that various aspects of the welfare state operate under a coherent set of values representative of each state's 'welfare package' (Kasza 2002). Kasza makes the case, however, that this assumption is inherently flawed. The United Kingdom (UK) is one often cited example of such "internal policy inconsistency" within welfare states (Bambra 2005a, p. 32). While the UK's broader liberal welfare policies leave provision mostly to the market, the National Health System offers universal care and is primarily funded by general taxation. Perhaps as a result of these types of inconsistencies, the conceptualization of welfare states often glosses over health care or avoids it altogether (Olafsdottir and Beckfield 2011).

Since health care is often not incorporated in the classical welfare regime framework, there instead have been a number of different attempts at health care system classification.[3] However, there is little consensus in the literature over what the key comparative dimensions of health care systems should be, indeed even no "canon of the scientific literature" which sets the research agenda for the field (Marmor and Wendt 2012, p. 17). One common typology centers around the configuration of medical professionals, the state, and payers in terms of coverage, funding, and

[3]The reader is referred to an article by Beckfield et al. (2013) for an overview of the history of health care system classification.

ownership (Scheiber 1987). This classification proposes three different models of health care systems: national health service, social insurance, and private insurance systems (Burau and Blank 2006).[4] In the *national health service* model (e.g., the UK), coverage is universal, funding comes through general taxation, and there is public ownership of health care. In the *social insurance* model (e.g., Germany), coverage is universal through mandatory insurance, funding comes primarily through contributions from both employer and employee, and provision of care is either public or private. As a contrast to the previous two models, in the *private insurance* model (e.g., the US), coverage is through private health insurance purchased by the individual or the employer, and health care delivery is primarily in private ownership.

However, while classifications provide a necessary framework for understanding the structure and organization of health care systems (Burau and Blank 2006; Marmor and Okma 2003), typologies alone are not sufficient. Too much effort is arguably spent on the macro-level description of institutional structures, when it should be spent on evaluating how these varying arrangements influence health outcomes (Marmor and Wendt 2012; Olafsdottir and Beckfield 2011). Since access is a determinant of health outcomes (Whitehead and Dahlgren 2006), Wendt (2009) argues that the most important comparative dimensions for health care systems research should be the provision of health care and access to services. For women, health policy is an important determinant of access to health care (Bird and Rieker 2008). In particular, given the existing tensions in ensuring women's ties to the labor market, it is vital that health care system policies ensure that women have consistent and affordable access to health care which is independent of the labor market (Zimmerman and Legerski 2010).

Access to health care is widely discussed and applied as a yardstick to measure the success of health systems (van Doorslaer et al. 2006), but is a complex concept and often poorly defined. To begin, it is important to differentiate between 'having access' and 'gaining access' to health care. The former represents the possibility of utilizing care if necessary (i.e., presupposing the existence of an adequate supply of health care services), while the latter represents the actual utilization of health care (i.e., presupposing the ability and willingness to use health care services) (Gulliford et al. 2002). Penchansky and Thomas (1981) break this down even further by characterizing access as the goodness of fit between patients and the health care system, and this book makes particular use of two central dimensions which they propose: availability and affordability.[5] *Availability* refers to whether the supply of

---

[4]Another common classification refers to the national health service model and the social insurance model as the Beveridge model and the Bismarck model, respectively, after the founders of these systems in the UK and Germany (Stevens 2001).

[5]Penchansky and Thomas (1981) also suggest three further dimensions of access: accessibility, accommodation, and acceptability. Accessibility addresses the geographic proximity of health care providers to the population. Accommodation and acceptability focus on cultural and personal barriers to health care. These have to do with whether the health care provider offers services in a manner that is accommodating to patients' preferences, and whether patients are accepting of health care providers' characteristics. However, these are beyond the scope of this book.

health care providers and specialized services is sufficient for meeting the needs of the population. *Affordability* has to do with the financial costs of health care in relation to the patients' ability and readiness to pay for care. Particularly when looking at issues of equity, Whitehead (2000) also includes the concept of *entitlement* to health care. She argues that "equal access to available care for equal need implies equal entitlement to the available services for everyone, a fair distribution throughout the country based on health care needs… and the removal of other barriers to access" (Whitehead 2000, p. 8). Building on these ideas, a number of indicators deserve consideration when systematically comparing access to health care. Addressing the first dimension of *availability*, levels of inpatient and outpatient health care providers (i.e., physician density) should be considered. In terms of the second dimension of *affordability*, the level of private out-of-pocket payments is important to consider. Finally, related to the third dimension of *entitlement* to health care, the level of health coverage in the population captures the extent to which individuals are granted access to health care services (Pankratz 2012).

In the empirical literature assessing the impact of access to care, health care utilization is often measured as an outcome because it is thought to be a primary pathway to improved health outcomes (Allin et al. 2007; Gulliford et al. 2002; McLaughlin and Wyszewianski 2002; Quimbo et al. 2011). Thus, the following paragraphs contain a review of the literature around both utilization and health outcomes, particularly focusing on women where possible.

First, a study of rural women in the US found that living in a county with higher primary care physician availability reduces unnecessary trips to the emergency department (Simmons et al. 2008). A number of different studies have also shown that increasing out-of-pocket costs for patients presents financial barriers for access and reduces *utilization of health care*, especially for low-income households (Aaltonen et al. 2015; Hacker 2004; Plümper and Neumayer 2013; Rice and Morrison 1994; Thomson and Mossialos 2004). Finally, one of the most researched indicators of access to health care in the US is the level of health insurance coverage, which has been found to be a primary determinant of health care utilization. In the US, uninsured women are less likely to utilize health services (Simmons et al. 2008; Taylor et al. 2006), particularly preventative services like mammograms or screening for cervical cancer, and are at least twice as likely to skip treatment due to cost issues (Kaiser Family Foundation 2013).

But as previously hinted at, in comparing access across different health care systems, it is also vital to assess its impact on *health outcomes* themselves (Marmor and Wendt 2012; Olafsdottir and Beckfield 2011). There is an international body of evidence demonstrating that improved access to health care has a positive impact on health outcomes (Gilson et al. 2007; Pankratz 2012; Plümper and Neumayer 2013). Comparative research suggests that a strong primary care system which increases the supply of primary care physicians is linked to lower rates of avoidable hospitalizations (Gulliford 2002), lower mortality rates, and improved mental health outcomes (Arah et al. 2005; Or et al. 2005; Starfield et al. 2005).

Likewise, the level of health insurance coverage (as an indicator of entitlement to care) has been found to be related to health outcomes. Comparing nine OECD (Organisation for Economic Co-operation and Development) countries with varying health care systems, Zimmerman and Legerski (2010) found that universal access systems have better health outcomes among women, as demonstrated by longer life expectancy and fewer years lost to premature mortality. Likewise, other comparative studies of OECD countries show higher levels of health insurance coverage being related to lower levels of mortality (Arah et al. 2005; Berger and Messer 2002). When comparing women's health outcomes across US states, researchers have also discovered lower levels of mortality due to heart disease and breast cancer in states with expanded levels of Medicaid insurance eligibility and provision (Wisdom et al. 2005). Likewise, morbidity levels for chronic and acute conditions in the US are higher among adults without insurance than those with health insurance (Baker et al. 2001, 2002).

In summary, evidence exists which points toward the influence of systems on women's utilization of health care and on health outcomes. Generally speaking, those health systems with universal entitlement, widespread availability of providers, and affordable care tend to demonstrate better population health outcomes. However, it should also be taken into account that the studies linking mortality rates to health insurance coverage are not able to establish a causal link (Levy and Meltzer 2008) and the benefits of health insurance coverage tend to vary according to disease and population group (Hadley 2003). Moreover, Chung and Muntaner (2007) make the case that although health care services play a role in population health outcomes, the role of welfare state policies as whole may be larger. Thus, research on the welfare state's impact on health should also consider aspects that are not directly related to health systems and policies.

3.3 Linking Social Policies to Women's Health

There are a number of arguments supporting the investigation of the impact of broader welfare policy on women's health. Indicators of women's status in society and their participation in the labor market, both of which are mediated by social policy, have been shown to affect women's health. Studies demonstrate that social structural factors, like increased income, full-time employment, and caring for a family, play a larger role in determining women's health than men's health (Denton and Walters 1999; Denton et al. 2004; Malmusi et al. 2014). Even more broadly, a comparison of US states found that women's mortality and morbidity rates were lower in those states with greater levels of political participation and economic autonomy among women (Kawachi et al. 1999). A multicountry comparison of the welfare state as a determinant of women's health focused on childcare provision and community-based long-term care, and came to the conclusion that nations with a social welfare orientation are more likely to have policies that positively impact women's health than nations with market-driven policy approaches (Raphael and

Bryant 2004). Looking more broadly at populations as a whole, a review of studies using a welfare regimes framework revealed a positive correlation between welfare generosity and improved population health (Muntaner et al. 2011). In particular, the generous family policies and labor market decommodification of social democratic regimes seems to be related to better population and individual health outcomes (e.g., old age mortality, self-assessed health) (Bambra 2006; Eikemo et al. 2008; Ferrarini and Norström 2010; Lundberg 2008; Van de Velde et al. 2014).

Another related strand of research involves the impact of the welfare state on social inequalities in health. Higher social status is solidly linked to better health outcomes, so that health represents a noteworthy source of stratification in society (Olafsdottir 2007) which varies significantly across countries (Beckfield and Olafsdottir 2009; Beckfield et al. 2013). However, the research looking into the role of the welfare state in shaping social inequalities in health has generally proven inconclusive (Beckfield and Krieger 2009; Bergqvist et al. 2013; Muntaner et al. 2011). There is an implicit assumption that because the social democratic welfare states have better health outcomes overall, they should also demonstrate smaller health inequalities (Bambra 2013). Yet, it has been shown that countries with better health outcomes tend to have larger relative inequalities in health (Huijts and Eikemo 2009), and that health inequalities are not at all systematically smaller in social democratic welfare states (Dahl et al. 2006). This is known in the literature as a 'public health puzzle' and 'paradox', which has garnered a number of attempts at explanation (see for example, Bambra 2011; Hurrelmann et al. 2011; Mackenbach 2012). One key factor to consider is the difference between *absolute* and *relative* inequalities. Since the overall levels of health in the social democratic welfare states are already high, the very high levels of health in the middle–upper classes ensure that relative inequalities remain. However, the lowest socioeconomic classes in the social democratic regimes are still better off in absolute terms as compared to the lowest socioeconomic classes in other welfare state regimes. According to Bambra (2013), this debate should raise political and normative questions as to whether the welfare state should aim to improve the lives of the most vulnerable in society, or to improve equality overall.

If one takes a closer look at gender differences in health outcomes and inequalities according to welfare or social policy regimes, there are relatively few studies to draw upon. In their review of the existing studies on this topic, Borrell et al. (2014) found partial support for the claim that social democratic welfare regimes and dual-earner family policies are related to fewer gender inequalities in health (see, for example, Backhans et al. 2012; Boye 2011). Additionally, a comparison of 26 European countries found that among countries with family policy models oriented toward gender equality, gender inequalities in self-assessed health were less than in countries with more traditional family policy models (Palència et al. 2014). However, when accounting for the influence of socioeconomic differences between men and women, Bambra et al. (2009) did not find conclusive evidence of a welfare regime pattern for gender differences in self-assessed health. She and her colleagues suggest that more research on the gendered nature of welfare states is necessary before conclusions can be drawn regarding welfare regime impact on gender differences in health.

Furthermore, very few studies attempting to explain social inequalities in health focus on the effects of the health care system itself (Beckfield and Krieger 2009). Thus, it has been suggested that future research should not solely compare regime types, but rather seek to illuminate the mechanisms and pathways through which specific social and health policies impact health inequalities (Beckfield et al. 2013). It has also been called into question whether it is more fruitful to abandon the welfare regimes approach and instead analyze health inequalities from more of an institutional approach, focusing on specific policies and benefits (Bergqvist et al. 2013; Brennenstuhl et al. 2012). It has also been suggested that comparing health among "the most marginalised, poorest and vulnerable" *across* welfare states would benefit the discussion of how to reduce inequalities *within* welfare states (Bambra 2013, p. 714). It is with this in mind that I introduce a conceptual framework attempting to make explicit the mechanisms connecting the social and policy context to health outcomes and inequities. Later in this chapter, this conceptual framework will be adapted for the case of health inequities for IPV survivors.

3.3.1 A Conceptual Framework: The Social Basis of Health Inequities

As alluded to in Chap. 1, Diderichsen et al. (2001) advanced a conceptual framework originally developed by Diderichsen and Hallqvist (1998) proposing that health inequities are shaped by the social and policy context through the interconnected mechanisms of *social stratification*, *differential exposure* to health risks, *differential vulnerability*, and *differential consequences* of ill health (see Fig. 3.1).[6] By identifying these mechanisms, the framework also proposes a number of points where policy could intervene in order to reduce inequities.

The framework begins with the social and policy context, defining it as the "structure, culture and function of a social system" which includes the "central engines in society that generate and distribute power, wealth and risks" (e.g., labor policies, gender norms, political systems) (Diderichsen et al. 2001, pp. 15–16). In turn, an individual's social position is partially defined by where he or she stands in relation to the social context, and could be informed, for example, by occupation, income, or gender. Thus, the social and policy context has the power to either equalize individual opportunities (e.g., universal access to health care) or to widen the gap (e.g., social benefits dependent on employment or occupation). This mechanism of *social stratification* allocates power and resources to members of society according to their social position. Reflecting back on the welfare state literature mentioned in

[6]The conceptual framework has been developed even further by Diderichsen et al. (2012), but the 2001 version remains the most relevant for this book.

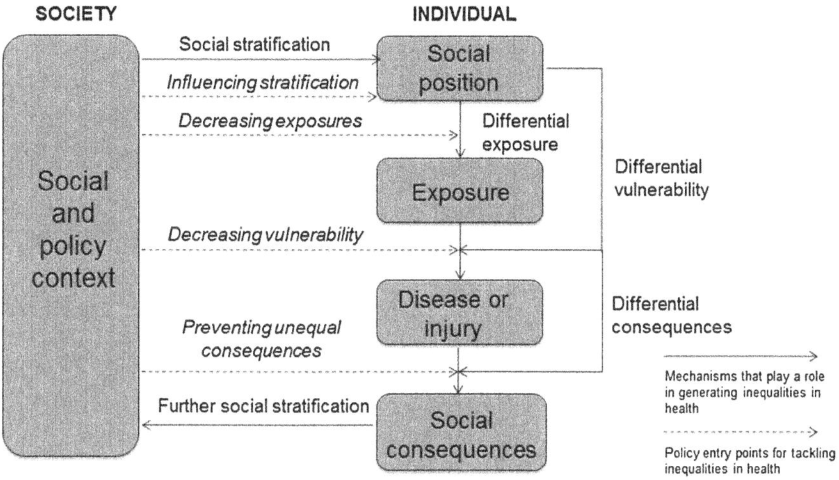

Fig. 3.1 Conceptual framework of pathways leading from social and policy context to health outcomes (adapted from Diderichsen and Hallqvist 1998; Diderichsen et al. 2001)

Chap. 1, stratification is one of the key dimensions in comparing welfare states and the empirical literature shows that through stratification, the welfare state does indeed shape an individual's social position. Those with more power and better social positions have greater possibilities for leading healthy lives, and thus structural inequities in the distribution of power and control over resources are central to the development of health inequities (Link and Phelan 1995).

The second mechanism of health inequity generation is that of *differential exposure* to ill health, which is based on the idea that exposure (e.g., type, amount, duration) to risk factors for disease and illness is inversely related to social position. "Other things being equal, these exposure differentials may explain excess risk of ill health associated with lower social positions across a wide range of specific diseases" (Diderichsen et al. 2001, p. 17). These advantages and disadvantages accumulate over the life course and can potentially be transferred from generation to generation (Bartley et al. 1997). Along these same lines, the health impact of a specific exposure is also dependent upon the presence of other risk factors. Given that individuals in lower social positions are often exposed to a variety of health risk factors, and that these may interact and compound one another, they are often more *differentially vulnerable* to ill health than those in higher social positions (Hallqvist et al. 1998). It is theorized that a risk factor's impact on health can be unevenly distributed because of fundamental differences among social groups in their susceptibility, even if the risk factor itself is evenly distributed across social groups. The final mechanism addressed in the framework is *differential consequences*, which refers to the differential impact that an ill health event may have on an individual's socioeconomic circumstances. Individuals in lower social positions may have access to fewer resources when faced with chronic illness or major health expenditures, which may put stress on their financial situation and put them at further risk of ill health. This may be particularly the case for countries without the social safety nets of universal access to health care, unemployment insurance, or disability benefits.

This framework also prioritizes the identification of interventions that address the special needs of disadvantaged populations in order to reduce the unequal consequences of poor health. In particular, it advocates *influencing stratification* by promoting labor market and family policies that aim at decreasing social inequalities and gender disparities. "Efforts to reduce differences in education or income between socioeconomic groups are likely to have a positive effect from a health equity perspective, as they increase the power of (and opportunities for) less privileged groups to avoid unhealthy living and working conditions" (Dahlgren and Whitehead 2007, p. 25). Second, *decreasing exposures* and *vulnerability* should be achieved by targeting policy, especially to reduce those key exposures which interact with many other types of exposures and therefore have broad impacts on health. Finally, in *preventing unequal consequences of ill health*, the framework proposes health policy that provides care according to need and equitable financing of health care, which protects those that become ill from being drained of all of their financial resources to cover their care.

In narrowing the focus to women specifically, several related studies have applied this conceptual framework to the examination of the production of health inequities among single mothers (i.e., Burstrom et al. 2010; Fritzell et al. 2007; Whitehead et al. 2000). They argue that focusing on a specific population group like single mothers, and the particular policies likely to directly affect them, is more effective than a one-size-fits-all strategy. Because the living conditions of vulnerable groups are "particularly sensitive to the setup of social policies," these groups therefore "may be among the first to be affected by any changes in welfare and employment policies" (Burstrom et al. 2010, p. 912). Using single within-country case and small N studies, the authors consistently found that health was significantly poorer for single mothers than for couple mothers across all countries. However, the mechanisms leading to poor health outcomes varied, with joblessness and poverty playing a larger role in countries with weaker social safety nets. It is with these results in mind that I seek to apply this conceptual framework to another group vulnerable to changes in social policies: female survivors of IPV. Thus, Sect. 3.4 provides background on where the lives of IPV survivors intersect with the welfare state and its social policies, then details a new conceptual framework applied specifically to IPV, and closes with the proposed research questions.

3.4 The Welfare State, IPV, and Health Inequities

Thus far, this chapter has provided the background necessary for a more focused examination of the close binds between the welfare state and women with histories of IPV. Disproportionate numbers of women receiving social assistance from the state have histories of violent relationships. In the US, anywhere from 50–60 % of women receiving state social assistance report past abuse, and as many as 20–30 % report abuse within the past year (Lown et al. 2006; Raphael et al. 1999; Tolman and Rosen 2001). These IPV prevalence rates among recipients of social assistance are approximately two to three times higher than those among non-recipients (Lown et al. 2006; Moe and Bell 2004). Likewise, in a nationally representative study of Norway, women were more likely to have experienced IPV if their main source of income was social security payments, unemployment benefits, or social assistance payments (Nerøien and Schei 2008). This is also the case in Germany, where women who receive social assistance either as a supplemental or primary source of income were more likely to have experienced physical or sexual abuse from a partner, and the severity of IPV increased with increased dependence on social assistance (Schröttle and Ansorge 2008). It is theorized that this is often because receiving state assistance is seen as the only option for economically dependent women to break the cycle of violence and transition into independent living arrangements (Bell 2003; Hughes and Brush 2011; Morrow et al. 2004; Scott et al. 2002). Indeed, researchers seem to concur that policies and programs that reduce financial difficulties and economic dependence on abusive partners are a critical resource for women to leave abusive relationships (Bornstein 2006; Golden et al. 2013; Scott et al. 2002).

Much of the literature on this topic has been written in reaction to broader reforms limiting social assistance provided by the welfare state. For example, Morrow et al. (2004) argue that the 'dismantling' of the Canadian social welfare state was resulting in a shift away from the view of social support as a right of social citizenship. They maintain that this reform was especially dangerous for women exiting violent relationships. Purvin (2007) makes the case that structural approaches, such as economic support, safe housing, transportation, and childcare which "better meet the needs of *all* low-income women, can be effective in reducing low-income women's vulnerability to domestic violence" (p. 205, emphasis added). Moreover, according to data collected through Ontario's shelter system, the elimination or reduction of many of these structural supports in Canada has left violence victims with fewer options, left them vulnerable to poverty, and exposed them to additional violence (OAITH, 1998 as cited in Morrow et al. 2004). In the US, it has also been shown that pushing women off of state support may indeed reduce reliance on social assistance, but in turn may increase their dependence on current and former abusive partners (Scott et al. 2002). Thus, feminist welfare state theorizing about the role of social policy in affecting women's 'voice' in relationships and their ability to 'exit' and establish autonomous households is directly relevant for women's exposure to IPV.

Moreover, given the wide spectrum of adverse health outcomes of IPV described in Chap. 2, it may not come as a surprise that women who have experienced IPV have a high need for health care services. Women who have been exposed to IPV generally do not always present with recognizable trauma, but rather with generalized symptoms (e.g., chronic pain, depression, PTSD) that are the result of the injuries, fear, and stress of long-term exposure to violence (Campbell 2002). Studies conducted in a number of different countries and health systems show that this leads to both higher health care utilization rates and higher average health costs among abused women than non-abused women. Among American health insurance plan members, women with histories of IPV were significantly more likely to be hospitalized, visit general clinics, and use mental health services, which cost the health plans approximately double that of female members who had not been abused (Ulrich et al. 2003; Wisner et al. 1999). Higher health care expenditures among IPV survivors also held true for poor women in the US eligible for Medicaid health insurance from the government (Coker et al. 2004). In Italy, these elevated utilization rates were found to persist several years after the violence has ended (Rivara et al. 2007). In addition to higher health needs, there is also evidence that these higher utilization rates are partially due to inefficient use of health services when health care providers are not aware of women's IPV experiences (Plichta 2007).

It is crucial to keep in mind that abused women have a high level of unmet need for health care, especially among women with acute injuries. A US population-based survey found that women who have been abused are twice as likely to have an unmet health care need as compared to women who have not been abused (Plichta and Falik 2001), with only about 17–34 % of women with injuries seeking health services (Plichta 2004). One study among abused women at a shelter in the US showed that only half reported having a community health clinic or primary care provider for preventative care, and only about one-third had had a preventative checkup in the previous year (Wilson et al. 2007). Moreover, in a nationally representative study in Germany, when asked about the worst experience of physical abuse from a current or former partner, 17 % of women with injuries said that had not sought medical care even though it had been necessary (Müller and Schröttle 2004). Even so, the health care system is among the most frequently accessed formal help system among women who have experienced IPV (Müller and Schröttle 2004; Postmus et al. 2009). Thus, the health care system presents itself as a 'window of opportunity' for providers to be a source of information and assistance for women in abusive relationships, particularly for women who find other forms of abuse-related assistance to be too stigmatizing (Petersen et al. 2003). Being able to overcome access barriers to the health care system is therefore key to addressing the health outcomes of IPV survivors and potentially reducing women's exposure to partner violence.

Therefore, this book adopts the conceptual framework described in Sect. 3.3.1 and applies it specifically to the context of IPV, proposing mechanisms involved in producing inequities in health outcomes, as well as points where social policy could intervene to reduce these inequities (see Fig. 3.2). *Social stratification* is the first mechanism, with the social and policy context shaping the overall social position of women through varying degrees of redistribution of resources across society to ensure equality. Second, women in lower social positions may be *differentially exposed* to IPV if they do not have access to the financial resources necessary to end

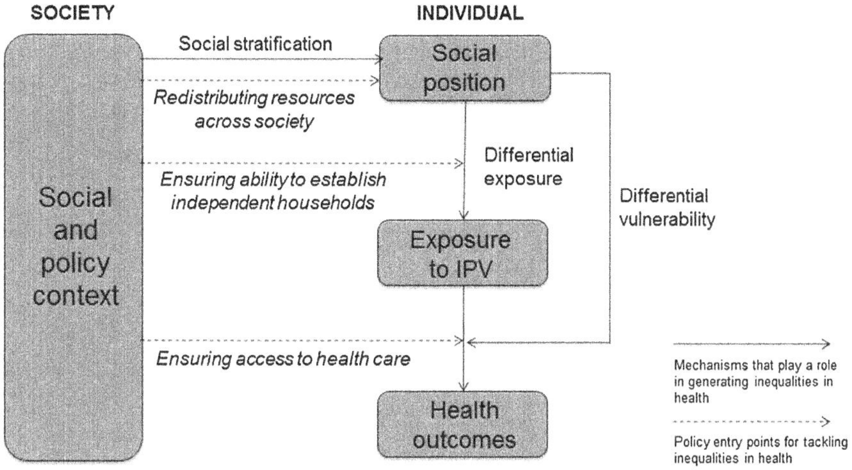

Fig. 3.2 Conceptual framework applied to IPV survivors (adapted from Diderichsen and Hallqvist 1998; Diderichsen et al. 2001)

an abusive relationship and establish an independent household.[7] Third, women in lower social positions who have experienced IPV may be *differentially vulnerable* to poor health outcomes if they are not able to access the health care system. Evidence shows that women in lower socioeconomic positions are generally vulnerable to poor health outcomes, especially if there exist barriers related to care (Wilson et al. 2007). Thus, adding the further health burden of IPV exposure may result in even greater vulnerability to poor health. This may particularly be the case for women who previously had access to health care through the health insurance of their abusive partner, but afterward find themselves in situations without health insurance and with fewer socioeconomic resources to seek health care than beforehand.

A central strength of this conceptual framework is that it also suggests where welfare state policy can intervene in each of these three mechanisms leading to health inequities for survivors of IPV. To begin, welfare policy which emphasizes a more equal *redistribution of resources across society* may serve to reduce the overall stratification of women. Following this, family policy can influence women's exposure to IPV by increasing *women's ability to establish independent households*. Policies allowing women to maintain strong ties to the labor market may ensure that women have the socioeconomic resources necessary to exit abusive relationships. Finally, health policy may reduce the social gradient in vulnerability to poor health outcomes for IPV survivors by ensuring *access to health care*. Given

[7]Although the conceptual framework suggests a unidirectional link between social position and IPV exposure, the literature is not so clear about which direction this relationship moves. For example, it is also possible that IPV exposure leads to a lower socioeconomic status, particularly after ending an abusive relationship. For the analytic purposes of this book, discussed in greater detail in Chap. 5, both directions are relevant.

the double health burden of lower socioeconomic status and IPV exposure, health policy may minimize vulnerability to poor health by removing barriers to availability, affordability, and entitlement to health care. If this conceptual framework holds true, then these intervention points are a potential means of reducing health inequities for survivors of IPV.

3.4.1 Research Questions

With this in mind, this book aims to address the significant gap in the understanding of health inequities experienced by survivors of IPV. To begin, there is limited research at the individual level regarding how social position, IPV, and health interact and produce susceptibilities to one another. Even though it seems probable that violence and poverty may magnify one another in their impact on health, the influences of social position are often not directly investigated. Furthermore, while there has been much written about the detrimental socioeconomic effects for IPV survivors of welfare state retrenchment, few studies have attempted to link these macro-level factors to health outcomes. Thus, whether the poorer health outcomes of IPV survivors are structurally produced through social policy remains unclear, as are the possibilities for reforming social policy in order to reduce these health inequities

Therefore, this book uses the conceptual framework described earlier in Sect. 3.4 as the guide for investigating the impact of welfare state policy on the generation of health inequities for women with histories of IPV. Examining the relationship between social position, IPV, and health at the individual level will aid in determining: whether there are *differences in exposure* to IPV related to social position; and whether women with IPV exposure are more *vulnerable* to social position's impact on health. Moreover, including the US, Germany, and Norway in the analysis as welfare states with varying institutional arrangements will further illuminate whether differences across countries at the individual level may be related to differences at the social policy level—particularly in reducing both exposure to IPV and vulnerability to poor health.

Thus, this book addresses the following two questions at the individual level (see Table 3.1). First, to what extent does social position impact IPV exposure? Variations in resource theory as well as dependency theory and family conflict theory posit that limited socioeconomic resources affect women's exposure to IPV. Moreover, overall empirical evidence links household income to the probability of experiencing IPV (e.g., Cunradi et al. 2002), as well as women's education and employment to women's ability to leave a violent partnership (e.g., Anderson and Saunders 2003), showing that social position is relevant regardless of whether IPV is conceptualized as situational couple violence or intimate terrorism. Thus, I hypothesize that a higher social position is related to lower exposure to IPV.

Second, to what extent are women with IPV exposure more vulnerable to social position's impact on health outcomes than women without IPV exposure? That is, does IPV exposure magnify the negative impact of social position on health? Evidence shows that both lower social position (e.g., Ansari et al. 2003; Raphael 2006) and IPV (e.g., Campbell 2002; Vives-Cases et al. 2011) are linked to poorer health outcomes. Therefore, based on the conceptual framework outlined in Sect. 3.4, it is hypothesized that: higher social position is related to better health; IPV negatively contributes to health outcomes above and beyond what can be explained by social position; and that social position's negative impact on health increases with IPV exposure.

Based upon the answers to the first two research questions for each of the countries under investigation, the third and fourth macro-level questions which focus on the comparison of institutional arrangements are proposed (see Table 3.1). Is social position's impact on IPV exposure reflective of national policies supporting women in establishing independent households? Both the conceptual framework and the empirical evidence suggest that women's access to economic resources can help reduce risk of IPV and increase women's ability to end an abusive relationship (e.g., Golden et al. 2013; Scott et al. 2002). Therefore, it is hypothesized that the amount of social inequalities in IPV exposure will be smaller in countries with social policies that support women with the economic resources necessary for establishing independent households (i.e., Norway). On the flip side, the amount of social inequalities in IPV exposure should be greater in countries without policies providing the necessary safety net for women to leave abusive relationships (i.e., the US and Germany).

Table 3.1 Research questions and hypotheses

Analysis focus	Research questions	Hypotheses
Individual level	RQ1. To what extent does social position impact IPV exposure?	H1. Higher social position is related to lower exposure to IPV
	RQ2. To what extent are women with IPV exposure more vulnerable to social position's impact on health outcomes?	H2a. Higher social position is related to better health H2b. IPV negatively contributes to health outcomes H2c. Social position's negative impact on health increases with IPV exposure
Macro level	RQ3. Is social position's impact on IPV exposure reflective of national policies supporting women in establishing independent households?	H3. Social inequalities in IPV exposure will be smaller in countries with social policies supporting women in establishing independent households, and greater in countries without such policies
	RQ4. Are vulnerabilities to social position's impact on health for IPV survivors reflective of national policies regarding access to health care?	H4. Vulnerabilities to social position's impact on health will be smaller in countries with policies ensuring access to health care, and greater in countries without such policies

Finally, are the vulnerabilities to social position's impact on health for IPV survivors reflective of national policies regarding access to health care? Although the literature demonstrates that abused women have increased health care needs, the lack of socioeconomic resources can be a barrier for seeking health care in countries which do not ensure access to health care (e.g., Wilson et al. 2007). In this case, IPV exposure may then serve to magnify social gradients in health (Ford-Gilboe et al. 2009). Therefore, it is hypothesized that these vulnerabilities to social position's impact on health will be smaller in countries with policies ensuring access to health care (i.e., Germany and Norway), and greater in countries without policies ensuring access to health care (i.e., the US).

These macro-level hypotheses are broken down even further after the presentation of the detailed case descriptions of each country in Chap. 4.

References

Aaltonen, K., Miettinen, J., Airio, I., Martikainen, J. E., Saastamoinen, L. K., Bell, J. S., et al. (2015). Cost-related barriers to use of health services and prescription medicines in Finland: A cross-sectional survey. *European Journal of Public Health, 25*(3), 368–372. doi:10.1093/eurpub/cku176

Allin, S., Masseria, C., Sorenson, C., Papanicolas, I., & Mossialos, E. (2007). *Measuring inequalities in access to health care: A review of the indices?* Brussels, Belgium: European Commission. http://eprints.lse.ac.uk/29837/. Accessed January 30, 2014.

Anderson, D. K., & Saunders, D. G. (2003). Leaving an abusive partner: An empirical review of predictors, the process of leaving, and psychological well-being. *Trauma, Violence, and Abuse, 4*(2), 163–191. doi:10.1177/1524838002250769

Ansari, Z., Carson, N. J., Ackland, M. J., Vaughan, L., & Serraglio, A. (2003). A public health model of the social determinants of health. *Sozial- und Präventivmedizin, 48*(4), 242–251.

Arah, O. A., Westert, G. P., Delnoij, D. M., & Klazinga, N. S. (2005). Health system outcomes and determinants amenable to public health in industrialized countries: A pooled, cross-sectional time series analysis. *BMC Public Health, 5*(1), 81–91. doi:10.1186/1471-2458-5-81

Backhans, M., Burström, B., de Leon, A. P., & Marklund, S. (2012). Is gender policy related to the gender gap in external cause and circulatory disease mortality? A mixed effects model of 22 OECD countries 1973–2008. *BMC Public Health, 12*(1), 969. doi:10.1186/1471-2458-12-969

Baker, D. W., Sudano, J. J., Albert, J. M., Borawski, E. A., & Dor, A. (2001). Lack of health insurance and decline in overall health in late middle age. *The New England Journal of Medicine, 345*(15), 1106–1112. doi:10.1056/NEJMsa002887

Baker, D. W., Sudano, J. J., Albert, J. M., Borawski, E. A., & Dor, A. (2002). Loss of health insurance and the risk for a decline in self-reported health and physical functioning. *Medical Care, 40*(11), 1126–1131. doi:10.1097/01.MLR.0000032192.46564.16

Bambra, C. (2005a). Worlds of welfare and the health care discrepancy. *Social Policy and Society, 4*(1), 31–41. doi:10.1017/S1474746404002143

Bambra, C. (2005b). Cash versus services: "Worlds of welfare" and the decommodification of cash benefits and health care services. *Journal of Social Policy, 34*(2), 195–213. doi:10.1017/S0047279404008542

Bambra, C. (2006). Health status and the worlds of welfare. *Social Policy and Society, 5*(1), 53–62. doi:10.1017/s1474746405002721

Bambra, C. (2007). Going beyond the three worlds of welfare capitalism: Regime theory and public health research. *Journal of Epidemiology and Community Health, 61*(12), 1098–1102. doi:10.1136/jech.2007.064295

Bambra, C. (2011). Health inequalities and welfare state regimes: Theoretical insights on a public health "puzzle". *Journal of Epidemiology and Community Health, 65*(9), 740–745. doi:10.1136/jech.2011.136333

Bambra, C. (2013). In defence of (social) democracy: On health inequalities and the welfare state. *Journal of Epidemiology and Community Health, 67*(9), 713–714. doi:10.1136/jech-2013-202937

Bambra, C., Pope, D., Swami, V., Stanistreet, D., Roskam, A., Kunst, A., et al. (2009). Gender, health inequalities and welfare state regimes: A cross-national study of 13 European countries. *Journal of Epidemiology and Community Health, 63*(1), 38–44. doi:10.1136/jech.2007.070292

Bardasi, E., & Gornick, J. C. (2008). Working for less? Women's part-time wage penalties across countries. *Feminist Economics, 14*(1), 37–72. doi:10.1080/13545700701716649

Bartley, M., Blane, D., & Montgomery, S. (1997). Health and the life course: Why safety nets matter. *BMJ, 314*, 1194–1196.

Beckfield, J., & Krieger, N. (2009). Epi + demos + cracy: Linking political systems and priorities to the magnitude of health inequities—Evidence, gaps, and a research agenda. *Epidemiologic Reviews, 31*(1), 152–177. doi:10.1093/epirev/mxp002

Beckfield, J., & Olafsdottir, S. (2009). Empowering health: A comparative political sociology of health disparities. *Perspectives on Europe, 39*(2), 9–12.

Beckfield, J., Olafsdottir, S., & Sosnaud, B. (2013). Healthcare systems in comparative perspective: Classification, convergence, institutions, inequalities, and five missed turns. *Annual Review of Sociology, 39*(1), 127–146. doi:10.1146/annurev-soc-071312-145609

Bell, H. (2003). Cycles within cycles. *Violence Against Women, 9*(10), 1245–1262. doi:10.1177/1077801203255865

Berger, M., & Messer, J. (2002). Public financing of health expenditures, insurance, and health outcomes. *Applied Economics, 34*(17), 2105–2113.

Bergqvist, K., Åberg Yngwe, M., & Lundberg, O. (2013). Understanding the role of welfare state characteristics for health and inequalities—An analytical review. *BMC Public Health, 13*(1), 1234–1253. doi:10.1186/1471-2458-13-1234

Bianchi, S. M., Casper, L. M., & Peltola, P. K. (1999). A cross-national look at married women's earnings dependency. *Gender Issues, 17*(3), 3–33. doi:10.1007/s12147-999-0001-0

Bird, C. E., & Rieker, P. P. (2008). *Gender and health: The effects of constrained choices and social policies*. New York, NY: Cambridge University Press.

Bittman, M., England, P., Sayer, L., Folbre, N., & Matheson, G. (2003). When does gender trump money? Bargaining and time in household work. *American Journal of Sociology, 109*(1), 186–214. doi:10.1086/378341

Bleijenbergh, I., de Bruijn, J., & Bussemaker, J. (2004). European social citizenship and gender: The part-time work directive. *European Journal of Industrial Relations, 10*(3), 309–328. doi:10.1177/0959680104047023

Bornstein, R. F. (2006). The complex relationship between dependency and domestic violence: Converging psychological factors and social forces. *American Psychologist, 61*(6), 595–606. doi:10.1037/0003-066X.61.6.595

Borrell, C., Palència, L., Muntaner, C., Urquía, M., Malmusi, D., & O'Campo, P. (2014). Influence of macrosocial policies on women's health and gender inequalities in health. *Epidemiologic Reviews, 36*(1), 31–48. doi:10.1093/epirev/mxt002

Boye, K. (2011). Work and well-being in a comparative perspective. The role of family policy. *European Sociological Review, 27*(1), 16–30. doi:10.1093/esr/jcp051

Brady, D., & Kall, D. (2008). Nearly universal, but somewhat distinct: The feminization of poverty in affluent Western democracies, 1969–2000. *Social Science Research, 37*, 976–1007. doi:10.1016/j.ssresearch.2007.07.001

Brennenstuhl, S., Quesnel-Vallee, A., & McDonough, P. (2012). Socioeconomic inequalities in health and the welfare state: A research synthesis. *Journal of Epidemiology and Community Health, 66*, 397–409. doi:10.1136/jech-2011-200277

Budig, M. J., Misra, J., & Boeckmann, I. (2012). The motherhood penalty in cross-national perspective: The importance of work-family policies and cultural attitudes. *Social Politics: International Studies in Gender, State, and Society, 19*(2), 163–193. doi:10.1093/sp/jxs006

Burau, V., & Blank, R. H. (2006). Comparing health policy: An assessment of typologies of health systems. *Journal of Comparative Policy Analysis: Research and Practice, 8*(1), 63–76. doi:10.1080/13876980500513558

Burstrom, B., Whitehead, M., Clayton, S., Fritzell, S., Vannoni, F., & Costa, G. (2010). Health inequalities between lone and couple mothers and policy under different welfare regimes—The example of Italy, Sweden and Britain. *Social Science and Medicine, 70*, 912–920. doi:10.1016/j.socscimed.2009.11.014

Campbell, J. C. (2002). Health consequences of intimate partner violence. *Lancet, 359*, 1331–1336. doi:10.1016/S0140-6736(02)08336-8

Christopher, K., England, P., Smeeding, T. M., & Phillips, K. R. (2002). The gender gap in poverty in modern nations: Single motherhood, the market, and the state. *Sociological Perspectives, 45*(3), 219–242. doi:10.1093/sp/9.1.60

Chung, H., & Muntaner, C. (2007). Welfare state matters: A typological multilevel analysis of wealthy countries. *Health Policy, 80*(2), 328–339. doi:10.1016/j.healthpol.2006.03.004

Coker, A. L., Reeder, C. E., Fadden, M. K., & Smith, P. H. (2004). Physical partner violence and Medicaid utilization and expenditures. *Public Health Reports, 119*, 557–567. doi:10.1016/j.phr.2004.09.005

Cook, L. P. (2010). The politics of housework. In J. Treas & S. Drobnic (Eds.), *Dividing the domestic: Men, women, and household work in cross-national perspective* (pp. 59–78). Stanford, CA: Stanford University Press.

Cunradi, C. B., Caetano, R., & Schafer, J. (2002). Socioeconomic predictors of intimate partner violence among White, Black, and Hispanic couples in the United States. *Journal of Family Violence, 17*(4), 377–389. doi:0885-7482/02/1200-0377/0

Dahl, E., Fritzell, J., Lahelma, E., Martikainen, P., Kunst, A., & Mackenbach, J. P. (2006). Welfare state regimes and health inequalities. In J. Siegrist & M. Marmot (Eds.), *Social inequalities in health: New evidence and policy implications* (pp. 193–222). New York, NY: Oxford University Press.

Dahl, E., & van der Wel, K. A. (2013). Educational inequalities in health in European welfare states: A social expenditure approach. *Social Science and Medicine, 81*, 60–69. doi:10.1016/j.socscimed.2012.12.010

Dahlgren, G., & Whitehead, M. (2007). *European strategies for tackling social inequities in health: Levelling up Part 2*. Copenhagen, Denmark: WHO Regional Office for Europe.

Denton, M., Prus, S., & Walters, V. (2004). Gender differences in health: A Canadian study of the psychosocial, structural and behavioural determinants of health. *Social Science and Medicine, 58*(12), 2585–2600. doi:10.1016/j.socscimed.2003.09.008

Denton, M., & Walters, V. (1999). Gender differences in structural and behavioral determinants of health: An analysis of the social production of health. *Social Science and Medicine, 48*(9), 1221–1235.

Diderichsen, F., Andersen, I., Manuel, C., Andersen, A.-M. N., Bach, E., Baadsgaard, M., et al. (2012). Health inequality—Determinants and policies. *Scandinavian Journal of Public Health, 40*(8 Suppl), 12–105. doi:10.1177/1403494812457734

Diderichsen, F., Evans, T., & Whitehead, M. (2001). The social basis of disparities in health. In T. Evans, M. Whitehead, F. Diderichsen, A. Bhuyia, & M. Wirth (Eds.), *Challenging inequities in health: From ethics to action* (pp. 12–23). New York, NY: Oxford University Press.

Diderichsen, F., & Hallqvist, J. (1998). Social inequalities in health: Some methodological considerations for the study of social position and social context. In B. Arve-Parès (Ed.), *Social inquality in health: A Swedish perspective* (pp. 25–39). Stockholm, Sweden: Swedish Council for Social Research.

Eikemo, T., Bambra, C., Judge, K., & Ringdal, K. (2008). Welfare state regimes and differences in self-perceived health in Europe: A multilevel analysis. *Social Science and Medicine, 66*(11), 2281–2295. doi:10.1016/j.socscimed.2008.01.022

Esping-Andersen, G. (1999). *Social foundations of post-industrial economies.* Oxford, UK: Oxford University Press.

Ferrarini, T. (2006). *Families, states and labour markets: Institutions, causes and consequences of family policy in post-war welfare states.* Cheltenham, UK: Edward Elgar Publishing.

Ferrarini, T., & Norström, T. (2010). Family policy, economic development and infant mortality: A longitudinal comparative analysis. *International Journal of Social Welfare, 19*(s1), S89–S102. doi:10.1111/j.1468-2397.2010.00736.x

Ford-Gilboe, M., Wuest, J., Varcoe, C., Davies, L., Merritt-Gray, M., Campbell, J. C., et al. (2009). Modelling the effects of intimate partner violence and access to resources on women's health in the early years after leaving an abusive partner. *Social Science and Medicine, 68*, 1021–1029. doi:10.1016/j.socscimed.2009.01.003

Fraser, N. (1994). After the family wage: Gender equity and the welfare state. *Political Theory, 22* (4), 591–618.

Freeman, R., & Moran, M. (2000). Reforming health care in Europe. *West European Politics, 23* (2), 35–58. doi:10.1080/01402380008425366

Fritzell, S., Ringback Weitoft, G., Fritzell, J., & Burstrom, B. (2007). From macro to micro: The health of Swedish lone mothers during changing economic and social circumstances. *Social Science and Medicine, 65*(12), 2474–2488. doi:10.1016/j.socscimed.2007.06.031

Gilson, L., Doherty, J., Loewenson, R., & Francis, V. (2007). *Challenging inequity through health systems.* WHO Commission on the Social Determinants of Health.

Golden, S. D., Perreira, K. M., & Durrance, C. P. (2013). Troubled times, troubled relationships: How economic resources, gender beliefs, and neighborhood disadvantage influence intimate partner violence. *Journal of Interpersonal Violence, 28*, 2134–2155. doi:10.1177/0886260512471083

Gornick, J. C., & Meyers, M. K. (2009). Institutions that support gender equality in parenthood and employment. In J. C. Gornick & M. K. Meyers (Eds.), *Gender equality: Transforming family divisions of labor* (pp. 3–64). London: Verso.

Gornick, J. C., Meyers, M. K., & Ross, K. E. (1997). Supporting the employment of mothers: Policy variation across fourteen welfare states. *Journal of European Social Policy, 7*(1), 45–70. doi:10.1177/095892879700700103

Graves, J. (2013). School calendars, child care availability and maternal employment. *Journal of Urban Economics, 78*, 57–70. doi:10.1257/aer.103.3.279

Gulliford, M. C. (2002). Availability of primary care doctors and population health in England: Is there an association? *Journal of Public Health Medicine, 24*(4), 252–254.

Gulliford, M. C., Figueroa-Munoz, J., Morgan, M., Hughes, D., Gibson, B., Beech, R., et al. (2002). What does "access to health care" mean? *Journal of Health Services Research and Policy, 7*(3), 186–188. doi:10.1258/135581902760082517

Gustafsson, S. S., & Bruyn-Hundt, M. (1991). Incentives for women to work: A comparison between the Netherlands, Sweden and West Germany. *Journal of Economic Studies, 18*(5/6), 30–65. doi:10.1108/EUM0000000000159

Hacker, J. S. (2004). Privatizing risk without privatizing the welfare state: The hidden politics of social policy retrenchment in the United States. *American Political Science Review, 98*(02), 243–260. doi:10.1017/S0003055404001121

Hadley, J. (2003). Sicker and poorer—The consequences of being uninsured: A review of the research on the relationship between health insurance, medical care use, health, work, and income. *Medical Care Research and Review, 60*(2), 3–75. doi:10.1177/1077558703254101

Hallqvist, J., Diderichsen, F., Theorell, T., Reuterwall, C., & Ahlbom, A. (1998). Is the effect of job strain on myocardial infarction risk due to interaction between high psychological demands and low decision latitude? Results from Stockholm Heart Epidemiology Program (SHEEP). *Social Science and Medicine, 46*(11), 1405–1415. doi:10.1016/S0277-9536(97)10084-3

Hirschman, A. O. (1970). *Exit, voice, and loyalty: Responses to decline in firms, organizations, and states*. Cambridge, MA: Harvard University Press.

Hobson, B. (1990). No exit, no voice: Women's economic dependency and the welfare state. *Acta Sociologica, 33*(3), 235–250. doi:10.1177/000169939003300305

Hobson, B. (1994). Solo mothers, social policy regimes and the logics of gender. In D. Sainsbury (Ed.), *Gendering welfare states* (pp. 170–187). London, Thousand Oaks, CA: Sage Publications.

Hook, J. L. (2006). Care in context: Men's unpaid work in 20 countries, 1965–2003. *American Sociological Review, 71*(4), 639–660.

Huber, E., Stephens, J. D., Bradley, D., Moller, S., & Nielsen, F. (2009). The politics of women's economic independence. *Social Politics: International Studies in Gender, State and Society, 16* (1), 1–39. doi:10.1093/sp/jxp005

Hughes, M. M., & Brush, L. D. (2011). Work, welfare, and protection orders: Modeling changing earnings in the context of group differences and institutional shifts. *Violence Against Women, 17*(3), 322–339. doi:10.1177/1077801211398562

Huijts, T., & Eikemo, T. A. (2009). Causality, social selectivity or artefacts? Why socioeconomic inequalities in health are not smallest in the Nordic countries. *European Journal of Public Health, 19*(5), 452–453. doi:10.1093/eurpub/ckp103

Hurrelmann, K., Rathmann, K., & Richter, M. (2011). Health inequalities and welfare state regimes: A research note. *Journal of Public Health, 19*(1), 3–13. doi:10.1007/s10389-010-0359-1

Jaehrling, K., Kalina, T., & Mesaros, L. (2014). A paradox of activation strategies: Why increasing labour market participation among single mothers failed to bring down poverty rates. *Social Politics: International Studies in Gender, State and Society, 22*(1), 86–110. doi:10.1093/sp/jxu017

Kaiser Family Foundation. (2013). *Women's health insurance coverage*. Menlo Park, CA. http://kaiserfamilyfoundation.files.wordpress.com/2013/11/6000-11-womens-health-insurance-coverage-factsheet1.pdf-sheet/. Accessed June 23, 2014.

Kasza, G. J. (2002). The illusion of welfare "regimes". *Journal of Social Policy, 31*(2), 271–287. doi:10.1017/S0047279401006584

Kawachi, I., Kennedy, B. P., Gupta, V., & Prothrow-Stith, D. (1999). Women's status and the health of women and men: A view from the States. *Social Science and Medicine, 48*(1), 21–32.

Kremer, M. (2007). *How welfare states care: Culture, gender and parenting in Europe*. Amsterdam: Amsterdam University Press.

Levy, H., & Meltzer, D. (2008). The impact of health insurance on health. *Annual Review of Public Health, 29*, 399–409. doi:10.1146/annurev.publhealth.28.021406.144042

Lewis, J. (1992). Gender and the development of welfare regimes. *Journal of European Social Policy, 2*(3), 159–173.

Link, B. G., & Phelan, J. (1995). Social conditions as fundamental causes of disease. *Journal of Health and Social Behavior, 35*, 80–94.

Lister, R. (1997). *Citizenship: Feminist perspectives*. London: Macmillan.

Lott, Y. (2009). Verwaltung und Entscheidung—Bestimmt das individuelle Einkommen die Machtverteilung in Paarbeziehungen? [Administration and decisions—Does the individual income decide the division of power in relationships?]. *Kölner Zeitschrift für Soziologie und Sozialpsychologie, 61*(3), 327–353. doi:10.1007/s11577-009-0071-8

Lown, E. A., Schmidt, L. A., & Wiley, J. (2006). Interpersonal violence among women seeking welfare: Unraveling lives. *American Journal of Public Health, 96*(8), 1409–1415. doi:10.2105/AJPH.2004.057786

Lundberg, O. (2008). Commentary: Politics and public health—Some conceptual considerations concerning welfare state characteristics and public health outcomes. *International Journal of Epidemiology, 37*(5), 1105–1108. doi:10.1093/ije/dyn078

Mackenbach, J. P. (2012). Public health and welfare. *European Journal of Public Health, 22*(1), 1. doi:10.1093/eurpub/ckr186
Malmusi, D., Vives, A., Benach, J., & Borrell, C. (2014). Gender inequalities in health: Exploring the contribution of living conditions in the intersection of social class. *Global Health Action, 7*. doi:10.3402/gha.v7.23189
Marmor, T., & Okma, K. G. H. (2003). Review essay: Health care systems in transition. Copenhagen: World Health Organization Regional Office for Europe, 1996. *Journal of Health Politics, Policy and Law, 28*(4), 747–755.
Marmor, T., & Wendt, C. (2012). Conceptual frameworks for comparing healthcare politics and policy. *Health Policy, 107*(1), 11–20. doi:10.1016/j.healthpol.2012.06.003
McLaughlin, C. G., & Wyszewianski, L. (2002). Access to care: Remembering old lessons. *Health Services Research, 37*(6), 1441–1443.
Misra, J., Budig, M. J., & Moller, S. (2007a). Reconciliation policies and the effects of motherhood on employment, earnings and poverty. *Journal of Comparative Policy Analysis: Research and Practice, 9*(2), 135–155. doi:10.1080/13876980701311588
Misra, J., Moller, S., & Budig, M. J. (2007b). Work family policies and poverty for partnered and single women in Europe and North America. *Gender and Society, 21*(6), 804–827. doi:10.1177/0891243207308445
Moe, A. M., & Bell, M. P. (2004). Abject economics. *Violence Against Women, 10*(1), 29–55. doi:10.1177/1077801203256016
Moran, M. (1999). *Governing the health care state: A comparative study of the United Kingdom, the United States and Germany*. Manchester, UK: Manchester University Press.
Moran, M. (2000). Understanding the welfare state: The case of health care. *The British Journal of Politics and International Relations, 2*(2), 135–160. doi:10.1111/1467-856x.00031
Morrow, M., Hankivsky, O., & Varcoe, C. (2004). Women and violence: The effects of dismantling the welfare state. *Critical Social Policy, 24*(3), 358–384. doi:10.1177/0261018304044364
Müller, U., & Schröttle, M. (2004). *Lebenssituation, Sicherheit und Gesundheit von Frauen in Deutschland: Eine repräsentative Untersuchung zu Gewalt gegen Frauen in Deutschland [Health, well-being and personal safety of women in Germany: A representative study of violence against women in Germany]*. Berlin: Bundesministerium für Familie, Senioren, Frauen und Jugend.
Muntaner, C., Borrell, C., Ng, E., Chung, H., Espelt, A., Rodriguez-Sanz, M., et al. (2011). Politics, welfare regimes, and population health: Controversies and evidence. *Sociology of Health and Illness, 33*(6), 946–964. doi:10.1111/j.1467-9566.2011.01339.x
Nerøien, A. I., & Schei, B. (2008). Partner violence and health: Results from the first national study on violence against women in Norway. *Scandinavian Journal of Public Health, 36*(2), 161–168. doi:10.1177/1403494807085188
O'Connor, J. S. (1993). Gender, class and citizenship in the comparative analysis of welfare state regimes: Theoretical and methodological issues. *The British Journal of Sociology, 44*(3), 501–518.
Olafsdottir, S. (2007). Fundamental causes of health disparities: Stratification, the welfare state, and health in the United States and Iceland. *Journal of Health and Social Behavior, 48*(3), 239–253. doi:10.1177/002214650704800303
Olafsdottir, S., & Beckfield, J. (2011). Health and the social rights of citizenship: Integrating welfare-state theory and medical sociology. In B. A. Pescosolido, J. K. Martin, J. D. McLeod, & A. Rogers (Eds.), *Handbook of the sociology of health, illness, and healing* (pp. 101–115). New York, NY: Springer. doi:10.1007/978-1-4419-7261-3_6
Or, Z., Wang, J., & Jamison, D. (2005). International differences in the impact of doctors on health: A multilevel analysis of OECD countries. *Journal of Health Economics, 24*(3), 531–560. doi:10.1016/j.jhealeco.2004.09.003
Orloff, A. (1993). Gender and the social rights of citizenship: The comparative analysis of gender relations and welfare states. *American Sociological Review, 58*(3), 303–328.

Orloff, A. (2009a). Should feminists aim for gender symmetry? Why a dual-earner/dual-caregiver society is not every feminist's utopia. In J. C. Gornick & M. K. Meyers (Eds.), *Gender equality: Transforming family divisions of labor* (pp. 129–157). London: Verso.

Orloff, A. (2009b). Gendering the comparative analysis of welfare states: An unfinished agenda. *Sociological Theory, 27*(3), 317–343. doi:10.1111/j.1467-9558.2009.01350.x

Palència, L., Malmusi, D., De Moortel, D., Artazcoz, L., Backhans, M., Vanroelen, C., et al., (2014). The influence of gender equality policies on gender inequalities in health in Europe. *Social Science and Medicine, 117*, 25–33. doi:10.1016/j.socscimed.2014.07.018

Pankratz, C. (2012). National health policies and population health outcomes in 17 OECD countries: An application of the welfare state regimes concept. The University of Manitoba. http://mspace.lib.umanitoba.ca/bitstream/1993/5311/1/curtis_pankratz.pdf. Accessed April 03, 2013.

Pearce, D. (1978). The feminization of poverty: Women, work, and welfare. *The Urban and Social Change Review, 11*(1–2), 28–36.

Penchansky, R., & Thomas, J. W. (1981). The concept of access: Definition and relationship to consumer satisfaction. *Medical Care, 19*, 127–140.

Petersen, R., Moracco, K. E., Goldstein, K. M., & Clark, K. A. (2003). Women's perspectives on intimate partner violence services: The hope in Pandora's box. *Journal of the American Medical Women's Association, 58*(3), 185–190.

Pettit, B., & Hook, J. (2005). The structure of women's employment in comparative perspective. *Social Forces, 84*(2), 779–801. doi:10.1353/sof.2006.0029

Pfau-Effinger, B. (1998). Gender cultures and the gender arrangement—A theoretical framework for cross-national gender research. *Innovation: The European Journal of Social Science Research, 11*(2), 147–166. doi:10.1080/13511610.1998.9968559

Pfau-Effinger, B. (2012). Women's employment in the institutional and cultural context. *International Journal of Sociology and Social Policy, 32*(9), 530–543. doi:10.1108/01443331211257634

Plichta, S. B. (2004). Intimate partner violence and physical health consequences: Policy and practice implications. *Journal of Interpersonal Violence, 19*(11), 1296–1323. doi:10.1177/0886260504269685

Plichta, S. B. (2007). Interactions between victims of intimate partner violence against women and the health care system: Policy and practice implications. *Trauma, Violence, and Abuse, 8*(2), 226–239. doi:10.1177/1524838007301220

Plichta, S. B., & Falik, M. (2001). Prevalence of violence and its implications for women's health. *Women's Health Issues, 11*, 244–258. doi:10.1016/S1049-3867(01)00085-8

Plümper, T., & Neumayer, E. (2013). Health spending, out-of-pocket contributions, and mortality rates. *Public Administration, 91*(2), 403–418. doi:10.1111/j.1467-9299.2012.02039.x

Postmus, J. L., Severson, M., Berry, M., & Yoo, J. A. (2009). Women's experiences of violence and seeking help. *Violence Against Women, 15*, 852–868. doi:10.1177/1077801209334445

Purvin, D. M. (2007). At the crossroads and in the crosshairs: Social welfare policy and low-income women's vulnerability to domestic violence. *Social Problems, 54*(2), 188–210. doi:10.1525/sp.2007.54.2.188

Quadagno, J. (2010). Institutions, interest groups, and ideology: An agenda for the sociology of health care reform. *Journal of Health and Social Behavior, 51*(2), 125–136. doi:10.1177/0022146510368931

Quimbo, S. A., Peabody, J. W., Shimkhada, R., Florentino, J., & Solon, O. (2011). Evidence of a causal link between health outcomes, insurance coverage, and a policy to expand access: Experimental data from children in the Philippines. *Health Economics, 20*(5), 620–630. doi:10.1002/hec.1621

Raphael, D. (2006). Social determinants of health: Present status, unanswered questions, and future directions. *International Journal of Health Services, 36*(4), 651–677. doi:10.2190/3MW4-1EK3-DGRQ-2CRF

Raphael, D., & Bryant, T. (2004). The welfare state as a determinant of women's health: Support for women's quality of life in Canada and four comparison nations. *Health Policy, 68*(1), 63–79. doi:10.1016/j.healthpol.2003.08.003

Raphael, J., Renzetti, C. M., & Edelson, J. L. (1999). Keeping women poor: How domestic violence prevents women from leaving welfare and entering the world of work. In R. A. Brandwein (Ed.), *Battered women, children, and welfare reform: The ties that bind* (pp. 31–44). Thousand Oaks, CA: Sage Publications.

Rice, T., & Morrison, K. R. (1994). Patient cost sharing for medical services: A review of the literature and implications for health care reform. *Medical Care Review, 51*(3), 235–287.

Rivara, F. P., Anderson, M. L., Fishman, P., Bonomi, A. E., Reid, R. J., Carrell, D., et al. (2007). Healthcare utilization and costs for women with a history of intimate partner violence. *American Journal of Preventative Medicine, 32*, 89–96. doi:10.1016/j.amepre.2006.10.001

Rogers, S. J. (2004). Dollars, dependency, and divorce: Four perspectives on the role of wives' income. *Journal of Marriage and Family, 66*(1), 59–74.

Sainsbury, D. (1994a). Introduction. In D. Sainsbury (Ed.), *Gendering welfare states* (pp. 1–7). London, UK: Sage Publications.

Sainsbury, D. (1994b). Women's and men's social rights: Gendering dimensions of welfare states. *Gendering welfare states* (pp. 150–169). London, UK: Sage Publications.

Sainsbury, D. (1999). Taxation, family responsibilities, and employment. In D. Sainsbury (Ed.), *Gender and welfare state regimes* (pp. 185–209). Oxford, UK: Oxford University Press. doi:10.1093/0198294166.003.0007

Sayer, L. C., & Bianchi, S. M. (2000). Women's economic independence and the probability of divorce: A review and reexamination. *Journal of Family Issues, 21*(7), 906–943. doi:10.1177/019251300021007005

Scheiber, G. (1987). Financing and delivering health care: A comparative analysis of OECD countries. Paris: Organisation for Economic Co-operation and Development. http://www.popline.org/node/354892. Accessed January 29, 2014.

Schröttle, M., & Ansorge, N. (2008). Gewalt gegen Frauen in Paarbeziehungen: Eine sekundäranalytische Auswertung zur Differenzierung von Schweregraden, Mustern, Risikofaktoren und Unterstützung nach erlebter Gewalt. [Violence against women in relationships: A secondary analysis of the differences between severity, types, risk factors and support after violence incidents]. Berlin: Bundesministerium für Familie, Senioren, Frauen und Jugend.

Scott, E. K., London, A. S., & Myers, N. A. (2002). Dangerous dependencies. *Gender and Society, 16*, 878–897. doi:10.1177/089124302237893

Simmons, L. A., Anderson, E. A., & Braun, B. (2008). Health needs and health care utilization among rural, low-income women. *Women and Health, 47*(4), 53–69. doi:10.1080/03630240802100317

Sorensen, A., & McLanahan, S. (1987). Married women's economic dependency, 1940–1980. *American Journal of Sociology, 93*(3), 659–687.

Starfield, B., Shi, L., & Macinko, J. (2005). Contribution of primary care to health systems and health. *The Milbank Quarterly, 83*(3), 457–502. doi:10.1111/j.1468-0009.2005.00409.x

Stevens, F. (2001). The convergence and divergence of modern health care systems. In W. C. Cockerham (Ed.), *The Blackwell companion to medical sociology* (pp. 158–179). Oxford, UK: Blackwell Publishers Ltd. doi:10.1002/9780470996447

Stier, H., & Lewin-Epstein, N. (2007). Policy effects on the division of housework. *Journal of Comparative Policy Analysis: Research and Practice, 9*(3), 235–259. doi:10.1080/13876980701494657

Stier, H., & Mandel, H. (2009). Inequality in the family: The institutional aspects of wives' earning dependency. *Social Science Research, 38*, 594–608. doi:10.1016/j.ssresearch.2009.01.008

Taylor, A. K., Larson, S., & Correa-de-Araujo, R. (2006). Women's health care utilization and expenditures. *Women's Health Issues, 16*(2), 66–79. doi:10.1016/j.whi.2005.11.001

Thomson, S., & Mossialos, E. (2004). *What are the equity, efficiency, cost containment and choice implications of private health-care funding in western Europe?* Copenhagen: World Health Organization.

Tolman, R. M., & Rosen, D. (2001). Domestic violence in the lives of women receiving welfare: Mental health, substance dependence, and economic well-being. *Violence Against Women, 7* (2), 141–158. doi:10.1177/10778012010070020003

Ulrich, Y. C., Cain, K. C., Sugg, N. K., Rivara, F. P., Rubanowice, D. M., & Thompson, R. S. (2003). Medical care utilization patterns in women with diagnosed domestic violence. *American Journal of Preventive Medicine, 24*, 9–15. doi:10.1016/S0749-3797(02)00577-9

Van de Velde, S., Bambra, C., Van der Bracht, K., Eikemo, T. A., & Bracke, P. (2014). Keeping it in the family: The self-rated health of lone mothers in different European welfare regimes. *Sociology of Health and Illness, 36*(8), 1220–1242. doi:10.1111/1467-9566.12162

Van Doorslaer, E., Masseria, C., & Koolman, X. (2006). Inequalities in access to medical care by income in developed countries. *Canadian Medical Association Journal, 174*(2), 177–183. doi:10.1503/cmaj.050584

Vives-Cases, C., Ruiz-Cantero, M. T., Escribà-Agüir, V., & Miralles, J. J. (2011). The effect of intimate partner violence and other forms of violence against women on health. *Journal of Public Health, 33*, 15–21. doi:10.1093/pubmed/fdq101

Wendt, C. (2009). Mapping European healthcare systems: A comparative analysis of financing, service provision and access to healthcare. *Journal of European Social Policy, 19*, 432–445. doi:10.1177/0958928709344247

Whitehead, M. (2000). *The concepts and principles of equity and health.* Copenhagen, Denmark: WHO Regional Office for Europe.

Whitehead, M., Burstrom, B., & Diderichsen, F. (2000). Social policies and the pathways to inequalities in health: A comparative analysis of lone mothers in Britain and Sweden. *Social Science and Medicine, 50*, 255–270. doi:10.1016/S0277-9536(99)00280-4

Whitehead, M., & Dahlgren, G. (2006). *Levelling up (part 1): A discussion paper on concepts and principles for tackling social inequities in health.* Copenhagen, Denmark: WHO Regional Office for Europe.

Wilson, K. S., Silberberg, M. R., Brown, A. J., & Yaggy, S. D. (2007). Health needs and barriers to healthcare of women who have experienced intimate partner violence. *Journal of Women's Health, 16*, 1485–1498. doi:10.1089/jwh.2007.0385

Wimbauer, C. (2003). *Geld und Liebe: zur symbolischen Bedeutung von Geld in Paarbeziehungen [Money and love: The symbolic meaning of money in intimate relationships].* Frankfurt: Campus Verlag.

Wisdom, J. P., Berlin, M., & Lapidus, J. A. (2005). Relating health policy to women's health outcomes. *Social Science and Medicine, 61*, 1776–1784. doi:10.1016/j.socscimed.2005.03.030

Wisner, C. L., Gilmer, T. P., Saltzman, L. E., & Zink, T. M. (1999). Intimate partner violence against women: Do victims cost health plans more? *The Journal of Family Practice, 48*(6), 439–443.

Zimmerman, M. K., & Legerski, E. (2010). The role of governments in health care: Implications for women's health and access to care. *Women's Health Issues, 20*, 87–91. doi:10.1016/j.whi.2009.11.001

Chapter 4
The Policy Context in the US, Germany, and Norway

Abstract The present chapter begins with a justification of the selection of the US, Germany, and Norway as country cases. Following this is a description of each country separately, beginning with background information on the prevalence of IPV and the history of policies on violence against women and the services available. Afterward is a brief overview of aspects of the welfare state insofar as they influence the first policy intervention point of the conceptual framework: the redistribution of resources across society. Specifically, this looks at institutional arrangements aimed at decreasing poverty and economic inequality among women, such as unemployment benefits, sickness benefits, and benefits directed at single, low-income mothers. Second, family policies influencing the second policy intervention point are highlighted: women's resources for establishing independent households. This details parental leave, childcare provision, and the organization of the school day, family, and child allowances, flexible working time arrangements, and taxation systems. Finally, the situation for each case in terms of the third policy intervention point is described: access to health care. This focuses on entitlement to care, availability of health care providers, and affordability of out-of-pocket payments by patients. The chapter closes with a comparison of the policy contexts as they may affect IPV survivors.

Employing a quantitative design allows for the investigation of the individual-level connections between social position and IPV exposure, and whether women with IPV exposure are more vulnerable to the social gradient in health. To a certain extent, however, these relationships are constrained or enabled by institutional arrangements at the national level. Thus, in order to be able to draw broader conclusions, the United States, Germany, and Norway were selected as country cases with highly varying conditions affecting the development of inequities in health. This chapter's description of each country serves as the basis for Chap. 9's cross-national comparison of the social policy context in relation to the quantitative analyses presented in Chaps. 6, 7, and 8. It is important to point out that these quantitative analyses make use of nationally representative surveys on violence and health in the selected case

© Springer International Publishing Switzerland 2016

M.M. Larsen, *Health Inequities Related to Intimate Partner Violence Against Women*, Social Disparities in Health and Health Care,
DOI 10.1007/978-3-319-29565-7_4

countries, conducted in 1995–96 in the US, 2003 in Germany, and 2003–04 in Norway (these surveys are discussed in greater detail in Chap. 5). Since social policy is subject to change and reform over time, the reader should be aware that the case descriptions presented in this chapter necessarily focus on the policy context most relevant at the period of data collection of the respective countries (i.e., the mid-1990s in the US, and the early 2000s in Germany and Norway). This allows for a discussion of whether social position's impact on IPV exposure is reflective of national policies supporting women in establishing independent households, and whether the vulnerabilities to social position's impact on health among IPV survivors are reflective of national policies regarding access to health care.

The present chapter begins with a justification of the selection of the country cases. The sections following describe each country separately, beginning with background information on the prevalence of IPV, and the history of policies on violence against women and the services available. Following this is a brief overview of aspects of the welfare state insofar as they influence the first policy intervention point of the conceptual framework: the *redistribution of resources across society*. Specifically, this looks at institutional arrangements aimed at decreasing poverty and economic inequality among women, such as unemployment benefits, sickness benefits, and benefits directed at single, low-income mothers. Second, family policies influencing the second policy intervention point are highlighted: women's resources for *establishing independent households*. This details parental leave, childcare provision and the organization of the school day, family and child allowances, flexible working time arrangements, and taxation systems. Finally, the situation for each case in terms of the third policy intervention point is described: *access to health care*. This focuses on entitlement to care, availability of health care providers, and affordability of out-of-pocket payments by patients. The chapter closes with a comparison of the policy contexts as they may affect IPV survivors.

4.1 Case Selection

In general, research using case studies attempts to make connections between the phenomena of interest and the broader economic, social, and historical context (Ragin 1987). This book seeks to explore both outcomes *within* cases in the quantitative analysis, and to what extent differing institutional arrangements may be connected to differences *across* cases. To this end, a cross-case comparative design (Gerring 2007) is applied, using diverse cases to allow for maximum variance along the areas of interest. As much as possible, a diverse case study design should cover a "full range of variation" on the dimensions of theoretical interest in order to boost the representativeness of the cases selected (Seawright and Gerring 2008, p. 301). The conceptual framework, as described in Chap. 3, proposes mechanisms and corresponding policy intervention points between the policy context and the generation of health inequities for IPV survivors. Thus, the diversity of policy contexts across these dimensions is the foundation for the case selection (see Table 4.1).

Table 4.1 Case selection dimensions and descriptions

Mechanisms of health inequities	Policy intervention points	Cases		
		US (1995–96)	Germany (2003)	Norway (2003–04)
Social stratification	Redistribution of resources in society	Market dominated, assistance from state limited and means-tested	Earnings-related assistance, reinforces traditional social patterns	Comprehensive state intervention to promote equality and reduce poverty
Differential exposure to IPV	Establishing independent households	Prioritizes labor market ties, but little state intervention to balance role as carers	Prioritizes role as carers, but weakens ties to labor market	Prioritizes balance between labor market ties and role as carers
Differential vulnerability to poor health	Access to health care	Primarily through private sector, no entitlement to health care, high out-of-pocket costs	Universal care via social insurance contributions, minimal out-of-pocket costs	Universal care through social citizenship, minimal out-of-pocket costs

Exactly how these three cases vary along these dimensions is generally described in the following paragraphs.

In terms of *redistribution of resources* in society, the US, Germany, and Norway represent three different types of social stratification systems, both at the time of data collection of the national surveys (i.e., 1995 and 2003–2004, respectively) and at the time of this writing. While not directly addressed by the research questions, social stratification is the conceptual framework's initial mechanism linking the welfare state to health inequities and it would therefore be remiss not to consider where policy could intervene. Here, Esping-Andersen's (1990) typology of welfare states is useful for differentiating among social policy contexts in the production of health inequities. For example, the US represents a welfare state where the market dominates, benefits from the state are typically modest and means-tested, and little is done by the state in the way of preventing poverty and inequality. Germany represents a context with earnings-related assistance administered through employers, which typically reinforces traditional social patterns and inequalities, but reduces the role of the market. At the other end of the spectrum, Norway represents a welfare state providing generous benefits based upon social citizenship and state intervention to ensure full employment and income protection, thereby promoting equality and reducing poverty.

In addressing the dimension of women's access to resources for *establishing an independent household*, family policies affect the balance of power within relationships and also women's abilities to leave a relationship. These are primarily institutional arrangements supporting labor market participation, allowing women to avoid economic dependency on their partners, and helping women avoid poverty. Despite critical family policy changes over the past decade, the three countries discussed in this book typically fall into the same diverse patterns of family policy, regardless of the specific typology applied.[1] The US is an example of a welfare state whose policies prioritize women's roles in the labor market, but offer very little in terms of state support for their roles as caregivers within the home. This leaves women to arrange family support and childcare through the market. Germany is an example of a welfare state, on the other hand, which prioritizes women's roles as caregivers over their roles in the labor market. The traditional family structure of the male breadwinner/female part-time caregiver is preserved through tax benefits for the married and extensive family leave benefits for mothers. Norway represents a welfare state, however, which prioritizes balancing both women's labor market and family roles, with family-friendly employment policies and comprehensive subsidized childcare provision.

In terms of *access to health care*, health policy should be understood in its relation to how health care systems serve those in need, since differences in access have the potential to prevent or create differentials in vulnerability to poor health (Richardson and Norris 2010). The three selected cases represent great diversity in their institutional arrangements affecting availability, affordability, and entitlement to care. Before the enactment of the Patient Protection and Affordable Care Act (PPACA) in 2010, the US was an example of a health care system that was primarily associated with the private sector and linked to either the individual's employment or the employment of a family member, with large numbers of under- or uninsured, relatively high out-of-pocket costs, and relatively limited availability of providers in rural areas of the country. On the other hand, Germany represents a universal system of health care that is based on mandatory social insurance contributions, although certain groups are eligible for private health insurance. In this type of system, out-of-pocket costs are relatively modest and patients are free to access both primary care providers and specialists at will. Finally, Norway is an example of a universal health care system based on social citizenship, where out-of-pocket costs are held to a minimum, with primary care providers serving as the gatekeepers to specialists.

In addition to background on the prevalence of IPV and the history of policies on violence against women, the specifics of these proposed policy intervention points of social stratification, women's access to resources for establishing an independent household, and access to health care are explored in greater depth in the following country sections.

[1]See Sect. 3.1 for a discussion of various family policy typologies.

4.2 The United States

The battered women's movement in the US began in the early 1970s amid the civil rights, antiwar, and feminist movements, focusing primarily on providing shelter and crisis services (Lehrner and Allen 2009). The first known women's shelter in the US opened in 1973 in Phoenix, Arizona, followed by a shelter in Pasadena, California in 1974 (Tierney 1982). Just a few years later, there were already hundreds of local battered women's programs that had been established across the country, as well as the formation of both state and national coalitions (Dobash and Dobash 1992; Lehrner and Allen 2009). The battered women's movement in the US, along with law enforcement and the courts, also played a significant role in getting violence against women recognized by lawmakers, with Congress enacting the Violence Against Women Act (VAWA) in 1994 (Brandwein 1999; Modi et al. 2014). With its passing, VAWA established the federal Office on Violence Against Women within the Department of Justice and delivered $1.6 billion for investigating and prosecuting violent crimes against women (Modi et al. 2014). VAWA and its subsequent reauthorizations demonstrated the federal government's commitment to funding programs to combat domestic violence, sexual assault, and stalking.[2] This funding goes toward shelters for abused women, support groups, and state grants for prevention and community-based services for survivors.

A recent national survey revealed that almost 33 % of women in the US reported being physically assaulted by a current or former spouse, cohabiting partner, or date, and nearly 10 % have been sexually assaulted by an intimate partner over the course of their lifetime (Black et al. 2011). Nearly 6 % of women reported physical or sexual IPV within the past 12 months. Of these women, 42 % reported experiencing injuries due to physical or sexual violence. The National Network to End Domestic Violence (NNEDV) (2012) estimates that there are over 1900 domestic violence programs in the US and that on any given day, more than 60,000 survivors and their children seek services from these programs. Over half of those seeking help are looking for emergency shelter or transitional housing, and approximately one-third call a local, state, or national domestic violence hotline (NNEDV 2012). However, there is still a large unmet need for services, and on any given day, nearly 7000 requests for shelter are denied due to lack of available space. Given that shelters are typically a last resort for women in abusive relationships (Haj-Yahia and Cohen 2009), this unmet need at the national level critically reduces the chance for women in abusive relationships to separate from their partners if they do not have other resources to do so.

---

[2]VAWA was reauthorized in 2000, 2005, and 2013. Although put up for reauthorization in 2012, there was not enough bipartisan support for VAWA to pass (Modi et al. 2014). The bill stalled due to Republicans' objection to additional measures protecting same-sex couples and undocumented immigrants. While the 2013 reauthorization included expanded measures for Native Americans, lesbian, gay, bisexual, transgender, gay, and queer individuals, and victims of human trafficking, it does not protect IPV survivors who are undocumented immigrants.

VAWA legislation also focuses heavily on law enforcement strategies, criminalization of violence against women, and prosecution of perpetrators. This includes turning IPV into a federal crime with the crossing of state borders, increasing federal penalties for repeat sex offenders, and having every state enact laws criminalizing stalking. These legal reforms have arguably had a positive effect in shifting the public discourse away from victim blaming (Brandwein 1999), making VAWA one of the successes of the battered women's movement (Lehrner and Allen 2009). However, as will be described in the following sections, they do not provide the reasonable social provisions needed for women to leave violent relationships, and are therefore limited in their scope of impact (Peter 2006).

4.2.1 Redistribution of Resources

In the mid-1990s as well as today, the US as a welfare state has not provided much in the way of social assistance as a right of social citizenship, offering instead very limited services and income benefits (see Table 4.2). As Olsen (2007) explains, this "restricted nature of the US welfare state reflects a commitment to a narrow conception of equal opportunity, [which is] a negative expression of liberty—freedom *from* the state—and limited government" (p. 145, emphasis in the original text). Under certain restrictions, those with full-time positions who become *unemployed* through no fault of their own are entitled to a percentage of their previous income (typically 50–60 %), with the duration of the benefit varying by state (typically up to 26 weeks) (US Department of Labor 2013). However, there are no federal laws requiring employers to pay their employees for time off due to illness (US Department of Labor, n.d.). Instead, *sickness leave* allowances vary by employers and employment status.

Prior to 1997, the social assistance most relevant for *single mothers* with weaker ties to the labor market included a means-tested and subsidized food program and income assistance through the Aid to Families with Dependent Children (AFDC) program (also known simply as 'welfare' in the American vernacular). Established in 1935, AFDC offered federal social assistance to women in poverty and their children for as long as necessary until the children were grown (Brandwein 1999). However, these programs had a reputation for being "politically less legitimate, less

Table 4.2 US: welfare policy related to redistribution of resources (mid-1990s)

Welfare policy dimensions	US
Unemployment benefits	Compensation and duration varies by state. Typical benefits: partial compensation of 50–60 % income for up to 26 weeks
Sickness leave	No entitlement. Varies by employer
Poverty protection for single mothers	Social assistance and food benefits: means-tested, available until children are 18

Table 4.3 US: family policy related to establishing independent households (mid-1990s)

Family policy dimensions	US
Parental leave	No entitlement to paid leave. Family and Medical Leave Act: 12 weeks of unpaid leave
Childcare	No entitlement. Arranged through family or market
School arrangements	33 h/week; continuous school day; 185 days/year
Family and child allowances	No entitlement to allowances. Earned income tax credit available for taxpayers
Working time regulations	Minimal regulation. Fair Labor Standards Act: standard 40-h workweek (27 % of workers are exempt); minimum wage for part-time work
Taxation systems	Choice of joint or individual filing. System favors households with sole breadwinner

generously funded, and more oriented to monitoring clients' behavior and income" (Orloff 1993, p. 315) than those programs serving unemployed and retired men. The public discourse around AFDC was that it created dependency among 'undeserving' women and hindered their ability to provide for themselves through employment (Brandwein 1999). This discourse fueled the passing of the Personal Responsibility and Work Opportunity Reconciliation Act in 1996 (also referred to as 'welfare reform'), which drastically reduced the social assistance available to single women with children.[3] Further policies affecting women with children in the US are described in the following section.

4.2.2 *Establishing Independent Households*

The US is one of the few advanced industrialized nations without an explicit set of comprehensive family policies in place (see Table 4.3). Yet in the mid-1990s, like today, there were implicit social policies which had a direct impact on families, although these tended to be "limited in scale, coverage, and generosity and [were] usually categorical and narrowly focused" (Kamerman and Kahn 2001, p. 69).

Then, as well as now, there existed no universal paid *parental leave* in the US. Instead, the Family and Medical Leave Act (FMLA) of 1993 established that employers with more than 50 employees must allow for 12 weeks of unpaid,

[3]In 1997, 'welfare reform' replaced AFDC with block grants to individual states, known as the Temporary Assistance for Needy Families (TANF) program. TANF became an assistance program with a maximum 5-year lifetime limit, designed to reduce the 'dependency' of low-income families on governmental cash assistance (Christopher 2004; Kamerman and Kahn 2001; Olsen 2007). Beneficiaries were required to be employed within 2 years of qualifying for TANF benefits, and low-income women with children were expected to be in the labor force as soon as three months after a child's birth (Kamerman and Kahn 2001).

job-protected leave for those caring for a newborn or newly adopted child, as well as for those taking care of family members with serious health conditions (US Department of Labor 2012). In order to take advantage of FMLA from the employers mandated to provide it, the individual must have been employed there for at least one year and must have first exhausted their accrued sick and vacation leave. Additionally, 13 states offered expanded versions of FMLA or other types of disability leave for new mothers (Ray 2008). While employers may choose to offer additional parental leave benefits at their own discretion, there are still no federal regulations governing this. Thus, many employed women return to work relatively soon after the birth of their child. Approximately, half of women with children under the age of one work outside the home—and of these, about one-third return to work within the first 3 months, and two-thirds are back at work within 6 months (Fujii 2011).

While nearly 62 % of women with children under the age of 6, and 59 % of women with children under the age of 3, were active in the American labor force in 1995 (US Department of Labor 2009), in the mid-1990s as well as today, the US has had no national *childcare* legislation. Instead, private childcare accessed through the market has remained the norm and "informal unlicensed, unregulated" childcare is widespread, more so than in many other developed countries (Olsen 2007, p. 151). High quality care is difficult to find and given that the costs are covered directly by families, it is out of the financial reach of many. For example, in some low-income families, childcare costs made up at least 20 % of the family's budget (Adams and Rohacek 2002; Christopher 2004). To offset a portion of these costs, a Child and Dependent Care Tax Credit has existed since 1976 for working parents who earn enough to pay taxes which allows taxpayers to claim credit up to a certain percentage of childcare expenses (Internal Revenue Service [IRS] 2013). However, critics argue that this type of tax credit disproportionately favors families who earn higher levels of income because it does not directly pay for childcare or address issues of access (Olsen 2007). While the Childcare and Development Block Grant of 1990 offered states federal funding to provide childcare services for families whose income falls below 85 % of the state median income, states are not obliged to provide this assistance to families and/or may adopt even more stringent income eligibility criteria (Kamerman and Kahn 2001). In fact, one study found that only 14 % of eligible low-income children received this type of assistance from states (Mezey et al. 2002). Thus, in order to address this gap in affordability, the majority of low-income families instead have looked to childcare solutions involving relatives or other types of informal care (Christopher 2004; Henly and Lyons 2000).

On the other hand, the organization of the *public school arrangements* in the US has been supportive of women's employment once children reach school age (Gornick et al. 1997). The start of formal schooling in the US starts around ages 5 or 6. Children spend a relatively high number of hours per week in school (33 h) and the school day is continuous (as opposed to children being sent home for lunch). However, this has been balanced out by spending fewer days per year in school

(185 days) than other OECD countries (e.g., 220 days in Italy, Luxembourg, and the Netherlands) (Gornick et al. 1997).

In the mid-1990s, as well as now, there were no universal *child or family allowances* in the US. Instead, financial assistance remains tied to income and other strict eligibility requirements. However, for those parents who earn enough to pay taxes, there are a number of tax credits meant to benefit families, such as the Earned Income Tax Credit established in 1975 (IRS 2014). It is important to note that such forms of assistance can be problematic. First, they require that families earn enough to pay taxes (Kamerman and Kahn 2001). Second, parents must have enough money up front to cover the costs of raising a family in order to claim the tax credits at the end of the year. For these reasons, such tax credits may be more beneficial for those already in the middle class and less beneficial to families already living in poverty.

In the US, there continues to be very few *working time regulations* allowing for flexible arrangements which would make it easier for women with children to balance employment and caregiving responsibilities. The typical workweek has remained at 40 h since the Fair Labor Standards Act of 1938 mandating overtime pay above a weekly threshold (US Department of Labor 2011), however 27 % of full-time workers are exempt (Gornick and Meyers 2003). The Fair Labor Standards Act also guarantees that part-time workers earn the minimum wage. However, there remains no legislation regarding maximum number of weekly working hours allowed, equal benefits for part-time work, rights to work a flexible schedule, or rights to a minimum number of paid vacation days per year (Gornick and Meyers 2009). Each employer determines for itself how working time is arranged and what it offers to employees. In practice, this means Americans traditionally have spent a large amount of time at work. For example, nearly two-thirds of couples with children in the US worked at least 80 h per week combined (Gornick and Meyers 2003). In 1995, 67 % of part-time jobs were held by women, with 20 % of employed women working part-time, as compared to 8 % of employed men (OECD 2014).

Finally, while married couples in the US have the option of filing taxes either jointly or separately, the *taxation system* essentially works more to the advantage of those filing jointly (Sainsbury 1994). Basically, better tax rates are offered to those filing jointly and tax breaks are more advantageous for households with a sole earner. Moreover, regardless of whether there are one or two earners in the household, everyone receives the same tax exemptions. Additionally, sole providers without a partner (i.e., single parents) do not enjoy the same tax privileges as those sole providers with a partner. Bergmann (1986) summarizes these aspects of the US tax system in the following way: (1) the dual-earner marriage penalty; (2) the housewife bonus; and (3) the single parent penalty. In other words, dual earners may be penalized, while sole providers with partners are favored. The lack of policy intervention in terms of women's resources for independent households is also reflected in other areas of policy, as is seen in the following section on access to health care.

Table 4.4 US: health policy related to access to health care (mid-1990s)

Health policy dimensions	US
Entitlement to care	Based primarily on private payment. Health insurance coverage for women, 18–64 years: Employer-based (58 %); private (7 %); Medicaid (12 %); uninsured (19 %)
Availability of providers	Gatekeeping depends on health insurance; PCP shortage; uninsured rely on community health centers or emergency departments
Affordability of care	Out-of-pocket costs vary by health plan and coverage. All services may be subject to co-payments. High deductibles not uncommon

4.2.3 Access to Health Care

When it comes to access to health care, the US is one of the few industrialized countries which, until the PPACA was passed into law on March 23, 2010, had not prioritized entitlement to care (see Table 4.4) (Rice et al. 2013).[4] Rather than one unified system, health care in the US is pluralistic and consists of multiple, independent systems which evolved primarily through the private sector with quite a low level of government input. Coordinated system-level planning in the US is minimal and has traditionally been frowned upon, resulting in an absence of centralized control over health care prices and no guaranteed insurance coverage (Rice et al. 2013). In the mid-1990s, the US spent 14 % of its Gross Domestic Product (GDP) on health care, the highest among Western industrialized countries (WHO 2014). Likewise, the US's per capita health expenditure was second only to Switzerland. During this same time period, about 48 % of the US's total spending on health care came from public sources, 40 % from third party payer sources, and 12 % from private out-of-pocket payments by patients (Rice et al. 2013).

Even after PPACA, *entitlement to health care* in the US for the non-elderly and non-poor continues to be based upon either private payment or employer contributions. In comparison to other industrialized countries, the private sector plays a large role in the US and was involved in the very beginnings of the US's health insurance system. Private health insurance began in the early 1930s with nonprofit hospital care plans and physician care plans (e.g., Blue Cross and Blue Shield) (Rice et al. 2013). Most commonly, adults of working age acquire health insurance through employment, although these levels have decreased as health care premiums and costs have increased for employers (Feder et al. 2001; Hoffman and Paradise 2008). Furthermore, in the mid-1990s, employer-sponsored health coverage was

[4]A number of important reforms to US health care were enacted with this law. At the time of this writing, these reforms are still in the process of being rolled out, the most central tenets of which essentially require all Americans to have health insurance, as well as the regulation and reduction of health care costs, which aim to improve access. However, since the effects of PPACA are not yet clear and because the US data used in the analysis were collected in the mid-1990s, this case description focuses solely on health care in the US prior to PPACA.

not guaranteed to everyone who was employed.[5] Qualifying for coverage necessitated that a number of requirements be met: (1) being employed or an employee's family member; (2) having an employer that (voluntarily) offers health care coverage, which was only the case in 68 % of firms with less than 200 employees; (3) meeting the employer's eligibility requirements, which usually involved working full-time; and (4) being willing to pay the employee's share of premiums, which could be quite high (Rice et al. 2013).

Another option prior to PPACA was to purchase individual health insurance on the private market, but gender-based premiums were common and could increase costs dramatically for women (Codispoti et al. 2008). Moreover, since regulation of private insurance was minimal compared to employer-based insurance, applications for coverage could be denied, benefits could be limited in scope, and costs could be higher (Feder et al. 2001). For example, private health insurance companies were not required to provide maternity coverage and could reject women's applications based on histories of cesarean sections or domestic violence (Codispoti et al. 2008).

If employer-sponsored or private health coverage was not feasible, women faced two choices: either apply for Medicaid coverage (if they qualified) or remain uninsured. Major federal government health insurance programs were not developed until the mid-1960s in the form of Medicaid for the poor and Medicare for the elderly and disabled. Prior to PPACA, Medicaid remained a strictly means-tested program offering coverage for low-income individuals falling into the following categories: children, pregnant women, disabled persons, senior citizens, and parents of dependent children. This meant that other low-income adults who did not care for dependent children did not qualify for Medicaid.[6] States which fell along the median provided coverage for pregnant women up to 185 % of the Federal Poverty Level (Rice et al. 2013).[7] However, much stricter eligibility requirements were required of low-income parents of dependent children, with the median state covering parents living at up to 64 % of the Federal Poverty Level. While poor children were widely covered by Medicaid, over half of women living below 138 % of the Federal Poverty Level were without any insurance coverage (Rice et al. 2013). Before PPACA went into effect, nearly 65 % of the approximately 98 million women between the ages of 18 and 64 were covered by employer-sponsored or privately purchased coverage, 19 % were uninsured, and 16 % received either Medicaid or other government care (e.g., services for active and retired members of the military, or Indian Health Service coverage).

In the mid-1990s, as well as currently, *availability of providers* varied in the US according to health insurance status. For those with health insurance, primary care

[5]According to the PPACA's employer mandate, today employers with more than 50 employees are required to offer health insurance to their full-time employees or else face a financial penalty.

[6]PPACA has expanded Medicaid eligibility to also include individuals without dependent children, although individual states are able to opt out of Medicaid expansion if they choose.

[7]In 1995, the Federal Poverty Level was $7470 for an unmarried individual and $15150 for a family of four (US Department of Health and Human Services, n.d). This is approximately the equivalent of $11,658 and $23,643, respectively in 2015 (US Bureau of Labor Statistics, n.d.).

is the typical point of entry into the health care system. Depending on the type of health insurance an individual has, primary care providers (PCP) may serve as gatekeepers to accessing further medical specialists, or patients may directly seek out the specialist themselves. This primary care is typically delivered through private physician clinics or nonprofit community health centers, but there are nearly 65 million Americans living in areas with PCP shortages, making it ever more difficult to gain access to care (Bodenheimer and Pham 2010). These shortages are arguably due to the significant imbalance in the number of specialist physicians as opposed to PCPs (Rice et al. 2013). Between 1965 and 1992, the specialist physician-to-population ratio increased by 120 %, while the PCP-to-population ratio only increased by 14 % (Bodenheimer and Pham 2010). Visits to PCPs make up over one-half of all visits to the doctors in the US, yet only about one-third of physicians provide primary care (Bodenheimer and Pham 2010). There is evidence that this imbalance and shortage of PCPs has resulted in unwanted delays in care (Rice et al. 2013) and higher rates of emergency department visits and hospitalizations (Bodenheimer and Pham 2010). Those patients with Medicaid coverage may face their own set of difficulties accessing primary care, as only about half of all providers accept all or most patients seeking care with Medicaid coverage (Zuckerman et al. 2004). This is due in part to the very low physician payment rates in comparison to the payment rates from private insurers, which limits provider choice among those with Medicaid coverage (Feder et al. 2001).

Moreover, access to health care for the uninsured was very limited in the mid-1990s. Anywhere from one-third to one-half of the uninsured in the US declined care, deferred care, or were not able to access it when needed (Van Loon et al. 2002). Rather than seeking preventative care, the uninsured tend to access care at community health clinics offering services free of cost or on a sliding scale according to the ability to pay (Cheong 2007; Rice et al. 2013; Wilper et al. 2008). This occurs usually only when acute health issues arise (Van Loon et al. 2002). For some of the uninsured, hospital emergency departments in the US act as a safety net (Trzeciak and Rivers 2003). First of all, hospitals are required to treat underinsured and uninsured individuals with emergency health issues until they are stable, which potentially also involves in-patient admission and surgery. Although patients are legally bound to pay for their treatment, they are often not financially able to do so, and the hospital is left with unpaid debt. Indeed, the emergency department utilization rates of low-income individuals are higher than among those with greater levels of income (Rice et al. 2013). Second, it is still not uncommon for the uninsured to visit emergency departments for treatment of nonurgent issues, or to wait until they are seriously ill before seeking treatment at the emergency department (GAO 2009). Oftentimes, these more serious health issues could have been prevented or addressed through routine check-ups with a PCP. In other words, especially prior to PPACA, hospital emergency departments tended to be overburdened with nonemergency cases, leading to a decrease in quality of care, which manifested itself in overcrowding and much longer waiting times than recommended for emergency cases.

In additional to primary care, mental health care options also play an important role in access. Over the last four decades, mental health care in the US has evolved from primarily institutionalized care into mainly outpatient services (or short-term inpatient stays) with a heavy reliance on pharmaceuticals and fewer psychotherapy and mental health counseling services. Between 1977 and 1997, the prescription of outpatient antidepressants doubled (Marcus and Olfson 2010) and cases treated with psychotropic drugs increased by over 20 % (Rice et al. 2013). Patients with insurance typically receive treatment in private outpatient practices from psychiatrists, psychologists, or social workers. Those who do not have access to health insurance are generally treated in public mental health hospitals or community health centers. However, of those in the US with mental health issues, only about one-third were being treated prior to PPACA, predominantly because insurance coverage for mental health services was often limited or not available at all through some private plans (Rice et al. 2013).

In the US, out-of-pocket costs (e.g., direct payment for services, co-payments, premiums, and deductibles) were generally not regulated prior to PPACA and *affordability of care* remains a key obstacle to accessing health care. Although on the rise internationally, the US has the second highest per capita out-of-pocket costs among OECD countries (Rice et al. 2013). One study found that cost was a barrier to care in the US for over 90 % of the uninsured and over 50 % of the insured (Strunk and Cunningham 2002). For example, high deductibles or co-payments were not uncommon among private health insurance plans, leaving some insured patients unable to afford the out-of-pocket expenses of care (Feder et al. 2001; Hoffman and Paradise 2008; Mendes 2012). As mentioned in the previous section, it was not always uncommon for women to be charged higher insurance premiums for private insurance than men, which could become a financial burden (Codispoti et al. 2008; Rice et al. 2013). Moreover, due to these barriers, those without any health insurance coverage tended to forgo preventative check-ups altogether in order to avoid the costs of such visits (Rice et al. 2013; Van Loon et al. 2002). For those that sought treatment, the consequences of unaffordable health costs could be dire, with medical debt listed as the cause of nearly two-thirds of bankruptcies filed in the US (Himmelstein et al. 2009).

4.3 Germany

Like in the US, Germany's services for abused women originated within the nongovernmental organizations (NGOs) of the women's movement, which paved the way for state recognition of partner violence (Hanmer et al. 2006). In 1999, the German government developed a National Action Plan to combat violence against women (BMFSFJ 1999). The plan advocated change at the federal, state, and local levels, emphasizing prevention efforts, awareness building, legal reforms, strengthened cooperation between governmental and NGOs, and nationwide networking of services. In order to inform further policy and concrete actions, the plan called for a national prevalence survey on the topic of violence against women in Germany. The results of the survey demonstrated that one-in-four women had experienced physical or sexual violence from a current or former partner in their lifetime (Müller and Schröttle 2004). Nearly two-thirds of women who had experienced IPV were injured by the violence, and approximately one-third of these women were injured seriously enough to require medical assistance. Slightly over one-in-four IPV survivors reported experiencing very severe or life-threatening violence. As a response, a Second Action Plan (BMFSFJ 2007) was developed in 2007, prioritizing optimal medical treatment of women experiencing violence through greater physician awareness of IPV and better organized treatment to ensure women are appropriately cared for and supported (Hornberg et al. 2008).

The first shelters for survivors of IPV opened in 1976 in West Berlin and Cologne. Today there are 345 women's shelters nationwide offering 6812 shelter spaces. This is nearly 1400 spaces short of the recommendation for Germany's population according to the Council of Europe Task Force to Combat Violence Against Women, Including Domestic Violence (one space per 7500 inhabitants) (Stelmaszekn and Fisher 2012). The shelters offer 3–6 months of accommodation for female survivors of IPV and their children, and are primarily under the nonprofit coordination of the Association of Women's Shelters (*Frauenhauskoordinierung* e.V., FHK e.V.) and the Central Information Center for Independent Women's Shelters (*Zentrale Informationsstelle Autonomer Frauenhäuser*, ZIF). Sufficient financing of shelters in Germany is not regulated on a national level, but rather varies by region. Typically, women with enough income must pay for their residence in the shelter, while low-income women must apply for social assistance to cover the costs (ZIF, n.d.). In 2013, the multiple local and regional telephone hotlines for survivors of IPV were replaced with one national hotline number. It is against this background of services for IPV that aspects of Germany's welfare, family, and health policy circa 2003–04 are described in the following sections.

4.3.1 Redistribution of Resources

As a pioneer of the welfare state, Germany has a strong system of generous social benefits straddling the divide between the individualism found in liberal welfare states and the 'statism' found in social democratic welfare states (see Table 4.5) (Leisering 2001). This middle ground has often been termed a 'social market economy'. The largest portion of social benefits from the German welfare state are based on a social insurance system (*Sozialversicherung*) which protects against major risks (e.g., unemployment, sickness) by sharing risk collectively among the insured (Aspalter 2001). Social insurance is a pay-as-you-go system financed primarily by mandatory employee and employer contributions, making the employed middle classes the key beneficiaries of the German welfare state (Leisering 2001). In this way, the system tends to be stratified along occupational and class lines, so

Table 4.5 Germany: welfare policy related to redistribution of resources (early 2000s)

Welfare policy dimensions	Germany
Unemployment benefits	Partial compensation: 60 % of income; 67 % with dependent child (ren). 6–32 months, depending on age and employment record After unemployment benefits exhausted, partial compensation: 53 % of income; 57 % with dependent children. Unlimited duration
Sickness leave	Full compensation: first 6 weeks. Partial compensation: 70 % of income for up to 18 months thereafter
Poverty protection for single mothers	Minimal policy addressing single mothers specifically

that delivery of benefits perpetuate prevailing patterns of social inequality (Beckfield and Krieger 2009).

In cases of illness, since 1998 employees have been allowed 6 weeks of *sickness leave* at full salary, paid by the employer (Leisering 2001). After these 6 weeks are exhausted, employees are entitled to up to 18 months of sick leave at about 70 % of full salary, covered by health insurance. During the time period relevant for this book's analysis, *unemployment benefits* (*Arbeitslosengeld*) were available if employees had worked for at least 12 months and had contributed to social insurance for at least 12 months in the previous 3 years (OECD 2003a).[8] In cases of unemployment, those eligible received 60 % of their post-tax income (or 67 % for those with at least one dependent child), up to a specified monthly ceiling of gross earnings. Length of benefit receipt varied according to age and employment record, ranging from 6 to 32 months (OECD 2003a). For those who exhausted their unemployment insurance benefits, they were then eligible to receive unemployment assistance (*Arbeitslosenhilfe*) for an unlimited duration at 53 % of their post-tax income (or 57 % for those with at least on dependent child), up to a monthly ceiling.

In addition to the social insurance system, needs-based social assistance (*Sozialhilfe*) was also available, providing financial support to guarantee a minimum income level. This social assistance was means-tested, unlimited in duration, and available to all of those who were not able to adequately cover the costs of living (OECD 2003a). These benefits were based on a standard cost-of-living rate appropriate for the household size, as well as benefits incorporating additional

[8] As of January 2005, the Hartz IV Reforms created a differentiation known as *Arbeitslosengeld I* and *Arbeitslosengeld II*. *Arbeitslosengeld I* remained similar to the above described 'unemployment benefits'. However, *Arbeitslosengeld II* combined the previous unemployment assistance benefits (*Arbeitslosenhilfe*) with social assistance benefits (*Sozialhilfe*) to create a single means-tested income-replacement benefit for those unable to work (OECD 2006). The reform also created stricter means testing and time limitations on *Arbeitslosengeld II* for long-term unemployed workers. However, since the German data used in the analysis were collected in 2003–2004, this case description focuses on policy prior to the Hartz IV Reforms.

needs and housing costs. Here another cornerstone of the German welfare state came into play: the principle of subsidiarity. In essence, assistance from the family is given priority consideration over assistance from the state. This means that social assistance is only provided if the individual's own resources and their family's resources do not adequately cover the costs of living (Aspalter 2001; Leisering 2001; OECD 2003a). It should be mentioned that those taking advantage of the means-tested social assistance in Germany are usually those who fall outside of the 'typical' employment patterns, such as single mothers, whose income loss may not be generally covered by social insurance benefits (Daly 2000; Hansen et al. 2006).

Traditionally, *single mothers* in Germany "have no policy domain as either full-time carers or as paid workers. Within the gender logic of the German policy constellation that is organized around marital status or paid work, solo mothers are a residual category" (Hobson 1994, p. 182). In this sense, they are not necessarily identified as a special group needing their own benefits, but rather "benefits are offered to them in respect of their being either a parent (child benefits, parental leave), in need of income support (social assistance), or a worker (unemployment benefits)" (Hansen et al. 2006, p. 270). They are also provided with a tax allowance which attempts to level the playing field between them and married couples who can take advantage of joint taxation (Leitner et al. 2008). However, research seems to indicate that the German welfare state's prioritization of social insurance benefits leave single mothers at a disadvantage, both due to inadequate employment support for working mothers and relatively low social assistance payments. As a result, single mothers in Germany tend to have higher poverty rates as compared to married mothers and these rates also tend to be higher than those in other European countries (Christopher 2002; Hansen et al. 2006). In other words, "the German welfare state, with a high wage replacement, a social insurance-based transfer system…and policies that tend to treat lone parent households as residual and atypical, seems to be a system less suited to protecting single parents from experiencing poverty" (Hansen et al. 2006, p. 277). These critiques continue to be explored in the following section on family policy.

4.3.2 Establishing Independent Households

Generally, family policy in today's Germany is a product of the unification of the former East German dual-earner model of family policy and the former West German male breadwinner/female carer model (see Table 4.6) (Leitner et al. 2008; Ostner 2010). Following World War II, West German family policy resolutely rejected government intrusion into family life, in part as a reaction to both the Nazi population policies and the developing socialist regime in East Germany. Privacy within marriage and the family was held sacred, and the state encouraged families to follow a male breadwinner/female carer pattern founded on ideas of gender roles that were 'different but equal'. In contrast, East German family policy sought to encourage both women's full-time employment and their motherhood by having the

Table 4.6 Germany: family policy related to establishing independent households (early 2000s)

Family policy dimensions	Germany
Parental leave	14 weeks maternity leave (100 %). Three years job-protected parental leave without income replacement
Childcare	Publicly subsidized childcare: part-time care for ages 3–6.5 years. Limits on private costs. Tax deduction available
School arrangements	20–27 h/week; mornings only; 188 days/year; limited opportunities for full-day school
Family and child allowances	Universal allowance for each child under 18 years Allowance for children ages 1–3 not attending publicly subsidized childcare. Means-tested, available for up to 24 months Tax deduction available
Working time regulations	EU Directive on working time: work week varies according to collective agreements; maximum 40 h/week allowed; 20 days annual leave EU Directive on part-time work: parents have right to part-time work if approved by employer; equal pay rate as full-time; benefits proportional to hours worked
Taxation systems	Joint taxation

state step in to relieve women of their caring responsibilities. After reunification in 1990, the male breadwinner/female carer family model of West Germany was spread to the former East Germany, but it also underwent a process of evolution heavily influenced by the EU's emphasis on employment-friendly family policies (Leitner et al. 2008). Beginning in 2002, the government of unified Germany presented a paradigm shift with its 'sustainable family policy' (*nachhaltige Familienpolitik*), focusing on the continuous employment of women and early education of children outside the home (Leitner 2011). Family policy in Germany continues to undergo significant changes in this direction, but especially for the 2003–04 policy context relevant for this book, Germany can be referred to as promoting a male breadwinner/female part-time carer family model (Andreß et al. 2006; Honekamp 2008).

Germany's *parental leave* benefits have evolved significantly over the last three decades. What has remained relatively consistent is women's entitlement to 14 weeks of paid maternity leave (6 weeks prior and 8 weeks after childbirth), replacing 100 % of women's previous income if enrolled in a statutory health insurance plan (available through women's own employment, partners' employment, unemployment benefits, or enrollment in education) (Honekamp 2008; Leitner et al. 2008; Ray 2008). These costs are borne partially by the health insurance plan and partially by women's employers. During the early 2000s, parents were also entitled to up to 3 years of unpaid, job-protected leave after the birth of a child (plus the right to an income-tested allowance for up to 2 years, which will be discussed later in this section).[9] Thus, Germany came to have one of the longest periods of parental leave in Europe, but with little support to replace women's lost income wages (Ray et al. 2010).

Related to long parental leave is the provision of *childcare*. In 1995, children in Germany between the ages of 3 and 6.5 were given the right to publicly funded or subsidized childcare (*Kindergärten*), with the objective of encouraging children's social development as well as accommodating the needs of parents (Leitner 2011; Leitner et al. 2008). Referring back to the welfare principle of subsidiarity, the state is indeed one provider of childcare, but it is only one among many. Thus, regulations for provision of childcare vary across Germany's 16 federal states, as do costs, parental involvement, and opening hours. However, the right to childcare only stipulates a maximum of 3–4 hours per day of care, either in the morning or afternoon (Honekamp 2008). It is also important to mention that during the early 2000s, children under the age of 3 were not guaranteed access to childcare (*Krippen*) and the number of available places was extremely limited.[10] Generally, parents are asked to contribute to the costs of childcare according to their means, with reduced costs available to low-income parents, and no fee at all for those receiving social assistance (Honekamp 2008; Leitner et al. 2008). In the early 2000s, parents could also deduct the cost of childcare up to a maximum of €1500 per year for children under the age of 14 (OECD 2003a).[11]

In 2002, approximately 90 % of children between the ages of 3 and 6.5 were enrolled in childcare, with only 33 % enrolled in full-time care (Leitner et al. 2008). Only about 9 % of children under 3 years of age were enrolled in formal childcare in 2002, which was well below the OECD average of 20.5 % (OECD 2014).[12] Many critics have argued that this structure placed severe limits on women's abilities to maintain either full- or part-time employment (Andreß et al. 2006; Honekamp 2008; Leitner 2011). The lack of care for children under 3 years of age, and the limited number of hours per day of available childcare essentially assumed that at least one parent is able stay home or work flexible, part-time hours. As such,

[9]This version of parental leave (*Erziehungsurlaub*) changed dramatically in 2007 with the introduction of an income-replacement benefit (*Elterngeld*), which entitled parents to 67 % of their previous income (up to a ceiling of €1800/month) for 14 months (12 months reserved for the mother and two months for the father) (Honekamp 2008; Leitner 2011; Ray 2008). Alternatively, parents could opt for 33 % of their previous income for twice the usual length. Moreover, parents were also entitled to the entire 3 years of leave, but without income replacement for the second or third year, depending on the level of replacement chosen.

[10]Beginning in 2005, reforms were introduced to increase the number of childcare places available to children under the age of three, and establishing a right to childcare at the age of one (Leitner 2011).

[11]In 2006, this was increased to a tax allowance covering two-thirds of childcare costs up to a maximum of €4000.

[12]Since the 2005 reforms, the percentage of children under three in childcare has gradually increased to 25.4 % in 2011, exceeding the original goal of 17.4 % set out with the reform (Honekamp 2008; OECD 2014).

childcare served rather as a complement to family care work, instead of serving as a replacement of family care (Andreß et al. 2006).

This assumption of a male breadwinner/female (part-time) carer model was also reflected to some extent in the *organization of the school day* in Germany. Compulsory schooling begins with the age of 6 and continues until approximately 15 years of age before further secondary or tertiary education begins. In their first year of school, children spend approximately 20–22 h per week in school, and this increases to about 27 h per week by the fourth grade, for a total of 188 days per year (EURYDICE 2013). Typically, up to six lessons are held in the morning, with the school day coming to an end around midday. Although the number of all-day schools and after-school education is increasing across Germany, only 5 % of primary school students attended all-day schools in 2003 (Kultusministerkonferenz 2006). As with the limited hours of childcare availability, the typical school day in Germany places some restrictions on the working hours of at least one parent.

There are two different types of *allowances for families and children* relevant for the time period examined in this book. First, there exists a universal child benefit (*Kindergeld*) which intends to guarantee a basic income for children. It is paid monthly as a tax credit to families for each child under the age of 18 (Honekamp 2008; Leitner et al. 2008; OECD 2003a). The benefit can be extended to age 25 while children are enrolled in secondary education or to the age of 21 for children who are unemployed. The benefit is universally provided to all families at the same amount, regardless of income level. As an alternative to a cash allowance, the benefit can also be taken as an annual tax deduction, which puts higher income families at an advantage (Leitner et al. 2008). In addition to the possibility of taking the universal child benefit as a tax deduction, another tax deduction is offered to offset childcare and education costs for children up until age 25 (*Betreuung- und Erziehungsfreibetrag*). The deduction is a flat rate and independent of actual costs of childcare and education (Leitner et al. 2008). Moreover, an additional amount could be deducted for children attending higher education (ages 18–25) as long as they are not living at home (*Ausbildungsfreibetrag*).

Finally, there was also an income-dependent child-raising allowance (*Erziehungsgeld*) available to mothers or fathers caring for their young children at home. Parents could choose to receive either a monthly allowance for the first 2 years after a child's birth, or a slightly higher monthly amount for just the first year (but a lower total amount overall). If the family's household income was below a certain threshold, parents received the full allowance amount for the first 6 months and then a gradually reduced amount thereafter. However, families with incomes above the threshold were not eligible to receive the child-raising allowance at all. Due to the relatively low amount of the child-raising allowance (e.g., in 2004, €300/month for 24 months or €450/month for 12 months), it was generally not sufficient to make up for the income lost among employed women with middle or high incomes (Honekamp 2008). Moreover, the allowance was not enough to sustain families with primarily breadwinner fathers who would want to give up their employment for parental leave. In other words, the allowance did not serve as an incentive for fathers to take parental leave. Instead, it rather required a male breadwinner to provide for the family while the mother took parental leave (Leitner 2011; Misra et al. 2007). This served as the background for the 2007 replacement of the child-raising allowance with an income-replacement benefit (see Footnote 9 for information on *Elterngeld*).

Germany's *working time regulations* are comprehensive, generally following the EU directives on the topic and aiming to assist women with children balance work and family responsibilities. For example, the 1993 EU Directive on Working Time (93/104/EC) stipulates that states must "take the measures necessary to ensure that, in keeping with the need to protect the safety and health of workers," that weekly working hours do not exceed 48 h and employees are granted 4 weeks of paid vacation per year. With the exception of managers, German working time law does not allow the working day to exceed 8 h, although it can be extended to 10 h as long as the 6-month average does not exceed 8 h (Bosch 2009). Working on Sundays and public holidays is not allowed unless expressly approved by the authorities. Typically regulated in Germany through collective bargaining agreements, average collectively agreed weekly working hours in 2003 were 37.4 in the former West Germany and 39.0 in the former East Germany (Bosch 2009). Also as a result of the directive, paid annual leave in Germany was increased from 3 to 4 weeks. Moreover, Germany follows the 1997 EU Directive on Part-Time Work (97/81/EC), requiring the elimination of discrimination against part-time workers by paying the same hourly rates as full-time employees and offering social benefits proportional to working time (Bosch 2009). According to the Federal Law on Parental Allowance and Parental Leave (*Bundeselterngeld- und Elternzeitgesetz*), parents are allowed to request a reduction of working hours to 15–30 h per week during or after parental leave, as long as the following conditions are met: the employer has more than 15 employees; the parent has been employed there for more than half a year; and there are no urgent operational reasons against it (Lembke 2013).

About 45 % of employees in Germany report flexibility in their working time arrangements (OECD 2014). Regulations around part-time work especially impact women. In 2003, 83 % of part-time jobs were held by women, with 36 % of employed women working part-time, as compared to 6 % of employed men (OECD 2014). A 2004–05 survey of companies in Europe found that 18 % of women who took parental leave did not return to work after the leave period, while over half returned to work but asked for reduced hours (Anxo et al. 2007). On the one hand, these figures show the flexibility available to working mothers in Germany. On the other hand, they are also perhaps representative of the overall limited policy support for dual-earner families.

In terms of taxation, Germany has one of the most disadvantageous *taxation systems* for employed women as compared to other industrialized nations, essentially discouraging a dual-earner family model (Sainsbury 1999). Joint taxation (*Ehegattensplitting*) involves adding two incomes together, dividing it in half, applying the progressive tax rate to the halved amount, and multiplying it by two (Honekamp 2008). This results in a high marginal tax rate for women who typically earn less than their partners in part-time or lower income jobs, and may result in their decision to forgo employment altogether. For example, "in the lower and middle income groups…the average tax burden for married women is more than twice that of married men with the same income" (Bach 2014, p. 813). Some critics also argue that this also puts married couples and families with male breadwinners at an advantage over unmarried individuals, who have to pay similar amounts of tax (Leisering 2001).

4.3.3 Access to Health Care

Germany's health care system is one of the oldest universal systems in existence (see Table 4.7). It originated in 1883 when the parliament passed a law requiring health insurance for employees in certain sectors of the labor market (Altenstetter and Busse 2005; Busse and Riesberg 2004). The guiding principles of solidarity, decentralization, and nonstate operations continue to be foundational to Germany's health policy despite the country's history of repeated upheaval (e.g., two world wars, the collapse of multiple regimes, division into two different states, and reunification) (Altenstetter 2003; Moran 1999). The fundamentals of the system include: mandatory membership in statutory health insurance (*gesetzliche Krankenversicherung*) for everyone under a certain income threshold; contributions to health insurance (*Krankenkasse*) based on income level; and shared responsibility between both the employee and the employer for contributions towards health insurance. The federal government is responsible for overseeing policies regarding benefits, eligibility, coverage, and contributions, while the responsibility for administration and service provision falls to independent nonstate bodies at the regional and local levels (e.g., provider associations, hospital associations, insurance companies) (Altenstetter and Busse 2005). In the early 2000s, Germany spent 11 % of its GDP on health care, placing it third among OECD countries and sixth in terms of per capita health expenditure (Busse and Riesberg 2004; WHO 2014). About 75.2 % of Germany's health care spending at the time came from public sources (e.g., taxes, insurance contributions), 12.5 % came from private sources like

Table 4.7 Germany: health policy related to access to care (early 2000s)

Health policy dimensions	Germany
Entitlement to care	Based on social insurance contributions. Health insurance coverage: Statutory (88 %); private (10 %); special governmental coverage (2 %); uninsured (0.2 %)
Availability of providers	No gatekeeping; imbalance in proportion of PCPs and specialists; minimal wait times
Affordability of care	Co-payments on prescription medications and hospital care. Exempt from costs: children under 18; pregnant women; poor; severely ill. Annual ceilings on out-of-pocket costs

private insurance companies and employers, and the remaining 12.2 % came from private out-of-pocket spending by patients (Busse and Riesberg 2004; WHO 2014).

As mentioned above, *entitlement to health care* in Germany is based on mandatory contributions through employers and employees to a statutory health insurance (SHI) plan, providing the overwhelming majority of the population with health care coverage. Dependent spouses and children (up to 18 years) are also covered by the employee's SHI. Furthermore, SHI covers university students, the retired, and the unemployed. Thus, while 62 % of the population in 2003 contributed to SHI, approximately 88 % of the population was covered by SHI (about 78 % compulsorily and 10 % voluntarily) (Busse and Riesberg 2004; Gerlinger 2010). With over 250 (nonprofit) insurance plans from which to choose, coverage is portable across hospitals, doctors, and federal states, and everyone is entitled to the same coverage, regardless of contribution amount or length of membership. Covered services include, among others: outpatient care offered by physicians and allied health professionals, hospital care, prescription medications, neonatal care for mothers, preventative visits for children, emergency and rescue care, and cancer screening for women over 20 years of age (Altenstetter 2003). In 2003, about 10 % of the population opted for private health insurance (available to civil servants, the self-employed, and those with incomes exceeding the ceiling for mandatory SHI enrollment) and 2 % were covered by other governmental schemes (e.g., for military personnel, police, asylum seekers) (Busse and Riesberg 2004). This system, however, does result in a minimal gap in coverage. In 2003, a very small percentage (0.2 % or 170,000 individuals) of the population was without health insurance, consisting of the self-employed and/or those who failed to pay SHI contributions or private health insurance premiums.

Overall, the *availability of providers* in Germany is quite high. Primary care is provided overwhelming by PCPs in private, for-profit, office-based settings (Schlette et al. 2009). As with PCPs, specialists also predominantly provide care in private practices and make up half of all office-based physicians. Traditionally, PCPs do not play a formal gatekeeping role and patients are able to freely choose their own physicians, psychotherapists, dentists, pharmacists, and nursing care providers (Busse and Riesberg 2004). While some claim that free access is related to increased patient satisfaction (Grol et al. 2000), critics argue that this lack of a gatekeeping function leads to uncoordinated, fragmented care and 'doctor hopping' among patients in Germany (Schlette et al. 2009). A potential consequence is that physicians treat acute illnesses and complaints separately, rather than managing the complexities of health conditions as a whole.

Generally, the number of physicians has increased at a steady pace over the decades. In 2003, Germany had a ratio of 3.4 physicians per 1000 population, slightly higher than the EU average of 3.1 and the OECD average of 2.9 (OECD 2005; WHO Regional Office for Europe 2014). However, there have been issues with decreasing numbers of PCPs and rapidly increasing numbers of specialists (both in proportion to the population and overall number of physicians) (Busse and Riesberg 2004). As a response to this imbalance, incentives were offered to physicians with specialties in internal medicine and pediatrics to shift their practices to primary care. As of 2003, the proportions had more or less balanced out, with PCPs representing approximately half of all practicing physicians in Germany (Bundesärztekammer 2004). Compared to other Western countries, Germany's waiting times are quite reasonable and are generally not considered to be an issue (Riesberg and Wörz 2008). In 2005, one-in-five patients reported a waiting time of 4 or more weeks to see a specialist (as compared to more than half of patients in Canada, Norway, and Sweden) (OECD 2012). Moreover, only 6 % reported waiting times of over 4 months for elective surgery (as compared to 41 % in the UK and 33 % in Canada).

Reform of mental health care in Germany began later than in other industrialized nations, partially because psychiatric hospitals were not overcrowded, resulting in much less of a push to improve the system (Salize et al. 2007). Gradually, beginning in the mid-1970s, long-term mental health care in Germany began shifting away from mental hospitals towards services integrated into the community. For instance, "psychiatric day hospitals were introduced, the number of office-based psychiatrists increased, and hospital-based outpatient services and social psychiatric services were implemented" (Salize et al. 2007, p. 93). Furthermore, Germany also offers more psychosomatic inpatient care than most other Western countries. For those patients requiring acute inpatient care, care is offered either in the psychiatric wards in general hospitals (Busse and Riesberg 2004) or in regionalized, significantly reformed psychiatric hospitals (Salize et al. 2007). Mental health counseling performed by psychiatrists, psychoanalysts, or psychologists is covered under SHI (Riesberg and Wörz 2008). Despite the wide variety of services, critics argue that the complexity and fragmentation of Germany's outpatient mental health care provision "is a serious obstacle to the identification of trends, the quality of care, interdependencies, overlapping care systems, or undersupply" (Salize et al. 2007, p. 99), leading potentially to competition among providers who should be cooperating to improve patient health.

As mentioned earlier in this section, enrollment in (and contribution to) SHI is mandatory for employees up until a certain income ceiling. However, there are certain mechanisms in place to distribute the cost burden and ensure *affordability of care*. For example, SHI contributions are based on income level rather than risk level, and in 2003, contributions were shared equally between the employer and employee. The overall contribution level in 2003 was 14.2 % of gross wages, meaning employees were obligated to contribute 7.1 % of their annual income up to a fixed maximum (Busse and Riesberg 2004). To ensure that nearly everyone is able to afford health insurance, employees whose monthly earnings are below a certain income threshold are not required to contribute, but they remain eligible for SHI. Likewise, dependent spouses and children (up to 18 years) are covered by the employee's SHI without any additional cost. Furthermore, in 2003, the government paid half of the contributions for artists and university students, and the retired and unemployed were covered by SHI through full contributions made by the retirement funds and the Federal Agency for Employment (*Bundesagentur für Arbeit*), respectively.

Other cost-sharing mechanisms have been part of the German health system since 1923, but at the same time, so have exemptions to protect vulnerable groups from undue financial burdens (Gericke et al. 2004). Reforms taking place over the last decades in Germany have required patients to cover increasing proportions of health care costs themselves in order to increase revenues and incentivize preventive behavior through lower co-payments. In 2002, approximately 12.2 % of total health expenditure was financed through private out-of-pocket payments by patients (Busse and Riesberg 2004). In the early 2000s, out-of-pocket costs in the form of minimal co-payments applied to prescription medications and hospital care.[13] Likewise, patients were responsible for a certain percentage of the costs of dental care, which decreased if they had engaged in regular annual checkups. Exempted from these costs were children under 18 years of age, pregnant women, the unemployed, and those with low incomes. Patients were also exempt from further co-payments once they had spent 2 % of the gross household income on co-payments in any given year (or 1 % for those with severe chronic illnesses). In practice, this meant that in 2000, approximately one-third of the population was exempt from out-of-pocket costs (Busse and Riesberg 2004). Moreover, the co-payments of nearly half of prescriptions filled in 2001 were under exemption (Gericke et al. 2004). For those costs not covered by SHI, patients could also be granted a tax deduction for health expenses exceeding a certain amount and a certain percentage of household income.

All in all, these cost-sharing and protective mechanisms led to a rather low out-of-pocket costs for patients. In 2003, 2 % of household consumption was devoted to out-of-pocket health expenditures in Germany, which was below the OECD average of 3 % (OECD 2003b). In terms of unmet health needs due to cost, only a small percentage (3.7 %) of the population in 2005 reported that they did not seek medical treatment because it was too expensive (Eurostat 2014). However, it is important to note that a social gradient in unmet need did indeed exist, with 15.7 % of those in the lowest income quintile reporting an unmet health need due to cost, as compared to 2.9 % of those in the highest quintile.

4.4 Norway

Norway is one of the most gender equal countries is the world (Bekhouche et al. 2013). Nevertheless, according to the first national survey on violence against women, 27 % of ever-partnered women in Norway have experienced violence from a partner in their lifetime and 6 % have experienced IPV within the past year (Nerøien and Schei 2008). Nearly one-third of these women were injured as a result

[13]Starting with the SHI Modernization Act of 2004, reforms included co-payments applied to outpatient doctor's visits (on a quarterly basis), prescription medications, and hospital care (Busse and Riesberg 2004). Reforms also eliminated exemptions based on poverty and made eligibility for partial exemptions stricter.

of the violence, and of those women injured, nearly half were injured severely enough to require them to take off time from work or school. Almost one-in-ten women who experienced IPV reported being exposed to life-threatening violence.

Attention to this issue in Norway was first initiated by activists of the women's movement in the 1970s and 1980s, and services were typically organized by private actors. Pressure from women's and feminist political groups helped place violence against women on the political agenda, pushing for action to also be taken in public services. Over the last decade and a half, the issue has increasingly been attracting the attention of policy makers, and most activities to combat violence now originate from a national political level through action plans (Saur et al. 2011). In 2003, the Norwegian government established their first national action plan against domestic violence, outlining a number of concrete political actions that could be taken to address violence again women in Norway (Ministry of Justice and the Police 2004). A series of follow-up plans have since been released (Ministry of Justice and Public Security 2012; Ministry of Justice and the Police 2008). The concrete actions described include improved services from the police, educational institutions, and state support services, particularly in their capabilities to identify, prevent and deal with violence against women and its consequences. Moreover, these plans focus on prevention by changing societal attitudes around violence (Saur et al. 2011).

The first women's shelter for survivors of abuse and rape in Norway opened in Oslo in 1978 (Saur et al. 2011). Spread throughout Norway's municipalities, today there are 46 shelters with a total of 815 shelter spaces. This greatly exceeds the 484 spaces recommended for Norway's population by the Council of Europe Task Force (one space per 7500 inhabitants) (Stelmaszekn and Fisher 2012). These shelters also offer crisis services for those not living in the shelter, and run regional helplines for IPV survivors. There is also a national helpline for all persons in crisis. Women's shelters offer low-threshold services which are nearly free of charge, they remain open 24 h a day, do not require a referral, and allow women and their children to stay as long as needed (Alsaker et al. 2011). While all of the shelters are run by independent women's NGOs, up until 2011, the shelters received 80 % of their funding from the Ministry of Children and Equality, with the remaining funding coming from the municipalities themselves (Stelmaszekn and Fisher 2012). While the shelters and helplines were not legislatively required provisions, they did depend on the parliament's (*Stortinget*) budget. Currently, however, shelters are now completely funded by the municipalities, mostly resulting in a reduction of shelter funding.

These shelters tend to serve women with lower levels of education, less access to paid work through employment, and minority backgrounds (Hutchinson and Weeks 2004). According to Jonassen and Skogøy (2010), the overrepresentation of women with minority backgrounds in Norway's shelters seems to be related to their limited access to personal income as compared with native Norwegians, as well as a lack of support from their social networks when fleeing an abusive situation. The authors claim that native Norwegian women, in contrast, are more economically independent, are aware of their rights, and hold fewer reservations about divorce. With

Table 4.8 Norway: welfare policy related to redistribution of resources (early 2000s)

Welfare policy dimensions	Norway
Unemployment benefits	Partial compensation: about 63 % for up to 24 months
Sickness leave	Full compensation: up to 12 months
Poverty protection for single mothers	Transitional allowance, financial support for childcare, and educational support

these help systems in place, the next sections explore Norway's social policy that could potentially be relevant for IPV survivors.

4.4.1 Redistribution of Resources

Norway's welfare state provides benefits based upon social citizenship, with state intervention ensuring full employment and income protection (see Table 4.8). The overall aim of the welfare state is to promote equality and reduce poverty. Social rights are universal and available to all those residing or working in Norway under the scope of the National Insurance Scheme (NIS), which is funded through contributions from employees, employers, and the government through taxation. The Norwegian Labor and Welfare Administration (NAV) oversees the provision of pensions (e.g., retirement, disability) and benefits related to accidents, illness, pregnancy, birth, and funerals. Since the 1990s there has been a shift in Norwegian welfare policies away from the former concept of *trygdelinje* (income maintenance for those not able to support themselves through paid work) towards *arbeidslinje* (employment strategy) (Kjeldstad 2000). In other words, policies supporting vulnerable populations tend to view employment as the best strategy to improve living standards, and "long periods with benefits and no employment should be avoided as it may obstruct future employment" (Kjeldstad 2000, p. 346). In cases of *unemployment*, the NAV offers benefits as partial compensation for loss of earned income if work time has been reduced by at least half, as long as wages previously earned are 1.5 times the NIS basic amount (Norwegian Labour and Welfare Administration [NAV] 2015a; OECD 2003c).[14] Unemployment benefits are available for up 2 years on the condition that one continues to search for employment during this period. At the time of this writing, as well as in 2003, in the case of illness, individuals receive *sickness benefits* paid at their current income level (but not to exceed 6 times the NIS basic amount) for up to one year (NAV 2015b; OECD 2003c). The first 16 calendar days are paid by the employer, with the NIS stepping in afterward.

[14]The NIS basic amount is adjusted annually to match inflation and is used for the calculation of many NIS benefits.

Within the context of the welfare state, *single parents* in Norway are treated as a group with special needs and are therefore entitled to extended benefits, including a transitional allowance, financial support for childcare, and educational support (Hansen et al. 2006). Established in the mid-1960s, the original aim of these benefits was to guarantee single mothers a minimum income by freeing them of the constraints of the labor market and allowing them to focus on their role as mothers and carers (Strand 2012).[15] However, after a reform in 1998, eligibility for these benefits has been tightened and more emphasis has been placed on employment activation (Syltevik 1999). In 2003, single parents with children under 8 years old were entitled to receive a transitional allowance (*overgangsstønad*) for 3 years of an amount 1.85 times the NIS basic amount (OECD 2003c). If the child was older than one year, the single parent must either be engaged in at least 50 % full-time employment, pursuing an education, or actively seeking work (ASD 2014).[16] In this sense, the transitional allowance has transformed into an 'in-work' benefit rather than as a benefit for care work (Strand 2012). That being said, single parents are also eligible for state assistance with childcare. In addition to receiving priority for available childcare center places (Vollset 2011), the cost of childcare is state subsidized up to 64 % as long as the parent does not earn more than 6 times the NIS basic amount. Moreover, in conjunction with the transitional allowance, single parents are eligible to receive state support for 3 years of full-time education, which covers tuition, school supplies, and additional living expenses. Thus, benefits for single parents allow for a multitude of different combinations of employment, education, and allowance—including using the transitional allowance as a supplement to employment income. According to Kjelstad (2000), these benefits have allowed quite a few single parents to "survive economically on part-time work, thus reducing the everyday time squeeze in these families" (p. 362). The principles reflected in the policies related to single mothers can also be seen in the family policies described in the following section.

4.4.2 Establishing Independent Households

While gender equality achieved through social policy has been a primary focus for the Nordic welfare states, Norway has historically differed slightly from its neighbors in that its institutional arrangements have rather underscored traditional family values and the importance of motherhood (see Table 4.9) (Duncan and Strell 2004; Ellingsæter 1998; Strand 2012). Even so, mothers in Norway began entering the labor force decades before any kind of supportive family policies were established (Ellingsæter 2003; Leira 1992). Perhaps due to these coexisting realities,

---

[15]These rights were extended to single fathers in 1980 (Syltevik 1999).

[16]The activity requirement may be waived if the parent or the child is sick, or no public childcare places are available.

Table 4.9 Norway: family policy related to establishing independent households (early 2000s)

Family policy dimensions	Norway
Parental leave	42 weeks (100 %) or 53 weeks (80 %); 4 weeks paternity leave
Childcare	Publicly subsidized childcare: full-time care for ages 1–5 years. Limits on private costs
School arrangements	30 h/week; continuous school day; 190 days/year; subsidized after-school activities
Family/child allowances	Allowance for each child under 18 years Allowance for children ages 1–3 not attending publicly subsidized childcare
Working time regulations	EU Directive on working time: standard 37.5-h workweek; maximum 40 h/week allowed; 21 days annual leave EU Directive on part-time work: right to part-time work if approved by employer; flexible working schedule
Taxation systems	Joint filing for breadwinner/caregiver couples and single parents. Individual filing for everyone else

Norway offers a high level of benefits important for dual-earner families (e.g., parental leave and publicly financed childcare), while at the same time offering benefits typically useful for male breadwinner/female carer households (e.g., cash transfers for children and/or care). In light of this dualism, Norway is sometimes referred to as 'ambivalent', 'double-track', or 'gender equality light' in the feminist welfare state literature, especially when compared to other Nordic countries (Leira 1992; Skrede 1999, 2004).

In support of dual-earner families, Norway offers *parental leave* benefits preventing income loss after the birth of a child. In the early 2000s, parents could take a total of either 42 (100 % compensation) or 53 (80 % compensation) weeks of parental leave (Gauthier 2011; Skevik and Hatland 2008). Moreover, 4 weeks of the parental leave were reserved specifically for the father. Using 'gentle force' to encourage fathers to make use of their leave, transferring the leave to the mother is not allowed, so if the father does not use the time, then parents lose their right to this leave completely (Brandth and Kvande 2003). Eligibility for parental leave is preconditioned on the mother's employment for 6 of the 10 months prior to delivery. If women are not employed or do not qualify for parental leave, they receive a flat payment in case of birth or adoption. In 2004, 4 out of 5 women who gave birth qualified for paid parental leave benefits (Skevik and Hatland 2008). Of these, 3 out of 4 elected to receive benefits for one year at 80 % compensation.

After parental leave comes to an end, *childcare* in Norway continues to be primarily provided through childcare centers financed by the state, municipalities, and parents. However, this was not always the case. Prior to 1975, the use of childcare centers (*barnehage*) was unusual, with only about 2 % of children under the age of 6 attending childcare (Skevik and Hatland 2008). The prevalent opinion at the time was that young children were best brought up by the family (Ellingsæter and Gulbrandsen 2007), although this was rather incongruous with the growing number of women participating in the labor force even then. The Day Care Institutions Act of 1975, which ensured that childcare centers were available for all families that required care, was controversial. A legacy of this controversy may be the rather heavy focus on providing younger children with opportunities for 'development and activity' (*utviklings- og aktivitetsmuligheter*), rather than on enabling women's employment: "Norwegian policies concerning pre-school children did not aim at facilitating mother's employment or accommodating the economy's demand for labour. Childcare policies were more exclusively oriented towards the socialisation of the child" (Leira 1992, p. 62). With the focus on improving the upbringing of children, the number of centers expanded throughout the 1980s and 1990s, and Norway established the legal right of care for children in 2009 (Eydal and Rostgaard 2011). While fees for childcare centers vary by municipality, there is a state-imposed maximum monthly fee and childcare centers are also required to offer reduced payments or exemptions for low-income families or families with more than one child in care. The overwhelming majority of children under 5 years of age attend a childcare center. In the early 2000s, 67 % of children aged 3–5, and 62 % of children between the ages of 1 and 2 attended childcare (Ellingsæter and Gulbrandsen 2007).[17] Almost 83 % of these children attended childcare full-time (i.e., 32 h a week or more).

At the age of 6, children begin school in Norway and compulsory schooling lasts for 10 years. Regarding the *organization of the school day*, children spend roughly 30 h per week in school with a continuous school day, totaling 190 days per year spent in school (Gornick et al. 1997). In order to ensure that younger school-aged children remain supervised and cared for during the gap between the end of the school day and the parents' workday, municipalities are obliged to provide supervised after-school activities (*skolefritidsordning*) for children from first to fourth grade (Skevik and Hatland 2008). The government limits the costs for such activities to the actual costs incurred by the program.

Additionally, Norway has *family and child allowances* which rather support a male breadwinner/female carer family model. All families receive an allowance (*barnetrygd*) for each child less than 18 years of age resident in Norway. Moreover, in order to address the shortage in childcare places at the time, Norway introduced its controversial cash-for-care scheme in 1998, which provides a cash benefit (*kontantstøtte*) to parents with children aged 1–3 who are not attending a publicly subsidized childcare center.[18] This benefit entitles parents to the monthly equivalent of the state's subsidy of a full-time place in a childcare center. While the uptake of the benefit was widespread after its introduction (e.g., in 1999, 75 % of children under 3 were cared for with the benefit), this decreased over time, partially due to

---

[17]This has since grown to 97 % of children aged three to five, and nearly 80 % of children between the ages of one and two. Approximately 93 % currently attend childcare more than 32 h per week (Statistik Sentralbyrå [SSB] 2013).

[18]However, as of 2012, only parents of one-year-old children are eligible (Ellingsæter 2012).

the increase in childcare availability (Ellingsæter and Gulbrandsen 2007).[19] Both proponents and opponents of the benefit expected that this would lead to a reduction in the time mothers spent in paid employment (Knudsen and Waerness 2001). However, evaluations demonstrated that in fact, employment among mothers was reduced only by about 6 % (Hardoy and Schøne 2010). It was found that instead of using the cash-for-care benefit to stay at home full-time, mothers more often used it to pay for private child minders or as a temporary solution until a childcare place became available (Ellingsæter 2012; Leira 2002).

In general, Norway has rather extensive regulations governing *working time and flexible arrangements*, falling in line with EU directives on the topic although it is not an EU member state. Norway has had a statute in place since 1919 limiting weekly working hours (Sterud 2009). Based on both collective agreements and labor law, the normal working week in Norway is 37.5 h, with a maximum of 40 h allowed (Gornick and Meyers 2009).[20] Moreover, statutes stipulate that employees must receive 21 days of paid leave per year. Norway also voluntarily implements the 1997 EU Directive on Part-Time Work (97/81/EC), granting employees the right to reduce working hours based on health or personal reasons if this is not a substantial inconvenience to the employer. Moreover, parents have the right to part-time work in order to care for their children until they reach 10 years of age, and breastfeeding mothers are allowed 2 paid working hours per day to breastfeed (Brandth and Kavande 2007). Generally, these regulations have had a positive effect on the working environment. Approximately 37 % of employees in Norway report that they have the possibility to adjust their hours according to their needs, as compared to an average of 24 % across the EU (Sterud 2009). The level of part-time work in Norway is high among women. In 2003, 75 % of part-time jobs were held by women, with 33 % of employed women working part-time, as compared to 6 % of employed men (OECD 2014).

Another area in which Norway diverges slightly from the path of its Nordic neighbors is in *systems of taxation*. Whereas the other Nordic countries began introducing individual taxation systems in the 1970s, Norway offers individual taxation as an option, but continues to hold onto joint taxation as well (Sainsbury 1999, 2001). There are two separate tax groups in Norway: one is geared toward couples with joint taxation, typically only used for couples in which one of the partners has little to no income, or for single parents with dependent children; the other group is geared toward everyone else (Skevik and Hatland 2008). Even so, the tendency leans toward individual taxation, and it is argued that having both joint and individual taxation has not created disincentives for women's employment (Ellingsæter 1998).

[19]Over a decade later, only about one-quarter of children under 3 years old are being cared for using the cash-for-care benefits (Ellingsæter 2012).

[20]Hours worked above the maximum may not be made compulsory.

4.4.3 Access to Health Care

According to the Health Systems in Transition report (Johnsen 2006), the key strengths of the Norwegian health system are: "provision of health care services for all based on need (regardless of personal income), local and regional accountability, public commitment and political interest in improving the health care system" (p. xvi) (see Table 4.10). Functioning under the auspices of the NIS, in the early 2000s as well as today, everyone who resides or works in Norway has access to health care. The system itself is considered to be semi-decentralized. The Ministry of Health and Care Services plays an indirect role by overseeing the health care sector at the national level (e.g., financing, legislation, allocation of resources), while specialist care (e.g., mental health care) is handled by the country's four regional health authorities, and primary health care is managed by the 428 local municipalities (Lindahl and Ringard 2013). Municipalities are independently governed and have a good deal of freedom in how they organize health services; however, certain measures are taken at the national level to ensure equal access to care. In the early 2000s, Norway spent 10.1 % of its GDP on health care, which was not an especially high proportion compared to other European countries (WHO 2014). However, since Norway has one of the largest GDPs per capita in the world, it has the second highest per capita health expenditure. Since 2003, about 85 % of Norway's spending on health care has been relatively consistently funded by taxes and transfers from the central government, with the remaining funding consisting mostly of out-of-pocket payments from patients (WHO 2014).

The *entitlement to care* in Norway has its foundations in the principle of "equal access to health care of good quality," made explicit in the 1999 Patients' Rights Act, regardless of social status, income, or geographical location (Ministry of Health 1999). Complementary principles are those: placing priority on care for those with the greatest health needs; treatments that will have the best efficacy; and a reasonable cost-to-benefit ratio (Ringard et al. 2013). Regardless of citizenship or residency status, everyone is entitled to acute emergency health services, including undocumented immigrants. Moreover, all pregnant women and children (again, regardless of legal status) are entitled to primary health care and immunization. There is no prescribed list of covered services in Norway per se, but these services

Table 4.10 Norway: health policy related to access to health care (early 2000s)

Health policy dimensions	Norway
Entitlement to care	Based on social citizenship. Universal coverage for all residing or working in Norway (100 %)
Availability of providers	PCPs gatekeepers to specialized care; moderate physician density; long wait times
Affordability of care	Co-payments on outpatient care and prescription medications. Exempt from costs: children under 18; ante- and postnatal care; HIV/AIDS patients. Annual ceilings on co-payments

tend to include: primary care services by PCPs; preventative services (e.g., check-ups, screenings, and immunization of children); preventive mental health services (primarily for children and youth); approved prescription drugs; the majority of specialist outpatient and hospital treatments; and dental care for children (Ringard et al. 2013). In addition to the statutory health insurance, about 5 % of Norwegians also hold private voluntary health insurance, primarily through their employers. Accounting for less than 1 % of total health expenditures, voluntary health insurance is usually used as a supplement to shorten waiting times for health care services and increase access to specialists in private facilities (Lindahl and Ringard 2013).

Although improving, Norway does have some issues with *availability of providers*. Contact with the health care system begins with PCPs, who are self-employed physicians contracting with the municipalities to offer services. Nearly the entire Norwegian population (99 %) is registered with a specific PCP of their choice, who serves as their gatekeeper to specialist care (Vikum et al. 2012). Typically, the PCPs are responsible for initial diagnoses, basic treatment, prescribing medications, and referring patients to specialist care. For patients who require more complex or specialized care, the PCP either makes an appointment with a specialist or provides the patient with a referral to the specialist. This gatekeeping system operates uniformly throughout the country and cannot be adapted or changed by the municipalities or the regional health authorities (Ringard et al. 2013).

After a physician shortage in the 1990s, Norway increased funding for medical education and increased the number of spaces for medical students (Ringard et al. 2013). This measure was successful and caused the level of health care providers in Norway to grow steadily over the last decades. In 2003, Norway had a rate of physician coverage at 3.1 physicians per 1000 inhabitants, slightly above the OECD average of 2.9 (OECD 2005).[21] Yet, despite this relatively average rate of health care professionals according to population, long waiting times for nonemergency health services continue to present themselves as a serious barrier to care. Much political will has been directed toward reducing waiting times in Norway for specialist care, including policies allowing patients to choose their own hospitals for treatment (in 2001), and guidelines on vertical waiting-time prioritization (in 2004). Even so, compared to other countries in Europe, data indicates that Norway has the largest proportion of the population (28 %) having to wait 2–5 days for a visit to their PCP (OECD 2012). Moreover, one-in-two respondents in Norway also reported having to wait more than 4 weeks to see a specialist, and one-in-five reported having to wait more than 4 months for nonemergency surgery (OECD 2012). Compared to other OECD countries, this places Norway behind only Canada and Sweden in terms of longest waiting times for these services.

[21]This rate has continued to rise and today Norway has a very high rate of physician coverage at 4.07 physicians per 1000 inhabitants (second in Europe only to Austria) (WHO Regional Office for Europe 2014).

In the last two and a half decades, the organization and content of mental health services have received increased political attention in Norway. The National Mental Health Plan in 1998 focused on care at the municipal level and increased social and occupational care services, representing a move away from institutionalized mental health care (Ministry of Health 1998). As such, the provision of mental health care begins with PCPs at the municipal level, where they are accountable for examining, evaluating, and treating patients. Patients requiring more intensive mental health care are referred to specialized mental health services which are based at the regional health authority level. In these cases, PCPs continue to play an important role through follow-up with the specialists in order to ensure continuity of care. These specialized services include mental health hospitals, private-practice psychiatrists and psychologists, and community mental health centers (Ringard et al. 2013). The community health centers offer low-threshold acute inpatient and outpatient care, rehabilitation, home visits, and coordination of primary care. Thanks to the implementation of the National Mental Health Plan, Norway has the third highest density of psychiatrists among OECD countries with 22.2 psychiatrists per 100,000 population (behind Switzerland and Iceland) (OECD 2012). However, despite this dramatic increase, unless patients pay for treatment completely out-of-pocket, issues of long waiting times face all patients without serious mental disorders.

Affordability of care is a central issue in Norway, with the health system grounded in the principle of equal access to care. Cost-sharing has been one of its features for the past three decades, aiming to "reduce the growth in public spending and to free up resources for high-priority areas. Another aim has been to curb demand from people with minor health-care problems" (Ringard et al. 2013, p. 64). As mentioned earlier, these cost-sharing mechanisms finance approximately 15 % of Norway's total health expenditure (ILO 2013). For the most part, out-of-pocket costs for patients in Norway stem from co-payments for PCP visits, prescription drugs, and the cost of adult dental care. In order to ensure that these out-of-pocket costs do not become a financial burden for patients, the government has put a number of mechanisms in place, including exemptions and cost ceilings, although there are certain services that are not subject to cost regulations (e.g., most dental care for adults).

All in-patient care provided at hospitals, including medications and treatments, is free of charge. Meanwhile, outpatient care by PCPs and specialists is subsidized by the NIS, with the exception of a co-payment. Approved prescription medications and outpatient hospital care are also subsidized and subject to co-payments. During the 1980s, yearly ceilings on co-payments were introduced, known as *egenandelstak 1* and *egenandelstak 2,* in order to limit annual cost-sharing for patients (Ringard et al. 2013). These ceilings are the same for everyone and do not depend on income levels. *Egenandelstak 1* applies to all private co-payments for physician and psychologist visits, approved medical prescriptions, and also includes transportation costs. Once the annual ceiling has been reached, which occurs for approximately 1.2 million people (i.e., 24 % of the population) each year, patients are exempt from further co-payments for the remaining calendar year (Directorate of Health 2012). Since dental care and physiotherapy are only partially covered by the NIS, the second ceiling (*egenandelstak 2*) limits certain approved out-of-pocket expenses for these covered services (Johnsen 2006).[22] Significantly fewer individuals reach this ceiling: approximately 46,000 residents in 2010 (Directorate of Health 2012). Moreover, there are certain groups of the population exempt from private out-of-pocket costs for health care (Lindahl and Ringard 2013). Children under 16 years of age receive physician care and approved prescription drugs free of charge, and children under 18 years of age also receive psychological care and dental care at no cost. Furthermore, all pregnant women receive free ante- and postnatal medical care. As of 2003, low-income elderly receive their prescription drugs and nursing care free of charge. Finally, patients with HIV/AIDS, as well as those with occupational injuries, receive free treatment and medications. Overall, out-of-pocket expenditure in Norway as a share of final household consumption was about 3.6 % in 2003 (slightly above the OECD average) (OECD 2003b). According to European survey data, less than one percent of those in Norway reported unmet health care needs due to cost considerations in 2004 (Eurostat 2014).

4.5 Contrasting Policy Contexts

Up to this point, each country's social and policy context was presented separately with a broad focus on women. This section narrows the focus and considers the potential impact on the lives of IPV survivors by comparing and contrasting the countries according to policy intervention points. Specifically, this serves as the background for the cross-national macro hypotheses made in Sect. 3.4.1.

The three cases under consideration present a number of differences in terms of how they approached redistribution of resources across society and protected against the risks of unemployment, illness, and status change during the examined time periods (i.e., mid-1990s for the US, and early 2000s for Germany and the US) (see Table 4.11). Although this is not directly addressed by the research questions, it does set the stage in terms of the degree of social inequalities faced by women. Of the three countries, Norway had at the time, and even today, perhaps the most supportive system in terms of redistribution of resources and protection against poverty. In cases of unemployment, individuals receive a portion of their income for up to 2 years, and full compensation in cases of illness for up to one year. In contrast, although Germany provides a strong system of benefits, it remains geared toward those with strong ties to the labor market. For example, in cases of unemployment, while everyone receives the same portion of their previous income,

[22]The adult dental services covered by the NIS are, however, limited. Therefore, the majority of dental care service still takes place on the private market with patients paying in full for treatment received. There is no regulation of dental care costs for adults (Johnsen 2006).

Table 4.11 Overview of potential impact of policies for IPV survivors

Mechanism	Intervention points and related policy dimensions	US (mid-1990s)	Germany (early 2000s)	Norway (early 2000s)
Social stratification	Redistribution of resources			
	Unemployment benefits	−	/	+
	Sickness leave	−	+	+
	Poverty protection for single mothers	/	−	+
Differential exposure	Establishing independent households			
	Parental leave	−	−	+
	Childcare	−	/	+
	School arrangements	+	−	+
	Family and child allowances	−	+	+
	Flexible working time	−	+	+
	Taxation systems	/	−	/
Differential vulnerability	Access to health care			
	Entitlement to care	−	+	+
	Availability of providers	−	+	−
	Affordability of care	−	+	+

+ potential positive intervention, / potential mixed intervention, − potential negative intervention

the length of the benefit depends on age and employment record. As opposed to the welfare policy in both of these countries, US welfare policy in the mid-1990s (as well as today) did very little to protect against risk. Unemployment benefits continue to vary by state and there is no federal entitlement to leave in cases of illness. These differences are perhaps most evident in the assistance provided to single mothers, which is a crucial consideration in the context of IPV survivors seeking to end abusive relationships. While Norway in the early 2000s recognized the special needs of single mothers and assisted them in balancing their roles as both earners and carers, IPV survivors with children in Germany at the same time may have found themselves falling between the cracks as a group that did not fit the traditional mold of social-insurance-based benefit provision. In contrast, social assistance in the US during the mid-1990s was provided only to the very poorest, was focused on child poverty, and was highly stigmatized. Against this background, IPV survivors may have been protected against the risk of poverty most in Norway, while facing greater risk in Germany if they did not have strong labor market ties, and may have been most at risk in the US.

The three countries also represent a great deal of variance in how family policies supported women's resources for establishing independent households. As research detailed in Chap. 3 made clear, family policies can support women in maintaining strong ties to the labor market, achieving economic independence, and avoiding poverty. Thus, based on resource and dependency theories, as well as empirical evidence linking economic vulnerability to IPV, policies which increase women's socioeconomic resources may either make women less susceptible to IPV in the first place by equalizing power relationships within families, or may serve as a stepping-off point to exit an already abusive relationship.[23] Thus, I argue that comprehensive family policies supporting women in establishing autonomous households can decrease women's exposure to IPV.

Although in relation to other Nordic countries, Norway is usually described as "gender equality light," it offered during the period under study the greatest amount of support for women in comparison to the other two countries highlighted in this book. Parental leave and childcare care policies supported women in maintaining their ties to the labor market through high levels of income replacement, full-time childcare for children starting at the age of one, and flexible working arrangements. In this sense, Norway helped women remain relatively economically independent by supporting them in their roles as both earners and carers, enabling women to exit a relationship if necessary. Moreover, Norway's high levels of income replacement during parental leave, universal allowances, as well as reduced childcare fees for low-income and single mothers, supported women in avoiding poverty once they had left a relationship (Hansen et al. 2006).

This is a dramatic contrast to both Germany and the US. On the one hand, Germany's policies in the early 2000s offered extensive benefits supporting families, but parental leave, childcare, and school arrangements were set up in such a way that assumed a male breadwinner, presenting obstacles for women's full-time work. On the other hand, the US in the mid-1990s provided next to no support for families, and required women to seek market solutions for balancing work and family responsibilities. For women with low-to-middle class incomes in the US, the costs of maintaining their ties to the labor market may have outweighed the financial benefits, leading them to instead rely on a partner's income. These policies (or lack thereof) in both countries may have fostered economic dependencies for women. Likewise, despite Germany's generous social benefits, economically dependent women with children who had left abusive relationships may not have fit the typical mold for benefits and may instead have had to rely on means-tested income assistance to avoid poverty. The same could also be said for economically dependent women in the US, although the access to social assistance was more restricted than in Germany. Furthermore, flexible working arrangements and benefits for part-time work in Germany may have put women at a greater advantage in avoiding poverty than women in the US, who may have faced difficulty seeking flexible working conditions which also provide equal pay and benefits.

Against the background of IPV, while family policy in Norway may support women in establishing an independent household free from poverty, it may instead serve as a barrier in the US and Germany for acquiring the resources necessary to

[23]As seen in Chap. 2, this may however, only prove to be the case as long as women's status does not exceed that of their partners'.

exit an abusive relationship. Based on this information, I would expect that social inequalities in IPV exposure would be less where institutional arrangements support women in establishing independent households. This is the reasoning behind my hypothesis in Sect. 3.4.1 that social position's effect on IPV exposure should be smaller in Norway, and greater in the US and Germany.

Regarding policies related to access to health care for women in the three countries, there was a great deal of differentiation in health policy arrangements during the time periods under examination. As described in Chap. 3, a wide range of international research has demonstrated that social inequalities in health exist across a wide variety of welfare and health systems. The literature also demonstrates that abused women have increased health care needs, but the lack of socioeconomic resources can be a barrier for seeking health care in settings which do not ensure access to health care. In this case, IPV exposure may then serve to magnify social inequalities in health. Thus, I argue that health policies supporting access to care reduce the additional burden of IPV exposure on the pre-existing social gradient in health outcomes.

The principle of equal access to services regardless of social status or income was in the early 2000s, and remains today, central to Norway's health policy, ensuring women's access to care without relying on a partner. While health care coverage was and is related to social insurance contributions via employment in Germany, there remains a safety net ensuring that nearly the entire population has health insurance. For instance, those employed part-time are entitled to health insurance; insurance contributions are relative to income earned; and the unemployed and those receiving social assistance are also covered. Furthermore, both countries ensure affordability of care and limit private out-of-pocket costs through annual ceilings, cost-sharing exemptions, and/or income-related contributions. While Germany has not implemented a gatekeeping system and waiting times have been minimal, PCPs in Norway serve as gatekeepers to specialist care and patients have faced much longer waiting times than in Germany or the US.

In contrast, entitlement to health care in the US has been linked to employment or private payment rather than being understood as a social right, and this introduced a number of complications to access for IPV survivors. As explored in Chaps. 2 and 3, women in the US who are economically dependent on their abusive partners may rely on partners' employment for health insurance. For these women, ending a relationship may have left them uninsured and unable to afford the premiums for private health insurance, or relying on the minimal coverage provided by Medicaid (Patchias and Waxman 2007). Related to this, these women may have faced obstacles to access presented by the high costs of care for both the insured and the uninsured in the US. Moreover, even those with health insurance may have faced delays in care related to a shortage of PCPs and various gatekeeping models.

Particularly focusing on the increased health needs of IPV survivors, health policy may have ensured women's access to health care in Germany and Norway irrespective of their partner or their socioeconomic resources, whereas it may have presented an obstacle for women with limited socioeconomic resources in the US. Based on these considerations, I would expect that vulnerabilities to social position's impact on health would be smaller in Germany and Norway with policies ensuring access to health care than in the US.

4.5.1 Summary

The aim of this chapter was to establish the social and policy context during the time periods under examination in each of the chosen countries as it relates to the following policy intervention points relevant for IPV survivors: redistribution of resources in society, resources for establishing independent households, and access to health care. Following a description of the research design and methods in Chap. 5, Chaps. 6, 7, and 8 will present the results of whether social position impacts IPV exposure (through differential exposure) and whether IPV survivors with low social positions are especially vulnerable to poor health (through differential vulnerability). Analysis of the potential links between the policy context and these outcomes will be presented in Chap. 9 against the hypotheses specified in Sect. 3.4.1.

References

Adams, G., & Rohacek, M. (2002). Child care and welfare reform. In A. Weil & K. Finegold (Eds.), *Welfare reform: The next act* (pp. 121–142). Washington, DC: Urban Institute Press.

Alsaker, K., Kristoffersen, K., Moen, B. E., & Baste, V. (2011). Threats and acts of intimate partner violence reported by users at Norwegian women's shelters. *Journal of Interpersonal Violence, 26*(5), 950–970. doi:10.1177/0886260510365864

Altenstetter, C. (2003). Insights from health care in Germany. *American Journal of Public Health, 93*(1), 38–44. doi:10.2105/AJPH.93.1.38

Altenstetter, C., & Busse, R. (2005). Health care reform in Germany: Patchwork change within established governance structures. *Journal of Health Politics, Policy and Law, 30*(1–2), 121–142. doi:10.1215/03616878-30-1-2-121

Andreß, H.-J., Borgloh, B., Brockel, M., Giesselmann, M., & Hummelsheim, D. (2006). The economic consequences of partnership dissolution: A comparative analysis of panel studies from Belgium, Germany, Great Britain, Italy, and Sweden. *European Sociological Review, 22* (5), 533–560. doi:10.1093/esr/jcl012

Anxo, D., Fagan, C., Smith, M., Letablier, M.-T., & Perraudin, C. (2007). *Parental leave in European companies: Establishment survey on working time 2004–2005*. Dublin: European Foundation for the Improvement of Living and Working Conditions.

Aspalter, C. (2001). *Different worlds of welfare capitalism: Australia, the United States, the United Kingdom, Sweden, Germany, Italy, Hong Kong and Singapore*. Discussion Paper No. 80. https://crawford.anu.edu.au/degrees/pogo/discussion_papers_previous/No80Aspalter.pdf. Accessed December 15, 2013.

Bach, S. (2014). Frauen erzielen im Durchschnitt nur halb so hohe Einkommen wie Männer [Average income of women only half that of men]. *DIW Wochenbericht, 35*, 803–813.

Beckfield, J., & Krieger, N. (2009). Epi + demos + cracy: Linking political systems and priorities to the magnitude of health inequities—Evidence, gaps, and a research agenda. *Epidemiologic Reviews, 31*(1), 152–177. doi:10.1093/epirev/mxp002

Bekhouche, Y., Hausmann, R., Tyson, L. D., & Zahidi, S. (2013). *The global gender gap report 2013*. Geneva: World Health Organization.

Bergmann, B. (1986). *The economic emergence of women*. New York City: Basic Books.

Black, M. C., Basile, K. C., Breiding, M. J., Smith, S. G., Walters, M. L., Merrick, M. T., et al. (2011). *The National Intimate Partner and Sexual Violence Survey (NISVS): 2010 summary report*. Atlanta, GA: CDC.

BMFSFJ. (1999). *Aktionsplan der Bundesregierung zur Bekämpfung von Gewalt gegen Frauen [Action plan of the federal government combating violence against women]*. Berlin: Bundesministerium für Familie, Senioren, Frauen und Jugend.

BMFSFJ. (2007). *Aktionsplan II der Bundesregierung zur Bekämpfung von Gewalt gegen Frauen [Action plan II of the federal government combating violence against women]*. Berlin: Bundesministerium für Familie, Senioren, Frauen und Jugend.

Bodenheimer, T., & Pham, H. H. (2010). Primary care: Current problems and proposed solutions. *Health Affairs, 29*(5), 799–805. doi:10.1377/hlthaff.2010.0026

Bosch, G. (2009). *Working time and working time policy in Germany*. Tokyo: In JILPT International Workshop on Working Time.

Brandth, B., & Kavande, E. (2007). Norway. In P. Moss & K. Wall (Eds.), *International review of leave policies and related research 2007*. London, UK: Department for Business, Enterprise and Regulatory Reform.

Brandth, B., & Kvande, E. (2003). *Fleksible fedre: maskulinitet, arbeid, velferdsstat [Flexible fathers: Masculinity, work, welfare]*. Oslo: Oslo University Press.

Brandwein, R. A. (1999). Family violence, women and welfare. In R. A. Brandwein (Ed.), *Battered women, children, and welfare reform: The ties that bind* (pp. 3–16). Thousand Oaks, CA: Sage Publications.

Bundesärztekammer. (2004). Ergebnisse der Ärztestatistik zum 31. Dezember 2003 [Results of the medical statstics for December 31, 2003]. Cologne. http://www.bundesaerztekammer.de/page.asp?his=0.3.1667.1678. Accessed May 14, 2014.

Busse, R., & Riesberg, A. (2004). Health care systems in transition: Germany. *Health Systems in Transition, 6*(9), 1–227. European Observatory on Health Systems and Policies.

Cheong, P. H. (2007). Health communication resources for uninsured and insured Hispanics. *Health Communication, 21*(2), 153–163. doi:10.1080/10410230701307188

Christopher, K. (2002). Welfare state regimes and mothers' poverty. *Social Politics, 9*(1), 60–86. doi:10.1093/sp/9.1.60

Christopher, K. (2004). Welfare as we [don't] know it: A review and feminist critique of welfare reform research in the United States. *Feminist Economics, 10*(2), 143–171. doi:10.1080/1354570042000217757

Codispoti, L., Courtot, B., & Swedish, J. (2008). *Nowhere to turn: How the individual health insurance market fails women*. Washington, DC: National Women's Law Center.

Daly, M. C. (2000). *The gender division of welfare: The impact of the British and German welfare states*. Cambridge, UK: Cambridge University Press.

Directorate of Health. (2012). *Nøkkeltall for helsesektoren 2011 [Key figures for the health care services 2011]*. Norway: Oslo.

Dobash, R. E., & Dobash, R. P. (1992). *Women, violence and social change*. London, UK: Routledge.

Duncan, S., & Strell, M. (2004). Combining lone motherhood and paid work: The rationality mistake and Norwegian social policy. *Journal of European Social Policy, 14*(1), 41–54. doi:10.1177/0958928704039789

Ellingsæter, A. L. (1998). Dual breadwinner societies: Provider models in the Scandinavian welfare states. *Acta Sociologica, 41*, 59–73.

Ellingsæter, A. L. (2003). The complexity of family policy reform: The case of Norway. *European Societies, 5*(4), 419–443. doi:10.1080/1461669032000127679

Ellingsæter, A. L. (2012). *Cash for childcare experiences from Finland, Norway and Sweden*. Berlin: Friedrich-Ebert Stiftung.

Ellingsæter, A. L., & Gulbrandsen, L. (2007). Closing the childcare gap: The interaction of childcare provision and mothers' agency in Norway. *Journal of Social Policy, 36*(04), 649–669. doi:10.1017/S0047279407001225

Esping-Andersen, G. (1990). *The three worlds of welfare capitalism*. London: Polity.

Eurostat. (2014). Self-reported unmet need for medical examination or treatment, by income quintile. http://epp.eurostat.ec.europa.eu/portal/page/portal/statistics/search_database. Accessed July 16, 2015.

EURYDICE. (2013). *The education system in the Federal Republic of Germany 2011/2012: A description of the responsibilities, structures and developments in education policy for the exchange of information in Europe*. Bonn: Secretariat of the Standing Conference of the Ministers of Education and Cultural Affairs of the Länder in the Federal Republic of Germany.

Eydal, G. B., & Rostgaard, T. (2011). Gender equality revisited—Changes in Nordic childcare policies in the 2000s. *Social Policy and Administration, 45*(2), 161–179. doi:10.1111/j.1467-9515.2010.00762.x

Feder, J., Levitt, L., O'Brien, E., & Rowland, D. (2001). Covering the low-income uninsured: The case for expanding public programs. *Health Affairs, 20*(1), 27–39. doi:10.1377/hlthaff.20.1.2.7

Fujii, M. (2011). *When to start working after giving birth? Impact on infant's health*. Madison, WI: University of Wisconsin, Madison.

GAO. (2009). *Hospital emergency departments: Crowding continues to occur, and some patients wait longer than recommended time frames*. Washington, DC.

Gauthier, A. H. (2011). *Comparative family policy database, Version 3 [computer file]*. Netherlands Interdisciplinary Demographic Institute and Max Planck Institute for Demographic Research.

Gericke, C. A., Wismar, M., & Busse, R. (2004). *Cost-sharing in the German health care system* (No. 2004/4). Berlin: Technische Universität Berlin.

Gerlinger, T. (2010). Health care reform in Germany. *German Policy Studies, 6*(1), 107–142.

Gerring, J. (2007). *Case study research: Principles and practices*. Cambridge: Cambridge University Press.

Gornick, J. C., & Meyers, M. K. (2003). *Families that work: Policies for reconciling parenthood and employment*. New York City: Russell Sage Foundation Publications.

Gornick, J. C., & Meyers, M. K. (2009). Institutions that support gender equality in parenthood and employment. In J. C. Gornick & M. K. Meyers (Eds.), *Gender equality: Transforming family divisions of labor* (pp. 3–64). London: Verso.

Gornick, J. C., Meyers, M. K., & Ross, K. E. (1997). Supporting the employment of mothers: Policy variation across fourteen welfare states. *Journal of European Social Policy, 7*(1), 45–70. doi:10.1177/095892879700700103

Grol, R., Wensing, M., Mainz, J., Jung, H. P., Ferreira, P., Hearnshaw, H., et al. (2000). Patients in Europe evaluate general practice care: An international comparison. *The British Journal of General Practice, 50*(460), 882–887.

Haj-Yahia, M. M., & Cohen, H. C. (2009). On the lived experience of battered women residing in shelters. *Journal of Family Violence, 24*(2), 95–109. doi:10.1007/s10896-008-9214-3

Hanmer, J., Gloor, D., Meier, H., Eriksson, M., Haller, B., Kavemann, B., et al. (2006). Agencies and evaluation of good practice: Domestic violence, rape and sexual assault. Coordination action on human rights violations. http://www.cahrv.uni-osnabrueck.de/reddot/D_16_Agencies_and_evaluation_of_good_practice_pub.pdf. Accessed January 19, 2011.

Hansen, H.-T., Jürgens, O., Strand, A. H. H., & Voges, W. (2006). Poverty among households with children: A comparative study of Norway and Germany. *International Journal of Social Welfare, 15*(4), 269–279. doi:10.1111/j.1468-2397.2006.00469.x

Hardoy, I., & Schøne, P. (2010). Kan billigere barnehage øke kvinners arbeidstilbud? [Can cheaper daycare increase women's employment?]. *Søkelys på arbeidslivet [Spotlight on Employment], 26*(4), 410–426.

Henly, J. R., & Lyons, S. (2000). The negotiation of child care and employment demands among low-income parents. *Journal of Social Issues, 56*(4), 683–706. doi:10.1111/0022-4537.00191

Himmelstein, D. U., Thorne, D., Warren, E., & Woolhandler, S. (2009). Medical bankruptcy in the United States, 2007: Results of a national study. *The American Journal of Medicine, 122*(8), 741–746. doi:10.1016/j.amjmed.2009.04.012

Hobson, B. (1994). Solo mothers, social policy regimes and the logics of gender. In D. Sainsbury (Ed.), *Gendering welfare states* (pp. 170–187). London, Thousand Oaks, CA: Sage Publications.

Hoffman, C., & Paradise, J. (2008). Health insurance and access to health care in the United States. *Annals of the New York Academy of Sciences, 1136*, 149–160. doi:10.1196/annals.1425.007

Honekamp, I. (2008). Family policy in Germany: Appraisal and assessment. *Journal of Family History, 33*(4), 452–464. doi:10.1177/0363199008323356

Hornberg, C., Schröttle, M., Bohne, S., Khelaifat, N., & Pauli, A. (2008). *Health consequences of violence, with special consideration of domestic violence against women*. Berlin: Robert Koch-Institut.

Hutchinson, G. S., & Weeks, W. (2004). Living conditions of women who experience violence from their partners: Norway and Australia comparisons. *Australian Journal of Social Issues, 39* (4), 393–407.

Internal Revenue Service [IRS]. (2013). Ten things to know about the Child and Dependent Care Credit. http://www.irs.gov/uac/Ten-Things-to-Know-About-the-Child-and-Dependent-Care-Credit. Accessed January 07, 2014.

International Labor Organization [ILO]. (2013). Percentage of health care expenditure NOT financed by private household's out of pocket payments. http://www.ilo.org/dyn/ilossi/ssiindic.viewMultiIndic?p_lang=en&p_indicator_code=H-1c&p_geoaid=578. Accessed January 07, 2014.

IRS. (2014). EITC income limits, maximum credit amounts and tax law updates. http://www.irs.gov/Individuals/EITC-Income-Limits,-Maximum-Credit–Amounts-and-Tax-Law-Updates. Accessed January 05, 2014.

Johnsen, J. R. (2006). Norway. *Health Systems in Transition, 8*(1), 1–167. European Observatory on Health Systems and Policies.

Jonassen, W., & Skogøy, E. (2010). *A home for us, a home for you... A study of change in user population and use of shelters for battered women*. Oslo, Norway: NKVTS, Nasjonalt kunnskapssenter om vold og traumatisk stress.

Kamerman, S. B., & Kahn, A. J. (2001). Child and family policies in the United States at the opening of the twenty-first century. *Social Policy and Administration, 35*(1), 69–84. doi:10.1111/1467-9515.00220

Kjeldstad, R. (2000). Employment strategy policies and lone parenthood. The case of Norway. *Social Politics: International Studies in Gender, State, and Society, 7*(3), 343–371. doi:10.1093/sp/7.3.343

Knudsen, K., & Waerness, K. (2001). National context, individual characteristics and attitudes on mothers' employment: A comparative analysis of Great Britain, Sweden and Norway. *Acta Sociologica, 44*(1), 67–79.

Kultusministerkonferenz. (2006). *Bericht über die allgemein bildenden Schulen in Ganztagsform in den Ländern in der Bundesrepublik Deutschland: 2002 bis 2004 [Report on the general schools in the all-day reforms in the states of the Federal Republic of Germany: 2002 to 2004]*. Bonn: Sekretariat der Ständigen Konferenz der Kultusminister der Länder in der Bundesrepublik Deutschland.

Lehrner, A., & Allen, N. E. (2009). Still a movement after all these years? Current tensions in the domestic violence movement. *Violence Against Women, 15*(6), 656–677. doi:10.1177/1077801209332185

Leira, A. (1992). *Welfare states and working mothers: The Scandinavian experience*. Cambridge, UK.

Leira, A. (2002). *Working parents and the welfare state: Family change and policy reform in Scandinavia*. Cambridge, UK.

Leisering, L. (2001). Germany—Reform from within. In P. Alcock & G. Craig (Eds.), *International social policy: Welfare regimes in the developed world* (pp. 161–182). London: Palgrave.

Leitner, S. (2011). Germany outpaces Austria in childcare policy: The historical contingencies of "conservative" childcare policy. *Journal of European Social Policy, 20*(5), 456–467. doi:10.1177/0958928710380482

Leitner, S., Ostner, I., & Schmitt, C. (2008). Family policies in Germany. In I. Ostner & C. Schmitt (Eds.), *Family policies in the context of family change: The Nordic countries in comparative perspective* (pp. 175–202). Wiesbaden: VS Verlag für Sozialwissenschaften. doi:10.1007/978-3-531-90895-3_9

Lembke, U. (2013). Germany. In S. Burri & H. Aune (Eds.), *Sex discrimination in relation to part-time and fixed-term work: The application of EU and national law in practice in 33 European countries* (pp. 128–144). Brussels: European Commission.

Lindahl, A. K., & Ringard, Å. (2013). The Norwegian health care system, In S. Thomson, R. Osborn, D. Squires, & M. Jun (Eds.), *International profiles of health care systems, 2013*. New York, NY: The Commonwealth Fund.

Marcus, S. C., & Olfson, M. (2010). National trends in the treatment for depression from 1998 to 2007. *Archives of General Psychiatry, 67*(12), 1265–1273. doi:10.1001/archgenpsychiatry.2010.151

Mendes, E. (2012). More Americans uninsured in 2011. *Gallup: Well-Being*. http://www.gallup.com/poll/152162/americans-uninsured-2011.aspx. Accessed May 29, 2013.

Mezey, J., Greenberg, M., & Schumacher, R. (2002). *The vast majority of federally-eligible children did not receive child care assistance in FY 2000*. Washington, DC: Center for Law and Social Policy.

Ministry of Health. (1998). *Om opptrappingsplan for psykisk helse 1999–2006 [The escalation plan for mental health]*. Norway: Oslo.

Ministry of Health. (1999). *Om verdiar for den norske helsetenesta (St. meld. nr. 26, 1999–2000) [Values in the Norwegian Health Care Services]*. Oslo, Norway.

Ministry of Justice and Public Security. (2012). *Action plan against domestic violence 2012*. Norway: Oslo.

Ministry of Justice and the Police. (2004). *Domestic violence action plan (2004–2007)*. Norway: Oslo.

Ministry of Justice and the Police. (2008). *Turning point: National action plan against domestic violence 2008–2011*. Norway: Oslo.

Misra, J., Budig, M. J., & Moller, S. (2007). Reconciliation policies and the effects of motherhood on employment, earnings and poverty. *Journal of Comparative Policy Analysis: Research and Practice, 9*(2), 135–155. doi:10.1080/13876980701311588

Modi, M. N., Palmer, S., & Armstrong, A. (2014). The role of Violence Against Women Act in addressing intimate partner violence: A public health issue. *Journal of Women's Health, 23*(3), 253–259. doi:10.1089/jwh.2013.4387

Moran, M. (1999). *Governing the health care state: A comparative study of the United Kingdom, the United States and Germany*. Manchester, UK: Manchester University Press.

Müller, U., & Schröttle, M. (2004). *Lebenssituation, Sicherheit und Gesundheit von Frauen in Deutschland: Eine repräsentative Untersuchung zu Gewalt gegen Frauen in Deutschland [Health, well-being and personal safety of women in Germany: A representative study of violence against women in Germany]*. Berlin: Bundesministerium für Familie, Senioren, Frauen und Jugend.

National Network to End Domestic Violence. (2012). *Domestic violence counts 2012: A 24-hour census of domestic violence shelters and services*. Washington, DC.

Nerøien, A. I., & Schei, B. (2008). Partner violence and health: Results from the first national study on violence against women in Norway. *Scandinavian Journal of Public Health, 36*(2), 161–168. doi:10.1177/1403494807085188

Norwegian Labour and Welfare Administration [NAV]. (2015a). Unemployment benefits. *Benefits and services*. https://www.nav.no/en/Home/Benefits+and+services/Relatert+informasjon/Unemployment+benefits.286402.cms#chapter-1. Accessed July 16, 2015.

Norwegian Labour and Welfare Administration [NAV]. (2015b). Sickness benefits for employees. *Benefits and services*. https://www.nav.no/English/English/Sickness+benefits+for+employees.283831.cms. Accessed July 16, 2015.

Norwegian Ministry of Labour and Social Affairs [ASD]. (2014). *The Norwegian social insurance scheme*. Norway: Oslo.

OECD. (2003a). *Benefits and wages: Germany 2003*. Paris: OECD Publishing.

OECD. (2003b). *Health at a glance: OECD Indicators 2003*. Paris: OECD Publishing.

OECD. (2003c). *Benefits and wages: Norway 2003*. Paris: OECD Publishing.

OECD. (2005). *Health at a glance: OECD Indicators 2005*. Paris: OECD Publishing.

OECD. (2006). Labour market reform should go on. In OECD Economic (Ed.), *Surveys: Germany 2006* (pp. 91–116). Paris: OECD Publishing.

OECD. (2012). *Health at a glance: Europe 2012*. Paris: OECD Publishing.

OECD. (2014). OECD family database. http://www.oecd.org/social/family/database. Accessed February 06, 2015.

Olsen, G. M. (2007). Toward global welfare state convergence? Family policy and health care in Sweden, Canada and the United States. *Journal of Sociology and Social Welfare, 34*(2), 143–164.

Orloff, A. (1993). Gender and the social rights of citizenship: The comparative analysis of gender relations and welfare states. *American Sociological Review, 58*(3), 303–328.

Ostner, I. (2010). Farewell to the family as we know it: Family policy change in Germany. *German Policy Studies, 6*(1), 211–244.

Patchias, E. M., & Waxman, J. (2007). *Women and health coverage: The affordability gap*. Washington, DC: The Commonwealth Fund.

Peter, T. (2006). Domestic violence in the United States and Sweden: A welfare state typology comparison within a power resources framework. *Women's Studies International Forum, 29*, 96–107. doi:10.1016/j.wsif.2005.10.001

Ragin, C. C. (1987). *The comparative method: Moving beyond qualitative and quantitative strategies*. Oakland, CA: University of California Press.

Ray, R. (2008). *A detailed look at parental leave policies in 21 OECD countries*. Washington, DC: Center for Economic and Policy Research.

Ray, R., Gornick, J. C., & Schmitt, J. (2010). Who cares? Assessing generosity and gender equality in parental leave policy designs in 21 countries. *Journal of European Social Policy, 20* (3), 196–216. doi:10.1177/0958928710364434

Rice, T., Rosenau, P., Unruh, L. Y., & Barnes, A. J. (2013). United States of America: Health system review. *Health Systems in Transition, 15*(3), 1–431. European Observatory on Health Systems and Policies.

Richardson, L. D., & Norris, M. (2010). Access to health and health care: How race and ethnicity matter. *The Mount Sinai Journal of Medicine, 77*(2), 166–177. doi:10.1002/msj.20174

Riesberg, A., & Wörz, M. (2008). *Quality in and equality of access to healthcare services: Country report for Germany*. Brussels: European Commission.

Ringard, Å., Sagan, A., Saunes, I. S., & Lindahl, A. K. (2013). Norway: Health system review. *Health Systems in Transition, 15*(18), 1–162. European Observatory on Health Systems and Policies.

Sainsbury, D. (1994). Women's and men's social rights: Gendering dimensions of welfare states. *Gendering welfare states* (pp. 150–169). London, UK: Sage Publications.

Sainsbury, D. (1999). Taxation, family responsibilities, and employment. In D. Sainsbury (Ed.), *Gender and welfare state regimes* (pp. 185–209). Oxford: Oxford University Press. doi:10.1093/0198294166.003.0007

Sainsbury, D. (2001). Gender and the making of welfare states: Norway and Sweden. *Social Politics, 8*(1), 113–143. doi:10.1093/sp/8.1.113

Salize, H. J., Rössler, W., & Becker, T. (2007). Mental health care in Germany: Current state and trends. *European Archives of Psychiatry and Clinical Neuroscience, 257*(2), 92–103. doi:10.1007/s00406-006-0696-9

Saur, R., Hustad, A. E., & Heir, T. (2011). *Violence prevention in Norway: Activities and measures to prevent violence in close relationships*. Oslo, Norway: Norwegian Centre for Violence and Traumatic Stress Studies (NKVTS).

Schlette, S., Lisac, M., & Blum, K. (2009). Integrated primary care in Germany: The road ahead. *International Journal of Integrated Care, 9*, 1–11.

Seawright, J., & Gerring, J. (2008). Case selection techniques in case study research: A menu of qualitative and quantitative options. *Political Research Quarterly, 61*(2), 294–308. doi:10.1177/1065912907313077

Skevik, A., & Hatland, A. (2008). Family policies in Norway. In I. Ostner & C. Schmitt (Eds.), *Family policies in the context of family change: The Nordic countries in comparative perspective* (pp. 89–107). Wiesbaden: VS Verlag für Sozialwissenschaften. doi:10.1007/978-3-531-90895-3_5

Skrede, K. (1999). Shaping gender equality—The role of the state: Norwegian experiences, present policies and future challenges. In H. Kitterød, R. Kjeldstad, T. Noack, & L. Østby (Eds.), *Livsløp i støpeskjeen: Utvalgte arbeide [Life in the melting pot: Selected works]*. Oslo, Norway: Statistisk Sentralbyrå.

Skrede, K. (2004). Familiepolitikkens grense - ved "likestilling light"? [Drawing the line for family policy—At "gender equality light"?]. In A. L. Ellingsæter & A. Leira (Eds.), *Velferdsstaten og familien [The welfare state and the family]* (pp. 160–200). Oslo, Norway: Gyldendal Akademisk.

Statistik Sentralbyrå [SSB]. (2013). Labour force survey. http://www.ssb.no/. Accessed November 01, 2014.

Stelmaszekn, B., & Fisher, H. (2012). *Country report 2012: Reality check on data collection and European services for women and children survivors of violence: A right for protection and support?* Vienna, Austria: WAVE Network.

Sterud, T. (2009). Working time in the European Union: Norway. *European Working Conditions Observatory*. http://www.eurofound.europa.eu/ewco/studies/tn0803046s/no0803049q.htm. Accessed March 07, 2013.

Strand, A. H. H. (2012). *The welfare state matters: On the economic consequences of partnership dissolution in Norway and Britain*. Bergen, Norway: University of Bergen. https://bora.uib.no/bitstream/handle/1956/6174/Dr.thesis_AnneHegeHendenStrand.pdf?sequence=1. Accessed April 11, 2014.

Strunk, B., & Cunningham, P. (2002). *Treading water: Americans' access to needed medical care, 1997–2001*. Washington, DC: Center for Studying Health System Change.

Syltevik, L. J. (1999). Endret velferdspolitikk for alenemødre—Fra relasjonelt til individualisert alenemoderskap [Changing welfare policies for lone mothers—From relational to individualistic lone motherhood]. *Tidsskrift for velferdsforskning, 2*, 85–101.

Tierney, K. J. (1982). The battered women movement and the creation of the wife beating problem. *Social Problems, 29*(3), 207–220. doi:10.2307/800155

Trzeciak, S., & Rivers, E. P. (2003). Emergency department overcrowding in the United States: An emerging threat to patient safety and public health. *Emergency Medicine Journal, 20*(5), 402–405.

US Bureau of Labor Statistics. (n.d.). CPI inflation calculator. http://www.bls.gov/data/inflation_calculator.htm. Accessed April 16, 2014.

US Department of Health and Human Services. (n.d.). Prior HHS poverty guidelines and federal register references. http://aspe.hhs.gov/poverty/figures-fed-reg.cfm. Accessed April 16, 2014.

US Department of Labor. (n.d.). Leave benefits: Sick leave. http://www.dol.gov/dol/topic/benefits-leave/sickleave.htm. Accessed April 15, 2014.

US Department of Labor. (2009). Labor force participation rate of mothers, 1975–2007. *The Economics Daily*. http://www.bls.gov/opub/ted/2009/jan/wk1/art04.htm. Accessed July 16, 2014.

US Department of Labor. (2011). The Fair Labor Standards Act of 1938, as amended. Washington, DC. http://www.dol.gov/whd/regs/statutes/FairLaborStandAct.pdf. Accessed July 16, 2014.

US Department of Labor. (2012). Fact Sheet #28: The Family and Medical Leave Act. Washington, DC. http://www.dol.gov/whd/regs/compliance/whdfs28.pdf. Accessed July 16, 2014.

US Department of Labor. (2013). State unemployment insurance benefits. Washington, DC. http://workforcesecurity.doleta.gov/unemploy/uifactsheet.asp. Accessed July 16, 2014.

Van Loon, R. A., Borkin, J. R., & Steffen, J. J. (2002). Health care experiences and preferences of uninsured workers. *Health and Social Work, 27*(1), 17–26.

Vikum, E., Krokstad, S., & Westin, Steinar. (2012). Socioeconomic inequalities in health care utilisation in Norway: The population-based HUNT3 survey. *International Journal for Equity in Health, 11*(48), 1–9. doi:10.1186/1475-9276-11-48

Vollset, G. (2011). *Familiepolitikkens historie—1970 til 2000 [The history of family policy—1970 to 2000]*. Oslo, Norway: NOVA.

WHO. (2014). Global health expenditure database. http://apps.who.int/nha/database/Select/Indicators/en. Accessed July 25, 2014.

WHO Regional Office for Europe. (2014). European health for all database (HFA-DB). Copenhagen. http://data.euro.who.int/hfadb/. Accessed July 25, 2014.

Wilper, A. P., Woolhandler, S., Lasser, K. E., McCormick, D., Bor, D. H., & Himmelstein, D. U. (2008). A national study of chronic disease prevalence and access to care in uninsured U.S. adults. *Annals of Internal Medicine, 149*(3), 170–176.

ZIF. (n.d.). Frauenhausfinanzierung. http://www.autonome-frauenhaeuser-zif.de/de/themen/frauenhausfinanzierung. Accessed October 03, 2014.

Zuckerman, S., McFeeters, J., Cunningham, P., & Nichols, L. (2004). Trends: Changes in Medicaid physician fees, 1998-2003: Implications for physician participation. *Health Affairs, Web Exclusive*. doi:10.1377/hlthaff.w4.374

Chapter 5
Research Design and Methods

Abstract The questions investigated in this book seek to understand both the individual- and macro-level factors involved in the health inequities of IPV survivors. At the individual level, three different national data sets on the topic of violence against women and health are quantitatively analyzed to examine the mechanisms of differential exposure to IPV and differential vulnerability to poor health among IPV survivors. At the macro level, the results from the quantitative analyses are qualitatively compared across the policy contexts of the US, Germany, and Norway using detailed case descriptions. With this in mind, the present chapter begins with a presentation of the three sets of national survey data, as well as a description of the sample selection, and the operationalization of the variables of interest. Finally, an account is given of the univariate, bivariate, and multivariate statistical analyses applied to answer Research Questions 1 and 2, as well as a description of the cross-national comparison to answer Research Questions 3 and 4.

The questions investigated in this book seek to understand both the individual- and macro-level factors involved in the health inequities of IPV survivors. At the individual level, three different national data sets on the topic of violence against women and health are quantitatively analyzed to examine the mechanisms of differential exposure to IPV and differential vulnerability to poor health among IPV survivors. At the macro level, the results from the quantitative analyses are qualitatively compared across the policy contexts of the US, Germany, and Norway using the detailed case descriptions presented in Chap. 4. With this in mind, the present chapter begins with a presentation of the three sets of national survey data, as well as a description of the sample selection, and the operationalization of the variables of interest. Finally, an account is given of the univariate, bivariate, and multivariate statistical analyses applied to answer Research Questions 1 and 2, as well as a description of the cross-national comparison to answer Research Questions 3 and 4.

© Springer International Publishing Switzerland 2016
M.M. Larsen, *Health Inequities Related to Intimate Partner Violence Against Women*, Social Disparities in Health and Health Care,
DOI 10.1007/978-3-319-29565-7_5

5.1 Quantitative Data

Quantitatively, a cross-national survey would be ideal for connecting the individual- and macro-level factors of interest for the research questions. At the time the analyses were conducted, however, such a data set was not available for industrialized nations including the US.[1] Even if such data had been available, it would still be vital to note the implications of using population survey data for measuring IPV. Recalling the debate presented in Sect. 2.1, such survey data is predisposed to revealing rather situational couple violence over intimate partner terrorism. At the same time, these surveys provide nationally representative data covering a broader spectrum of socioeconomic, IPV, and health outcomes than is often available in self-selected help-seeking samples.

For these reasons, this book makes use of data from the national prevalence surveys on violence against women conducted in the US, Germany, and Norway (see Table 5.1), with careful attempts to ensure that intimate partner terrorism is also captured in the analyses. It is important to note that while these surveys were informed by one another, they were not designed to be directly comparable and thus have methodological differences which require consideration in their comparison (Heise and García-Moreno 2012). "Sometimes even small differences in the details of data collection, time-frames, recorded acts and contexts seriously limit comparability" (Schröttle et al. 2006, p. 3). To increase the comparability of the three data sets, the approach recommended by the Co-ordination Action on Human Rights Violations (CAHRV) was applied for comparative secondary analysis of violence against women and health data (Schröttle et al. 2006). This structured approach included comprehensive documentation of: (1) the similarities and differences across surveys in sampling, methodology, and data collection; (2) the exact definitions of violence, health, reference groups, and age groups to be analyzed; and (3) consideration of methodological influences on the outcomes in the data. These points are addressed throughout this chapter.

For the analysis of the United States, the *National Violence Against Women Survey* was used (Tjaden and Thoennes 1999).[2] This survey was commissioned by

[1]Although, to be clear, international surveys on violence against women have been conducted. The WHO Multi-country Study on Women's Health and Domestic Violence Against Women covered: Bangladesh, Brazil, Ethiopia, Japan, Peru, Namibia, Samoa, Serbia and Montenegro, Thailand, and the United Republic of Tanzania (WHO 2005). The International Violence Against Women Survey covered: Australia, Costa Rica, the Czech Republic, Denmark, Greece, Hong Kong, Italy, Mozambique, the Philippines, Poland and Switzerland (Johnson et al. 2008). Additionally, the Demographic and Health Surveys also include items regarding violence and health, but do not systematically cover countries with functioning welfare states. Most promising is the data from a cross-national survey conducted by the EU Agency for Fundamental Rights (European Union Agency for Fundamental Rights [FRA] 2014) among 42,000 women in all 28 member states of the EU, which was made available for public use only in the second half of 2015.

[2]The National Intimate Partner and Sexual Violence Survey is a more recent national survey conducted in 2010 by the CDC, NIJ, and Department of Defense (Black et al. 2011). However, the data were not publically available when analysis for this book began.

Table 5.1 Overview of utilized nationally representative surveys on violence against women

Country	Survey year	N	Age	Data collection	Survey report
US	1995–96	8000[a]	18+	Computer-assisted telephone interviewing	Tjaden and Thoennes (2000)
Germany	2003	10,769	16–85	Face-to-face + self-administered	Müller and Schröttle (2004)
Norway	2003–04	2407[a]	20–55	Postal survey, self-administered	Haaland et al. (2005)

Adapted from Schröttle et al. (2006)
[a]The US survey additionally involved 8000 male participants, and the Norway survey 2211 male participants

the National Institute of Justice (NIJ) and the CDC and was led by researchers from the Inter-university Consortium for Political and Social Research (ICPSR) in Ann Arbor, Michigan (Tjaden and Thoennes 2000).[3] A random-digit dialing sample of telephone households in all 50 states and the District of Columbia was drawn. In order to control for varying response rates by region, the sample was stratified according to US Census region. A total of 8000 women, 18 years and older, were interviewed in either English or Spanish using a computer-assisted telephone interview system from November 1995 to May 1996, with an overall participation rate of 72 %. Respondents answered questions regarding their general fear of violence, physical abuse as a child or adult, sexual assault as an adult, and incidents of threatened violence. Interviews lasted approximately 25 min in English and 32 min in Spanish. When comparing the survey's sample to the US Census Bureau's 1995 Current Population Survey, there is an underrepresentation of the elderly, African Americans, and those without a high school diploma (Tjaden and Thoennes 2000).

The analysis of Germany made use of the *Health, Well-being, and Safety of Women in Germany Survey* commissioned by the Federal Ministry for Family Affairs, Senior Citizens, Women, and Youth (BMFSFJ) (Müller and Schröttle 2005). The survey was coordinated by a research team at the Interdisciplinary Center for Research of Gender and Women's Issues (*Interdisziplinäres Zentrum für Frauen- und Geschlechterforschung*, IFF) at the University of Bielefeld and conducted by the Institute for Applied Social Sciences (*Institut für angewandte Sozialwissenschaft*, infas).[4] A cross-sectional sample was randomly drawn from 250 registration offices (*Einwohnermeldämter*) throughout the country. The main survey took place from January to October 2003 and consisted of 10,264

[3]The original collector of the data (i.e., ICPSR) and the sponsoring agencies (i.e., NIJ, National Center for Injury Prevention and Control, and the CDC) bear no responsibility for uses of this collection or for interpretations or inferences based upon such uses.

[4]These data were made available by the Data Archive for Social Sciences at GESIS in Cologne. Neither the authors of the study, IFF, infas, nor GESIS bear any responsibility for the analysis or interpretation of the data presented here.

face-to-face interviews with adult, German-speaking women between the ages of 16 and 85. Of these participants, 94 % also completed an additional self-administered, written questionnaire to be either handed to the interviewer directly or submitted via post. During the face-to-face interview, which lasted an average of 64 min, respondents answered questions regarding their lifetime violence victimization experiences and their mental and physical health. The written questionnaire focused primarily on partner violence, stalking, and violence during childhood, and took an average of 18 min to complete. Overall, 52 % of those randomly drawn participated in the main survey (Fredebeul et al. 2004).

In order to ensure that the largest immigrant groups in Germany were adequately represented, a supplemental survey of 253 Turkish and 252 Eastern European women was conducted from July to December 2003. Of these interview participants, 92 % of Turkish women, and 98 % of Eastern European women also completed the written questionnaire. Women were interviewed either in Turkish, Russian, or German, and asked the exact same questions as those included in the main survey. In order to achieve the sample, women specifically of Turkish nationality or origins, and women from Russia or other former Soviet countries, were drawn from the 250 registration offices described above. The face-to-face interviews lasted an average of 74 min for the women of Turkish origin, and 72 min for the women of Eastern European origin, while the written questionnaires took an average of 27 and 23 min, respectively. Overall, 45 % of the women drawn participated in the supplemental survey (Fredebeul et al. 2004). When comparing the main and supplemental survey samples to the 2001 Microcensus in Germany, there is an underrepresentation of women over 70 years of age, women with a *Volks-* or *Hauptschulabschluss*, and women who are not employed.

For the analysis of Norway, the *Survey of Everyday Safety* was utilized, financed by the Norwegian Institute of Urban and Regional Research (*Norsk institutt for by- og regionforskning*, NIBR) and conducted by Statistics Norway (*Statistisk sentralbyrå*, SSB) (SSB 2003).[5] A nationally representative sample was drawn from Norway's central demographic and population database, which is updated several times per month with information from the National Population Register. Between October 2003 and January 2004, this sample of women between the ages of 20 and 55 years received self-administered, postal questionnaires (12 pages long, with 67 questions) in the *Bokmål* form of written Norwegian, with the option to request the survey be sent in the *Nynorsk* form.[6] Overall, 2407 women completed and sent back the survey, resulting in a response rate of 63 % (Flåte 2004). The questionnaire contained items pertaining to general safety, physical and mental health, and the extent and type of violence in relationships experienced. When

[5]These data were prepared and made available by the Norwegian Social Science Data Services (NSD). Neither the authors of the study, Statistics Norway, nor NSD are responsible for the analyses or interpretation of the data presented here.

[6]However, there were no requests to receive the survey in *Nynorsk*.

comparing the survey sample to the overall population, women under 24 years of age and those with migration backgrounds are underrepresented.

In sum, it is important to be aware of a number of differences in the data collection across these three surveys which could have affected the responses provided. On the one hand, the privacy of the written self-administered postal survey in Norway and the written self-administered questionnaire in Germany may have enhanced women's willingness to disclose sensitive information related to experiences of abuse, as compared to the telephone interview in the US survey and the face-to-face interview (also) in Germany (WHO 2001). On the other hand, in order to increase the likelihood of a response, the Norwegian questionnaire was necessarily shorter and simpler, as was the self-administered portion of the German survey. Meanwhile, the face-to-face interview of the German survey and the telephone interview of the US survey could collect more complex and detailed information than the written questionnaires. Finally, there was no opportunity for respondents to ask for clarification in the Norwegian survey as opposed to in the US and German surveys, which could have led to either errors in survey completion or to non-response (Flåte 2004). As much as possible, the harmonization of the three data sets detailed throughout this chapter attempts to account for these differences, but they should be kept in mind while interpreting the results.

5.2 Sample Selection

In order to increase the comparability of the data sets, the study populations were narrowed to women ages 20–56, which was the maximum age range available in the Norwegian data.[7] The conceptual framework of this book assumes a causal directionality leading from social position to IPV to health outcomes. Thus, due to the cross-sectional nature of the surveys, it was necessary to minimize the time between the respondents' social position and health at the time of the survey and the time of their last IPV incident (if applicable). Thus, the portion of each sample with IPV exposure was restricted to those with exposure within the past 5 years.[8] This resulted in an overall sample for each country of those without any IPV exposure and those with exposure within the past 5 years.[9] This narrowed, to a certain extent, the chance of significant changes in social position or health due to circumstances unrelated to IPV.

[7]Although the age range sampled in Norway was 20–55, some respondents turned 56 during the period of data collection (Flåte 2004).

[8]All three data sets also allowed for the narrowing of IPV exposure to within the past year. However, it would have resulted in sample sizes too small for the appropriate statistical analyses. For this reason, the time frame of the past 5 years was chosen.

[9]For clarity's sake, the reader should be aware that those women with IPV experiences more than 5 years ago were not included in the analysis.

5.3 Measurement

The present section offers a description of the creation and operationalization of the variables for the analytical models, starting with IPV exposure and health outcomes, and followed by the social position and control variables. Fitting with the CARHV guidelines, particular attention is paid to harmonizing the victim-perpetrator context, time span of violence, type of violence, and health outcomes (Schröttle et al. 2006). Where substantial differences in variables across the data sets existed, specific details regarding their harmonization are provided.

5.3.1 *IPV Exposure*

In Chap. 7, the effects of social position on the dependent variable of IPV exposure are analyzed, and in Chap. 8, the moderating effect of IPV exposure on health is also examined. Thus, the operationalization of *IPV exposure* as a variable and the key limitations imposed by data availability are important to understand. For the purposes of this book, this involved the combination of a number of key variables in the data, namely: type of violence (e.g., physical, sexual), perpetrator (e.g., current spouse, ex-spouse, current partner, or ex-partner), and when the violence occurred (see Table 5.2). To measure the occurrence of physical abuse, all three surveys partially adapted items from the frequently used Conflict Tactics Scales (CTS) (Straus 1979; Straus et al. 1996). The CTS measures specific acts of physical violence occurring between partners, such as being pushed, kicked, strangled, or threatened with a weapon. Therefore, *physical abuse* was defined in this study in a dichotomous variable as the occurrence of at least one of the physical victimization items perpetrated by a current or former partner. Despite the widespread use of the CTS, however, the controversy around this scale should not be ignored. It remains at the center of the debate regarding the gender symmetry of IPV (see, for example, Hamby 2014, 2015; Winstok 2015). It is argued that the CTS does not capture patterns of abuse, fear, or the outcomes of such acts and therefore more frequently finds gender symmetry in physical violence than other measures. In other words, it may be more adept at capturing situational couple violence than intimate partner terrorism. With this in mind, an additional measure of severity, which is detailed later on in this section, was deemed necessary for the analyses conducted in this book.

Sexual abuse was measured with the occurrence of attempted and/or completed forced sex by a current or former partner. For the US data, any attempted or completed occurrence of forced vaginal, oral, and anal intercourse or penetration by other means was coded as sexual abuse. Using the written questionnaire from the German survey, the measurement of sexual abuse was less explicit, with items asking about unwanted forced sexual relations, either attempted or completed. Finally, the Norwegian survey included only one item regarding attempted sexual

Table 5.2 Overview of IPV exposure variable

Type	Description	Operationalization		
		US	Germany	Norway
Dependent and independent	Categorical	0 = <1 incident physical/sexual abuse from current/former partner	0 = <1 incident physical/sexual abuse from current/former partner	0 = <1 incident physical/sexual abuse from current/former partner
		1 = ≥1 incident physical/sexual abuse from current/former partner in past 5 years, but no injury from *most recent* incidence	1 = ≥1 incident physical/sexual abuse from current/former partner in past 5 years, but no injury from *any* incident	1 = ≥1 incident physical/sexual abuse from current/former partner in past 5 years, but no injury from *most recent* incidence
		2 = ≥1 incident physical/sexual abuse from current/former partner in past 5 years, with injury from *most recent* incident	2 = ≥1 incident physical/sexual abuse from current/former partner in past 5 years, with injury from *any* incident	2 = ≥1 incident physical/sexual abuse from current/former partner in past 5 years, with injury from *most recent* incident

assault by an intimate partner, with no differentiation of incidences which were completed. For all three surveys, any incidence of attempted or completed sexual assault from a current or former partner was coded in a dichotomous variable as sexual abuse. These variables of physical abuse and sexual abuse were then combined into one overall dichotomous measure of whether the respondent had experienced IPV in her lifetime.[10]

In order to narrow down IPV exposure to the *past 5 years*, variables in the US and German surveys which specifically asked when the last incident occurred (US) or about incidents within the past 5 years (Germany) were used. With the Norwegian survey, the recency of the last IPV incident was calculated based on the respondent's age at the time of the survey and age at last incident. In sum, for measurement purposes, *IPV exposure* was defined as those who reported physical

[10]While psychological or emotional abuse (e.g., possessive behavior, humiliation, limiting contact with friends or family) is increasingly included in definitions of IPV, and it has been shown to have a negative effect on the health of IPV survivors (Nicolaidis and Paranjape 2009), key conceptual, definitional, and methodological problems remain in its measurement (Follingstad 2009; Follingstad et al. 2015; Maiuro 2001). This is unfortunately also the case for the data analyzed in this book. Along with differences in the items assessing psychological abuse across the three data sets, the German data only measured psychological violence for current partners, thus excluding all of the women not in partnerships at the time of the survey. For these reasons, psychological abuse was excluded from the definition of IPV exposure in the analysis.

or sexual violence from a current spouse, ex-spouse, current partner, or ex-partner within the past 5 years.

Finally, in measuring *IPV exposure*, the severity of the consequences of the violence was considered since this research operates under the theoretical assumption that not all violence is equal (Schröttle et al. 2006) and extensive research shows that greater severity is linked to worse health outcomes (Dillon et al. 2013). Thus, referencing a number of categorizations of IPV severity in the literature (Brzank 2012; Müller and Schröttle 2004; Straus 2001), a categorical measure which divided respondents into the following three groups was created: no IPV experience, at least one incident of IPV but no injury (i.e., 'minor'), and those who were injured during an IPV incident (i.e., 'severe'). This required first harmonizing the measurement of *injuries due to IPV* into a dichotomous variable. For both the US and Norway data, 'yes' was coded to injury if the respondent indicated that any one of a given list of possible injuries (e.g., bruising, broken bones, concussions) had occurred during the most recent incident of physical or sexual IPV. However, due to a difference in the surveys, for the German data 'yes' was coded if any one of a given list of injuries had occurred during *any* incident of physical or sexual IPV. This dichotomous injury variable was then combined with the dichotomous variable regarding IPV in the past 5 years to create the categorical measure of IPV exposure. Due to data limitations, this measure of IPV exposure unfortunately does not incorporate important factors like frequency, duration of exposure or fear. However, the categorization according to injury still reflects these factors to a certain degree when assuming that violence is an escalating cycle (Krantz and Garcia-Moreno 2005).

5.3.2 Health Outcomes

In Chap. 8, the results of the impact of social position and IPV exposure on health outcomes are presented for two different outcome variables (see Table 5.3). The first is a general rating of *self-assessed health* asking the respondents to rate their overall health according to a scale. Such self-assessed health ratings have been found to be associated with morbidity (Power et al. 1991) and to predict use of medical care and mortality (Idler and Benyamini 1997; Van Doorslaer and Gerdtham 2003). These associations likely reflect the knowledge individuals hold regarding factors that influence their health (e.g., family history, health behaviors) and captures elements of health that are usually difficult to capture with more specific measures (e.g., physiological state, vitality) (Au and Johnston 2014; Jylhä 2009; Manor et al. 2000). Moreover, it has been recommended by the WHO as a health indicator suitable for comparative research and is thus one of the most widely used measures of health (De Bruin et al. 1996). Because responses to self-assessed health in all three data sets are highly skewed toward the positive end of the scale, linear regression would not be recommended (Manor et al. 2000). Likewise, the skew toward good health left too few cases in the lowest categories to enable analysis as an ordinal variable. To accommodate these limitations, a dichotomous self-assessed health variable was created. Due to the slight differences in scaling across the three surveys, it is worth describing how the dichotomous variable was created for each. With the US's five-point scale stacked toward positive responses, 'excellent,' 'very good,' and 'good' were grouped together under good health, while 'fair' and 'poor' were grouped together under poor health. The German six-point scale, on the other hand, offered anchors of 'very good' (1) and 'very poor' (6) and asked the respondents to use their own judgment to assess the points in between. Thus, points 1, 2, and 3 were categorized under good health, and points 4, 5, and 6 under poor health. Finally, while the Norwegian scale used five points, it offered a true middle point. Because the overwhelming majority of respondents indicated 'very good' or 'good' health, 'neither good nor bad' was considered poor health, along with 'poor' and 'very poor'.

Finally, in order to also capture *mental health* outcomes, a count variable was developed which summed the number of symptoms common to depression, anxiety, and PTSD reported by the respondents. The list of symptoms in the US survey was based on a group of questions from the SF-36 Health Survey (Ware et al. 1993), while the Norway survey made use of a standardized short version of the Hopkins Symptom Check List for anxiety and depression (Derogatis et al. 1974). The questions used in all three surveys asked respondents to rate on a 4-point scale either how often respondents experienced such symptoms either in the past week (US) or past 12 months (Germany), or how bothered respondents have been by such symptoms in the past 14 days (Norway). For each respondent, I summed up the total number of symptoms experienced either 'some of the time' or 'most of the time' (US), 'frequently' or 'occasionally' (Germany), or which bothered her 'pretty much' or 'very much' (Norway).

Table 5.3 Overview of health outcome variables

Variable	Type	Description	Operationalization		
			US	Germany	Norway
Self-assessed health	Dependent	Dichotomous	0 = Excellent, very good, or good	0 = Very good (1), (2), (3)	0 = Very good, good
			1 = Fair or poor	1 = (4), (5), Very poor (6)	1 = Neither good nor bad, poor, very poor
Mental health complaints	Dependent	Count	Number of symptoms in past *week*, experienced some or most of the time	Number of symptoms in past 12 months, experienced frequently or occasionally	Number of symptoms in past 14 days which were pretty much or very much bothersome

5.3.3 Social Position

Variables on education, employment, personal income, and household income were conceptualized as independent variables of social position for models predicting IPV exposure and health outcomes (See Table 5.4). To aid in the comparison of *education* across the three countries, categorical variables of education were transformed into interval variables using the maximum number of years needed to attain the respondents' completed education. This transformation was rather straightforward for the US and Norwegian data. The German data, however, required the combination of two separate variables on general education and professional education, as well as the consideration of Germany's tiered system of education. The German Socio-Economic Panel Study's (SOEP) documentation on the transformation of German education into number of years completed was used as a guide (SOEP Group 2012, pp. 53–4). Another variable of social position was a dichotomous measure of the respondent's current *employment status*. If a respondent reported working either full- or part-time for pay (regardless of the number of hours), she was classified as employed. In the US data, military service was counted as employment, along with maternity leave in the German data.

As an additional measure of social position, an interval variable was constructed to represent equivalent annual *household income*. Due to variations in how the data were collected, the construction of this variable involved slightly different steps for each country. For the US data, household income was first transformed from a categorical to a continuous variable by assigning each observation to the midpoint

Table 5.4 Overview of social position variables

Variable	Type	Description	Operationalization		
			US	Germany	Norway
Education	Independent	Interval	Years of education completed	Years of general and professional education completed	Years of education completed
Employment	Independent	Dichotomous	0 = Not employed FT/PT	0 = Not employed FT/PT	0 = Not employed FT/PT
			1 = Employed FT/PT (including military service)	1 = Employed FT/PT (including maternity leave)	1 = Employed FT/PT
Household income	Independent	Interval	Equivalent household income, US Dollars	Equivalent household income, Euros	Equivalent household income, Norwegian Kroner
Personal income	Independent	Interval	Equivalent personal income, US Dollars	Equivalent personal income, Euros	Equivalent personal income, Norwegian Kroner

of the known income threshold bounds of each category (e.g., Bhat 1994). Since the needs of a household increase disproportionately with each added household member, the square root equivalence scale was applied, which divides the household income by the square root of the household size to create an equivalent household income (OECD n.d.). Then, household income was scaled down to $1000 increments. The construction of the household income variable for Germany involved the same steps as for the US data, with one notable exception. Since the German survey collected data on monthly income rather than annual, the monthly midpoint income information was multiplied by 12 to generate an annual midpoint household income before the equivalence scale was applied. This annual household equivalent income was then scaled down to €1000 increments. Finally, while the US and German data specifically collected household income information, for the Norwegian data it was necessary to combine both the respondent's and her partner's (if applicable) annual income. This involved establishing midpoints of the income categories and summing them together to create the gross annual household income. The equivalence scale was then applied and this annual household equivalent income was scaled down to increments of 10,000 Norwegian Kroner (NOK).[11] Variables measuring *personal income* followed the same process as described above. It should also be kept in mind that while the US and Norway surveys specifically collected information on income before taxes, the German survey specified income after taxes and social contributions.

5.3.4 Sociodemographic Control Variables

In order to control for their effects on IPV exposure and health outcomes, the following control variables were included in the analysis (see Table 5.5). First was a continuous variable of the respondent's *age* at the time of the survey, because older age is associated with poorer health but less frequent IPV (Bachman and Saltzman 1995; Band-Winterstein and Eisikovits 2009). Second was a dichotomous variable measuring whether a woman was currently *married or in a long-term partnership*, since marriage or partnership is associated with better health (Zheng and Thomas 2013). Also included was the *number of children* under the age of 18 in the household, since this may affect women's decision making in a violent relationship, either creating a stressor within the relationship or an additional form of dependency (DeMaris et al. 2003; Kaukinen 2004; Moxnes 1991). Given alcohol's association with poorer health and IPV exposure (Kaukinen 2004; Tolman and Rosen 2001), a dichotomous variable was included measuring whether the respondent *consumes alcohol* a couple of times per week or more. It should be noted that while the US and German surveys framed the question in terms of the past 12 months, the Norwegian survey did not provide a time frame. A dichotomous

[11]Which was equal to approximately €1376 in 2003 (European Central Bank 2014).

variable was used measuring whether a respondent had experienced *physical or sexual violence as an adult from someone other than a partner* (e.g., a stranger or relative), because this is often related to poorer health outcomes and experiences of partner violence (Casey and Nurius 2005; Scott-Storey 2011).

To take into account the structural prejudices in society, dichotomous variables were included regarding whether the respondent belongs to a *racial or ethnic minority* (for the US) or whether she has a *migration background* (for Germany and Norway) (Bent-Goodley 2007; Loya 2014; Sokoloff and Dupont 2005). In the US, if the respondent was non-white or Hispanic, then for the purposes of the analysis, she belonged to a racial or ethnic minority. In the German and Norwegian data, if the respondent was born outside of the country and both of her parents or caregivers were born outside of the country, then she was considered to have a migration background. Finally, in order to control for the effect of chronic health issues on mental health (Nash and McDermott 2011), a dichotomous measure of *health impairment* was used, looking at whether respondents were healthy enough to carry out their daily activities. Whereas the US and Norwegian surveys presented respondents with a dichotomous yes/no response category, the German survey included a scale of the degree to which respondents felt limited by their health. To transform the German scale into a dichotomous variable, 'very strongly,' 'strongly,' and 'fairly' limited were categorized as having a chronic health impairment, while 'a bit' and 'not at all' limited were categorized as not being impaired by health (e.g., Ahnquist et al. 2012).

5.3.5 Cross-National Data Comparability

In addition to the differences in overall data collection mentioned earlier, it is also worthwhile to make note of the slight differences in operationalization of the variables presented here. Specific attention should be paid to differences in measurement of household and personal income, sexual IPV, injuries due to IPV, and mental health complaints. While the measurement of income in the US and Norwegian surveys concentrated on income before taxes and social contributions, the German survey measured income after taxes and social contributions. Thus, the measurement of income in Germany already takes into account redistribution of resources and it may be expected that the social gradient in income is therefore reduced in the data. It is also important to keep in mind that the measurement of sexual abuse in the US survey is far more explicit than the measurement in the other two surveys, which may lead to a higher prevalence because it increases the likelihood of recalling specific acts (Schröttle et al. 2006). Another important difference is in the measurement of IPV injury, which asks respondents to refer to the *most recent* incidence of IPV in the US and Norwegian surveys, but to *any* incident in the German survey. This may lead to an increased rate of injury in the German data, and thus, may increase the number of respondents categorized as experiencing severe IPV exposure. Finally, the total number of mental health complaints reported

Table 5.5 Overview of sociodemographic control variables

Variable	Type	Description	Operationalization		
			US	Germany	Norway
Age	Control	Interval	Years	Years	Years
Married/partnered	Control	Dichotomous	0 = Not married/partnered	0 = Not married/partnered	0 = Not married/partnered
			1 = Married/partnered	1 = Married/partnered	1 = Married/partnered
Number of children	Control	Count	Number under 18 years in household	Number under 18 years in household	Number under 18 years in household
Frequent alcohol	Control	Dichotomous	0 = <1–2 times/week in *past year*	0 = <2–3 times/week in *past year*	0 = <Couple times/week
			1 = >1–2 times/week in *past year*	1 = >2–3 times/week in *past year*	1 = >Couple times/week
Other violence	Control	Dichotomous	0 = No physical/sexual abuse from non-partner	0 = No physical/sexual abuse from non-partner	0 = No physical/sexual abuse from non-partner
			1 = ≥1 incident physical/sexual abuse from non-partner	1 = ≥1 incident physical/sexual abuse from non-partner	1 = ≥1 incident physical/sexual abuse from non-partner
Racial/ethnic minority or migration background	Control	Dichotomous	0 = White or non-Hispanic	0 = No migration background	0 = No migration background
			1 = Non-white or Hispanic	1 = Respondents and parents born in another country	1 = Respondents and parents born in another country
Health impairment	Control	Dichotomous	0 = Health does not interfere with daily activities	0 = A bit or not at all limited by chronic illness or physical disability	0 = Mostly healthy enough to carry out daily tasks
			1 = Health interferes with daily activities	1 = Very strongly, strongly or fairly limited by a chronic illness or physical disability	1 = Generally not able to carry out daily tasks

by respondents in the US data refers to the previous week, while the Norwegian data refers to the previous 2 weeks, and the German data refers to the previous year. Thus, the simple counts of mental health complaints are not directly comparable across data sets. In sum, all of these differences, along with the differences in data collection, prevent a direct statistical comparison of the three surveys. However, the careful harmonization of the data does facilitate analysis of IPV exposure and health outcomes within each data set, producing specific national patterns of relationships between the variables. Thus, cross-national comparison rather takes place through the examination of these patterns in relation to the various policy contexts of the three countries.

5.4 Methods

This section reviews the analytical methods applied in this book. It begins with an overview of techniques used to cope with missing data, followed by a description of the univariate, bivariate, and multivariate statistical analyses. Stata 12 software was used to conduct all of the statistical analyses described (StataCorp 2011). The section ends with a description of the cross-national comparison.

5.4.1 Missing Data

Before beginning the analyses, individuals with missing data were excluded in order to ensure consistent sample sizes when comparing various models. However, in order to retain as many of the individuals as possible, values for non-IPV variables with extensive missing data were imputed.[12] This resulted in imputation of values for personal and household income for the US and Germany data, but not for Norway, due to its low level of missing data for non-IPV variables. For the imputations, a single imputation using predictive mean matching (PMM) was performed, taking into account the categorical nature of IPV exposure as a moderating variable by performing imputations for each level of IPV exposure separately (SSCC 2012a). PMM is a stochastic regression technique which replaces a "missing value with the value from a respondent whose regression-predicted score is closest to the regression-predicted score of the respondent for whom the value is missing" (Landerman et al. 1997, p. 4). The advantage of PMM over mean imputation or deterministic regression imputation is an improved standard error estimation and a more accurate distribution in the case that the imputed variable is

[12]The necessity of accounting for different levels of IPV exposure in the imputation models (due to its role as a moderator) created difficulties with imputing missing values for IPV-related variables. Thus, missing values for IPV-related variables were not imputed.

nonnormal (Landerman et al. 1997; SSCC 2012a; White et al. 2011). Before using the imputed values, graphs of kernal density estimates and distributions were used to determine whether the imputed data resembled the original data in overall distribution (SSCC 2012b). After these checks, the imputed values were used to replace the missing values in the dataset.

5.4.2 Univariate Analyses

The purpose of the univariate, or descriptive, analyses is to provide a brief overview of the study samples for each country in the context of the variables under examination. The mean and standard deviations of each of the variables were calculated, along with the minimum and maximum values. This offers insight into the central tendency of the variables and measures dispersion (Park 2008). The results of these analyses are presented in Chap. 6.

Since many statistical tests assume that interval variables are normally distributed, it was also important to test this assumption in order to avoid inaccurate interpretation of results. To begin, histograms were run to provide a visual picture of the distribution of the variables. This was then followed by a combination of statistical tests of normality. This included the Shapiro–Wilk for testing normality in sample sizes between 7 and 2000 (Shapiro and Wilk 1965) and the Shapiro–Francia test, which is a modification of the Shapiro–Wilk and is appropriate for sample sizes ranging from 5 to 5000 (Shapiro and Francia 1972). Finally, since the previous tests tend to reject the null hypothesis when the sample size becomes large (Park 2008), the Skewness–Kurtosis test was also used since it is especially appropriate for testing normality in large sample sizes (D'Agostino et al. 1990). The results of these tests revealed that all interval variables (i.e., age, number of children, income levels, years of education, and number of mental health complaints) violated the assumption of normality. This was taken into account in the selection of appropriate bivariate and multivariate analyses.

5.4.3 Bivariate Analyses

The next step of the analysis measures the relationship between the variables of interest for each country (see Chap. 6 for results). This was done using correlation techniques where the degree and the direction of the relationship was measured on a scale of −1 to +1, where −1 indicates a perfect negative correlation and +1 indicates a perfect positive correlation. The closer the correlation measure comes to either end point, the stronger the relationship between the two variables (Howell 2007). Further tests of independence were conducted to determine whether the variables are indeed dependent upon one another.

The appropriate measures of correlation and tests of independence varied according to the type of variables assessed (see Table 5.6). The Pearson Product-Moment Correlation (r) is a common measure of correlation assessing the proportion of variation that can be explained. Pearson's r is generally used when both variables are interval and where assumptions of normality can be made (Howell 2007). However, in cases of nonnormality, it can also be cautiously used as long as the sample is large enough (e.g., Bishara and Hittner 2012; Chok 2010). The Spearman Rank Correlation Coefficient (r_s; also known as Spearman's rho) was used to measure correlations between the ordinal variables (i.e., IPV exposure) and interval variables (i.e., age, number of children, income levels, years of education, and number of mental health complaints). It is effectively a form of Pearson's r which converts the data to rankings. The Point-Biserial Correlation (r_{pb}) was applied to measure the relationship between interval variables and dichotomous variables (i.e., employment, partnership status, minority/migration background, alcohol consumption, other violence, health impairments, and self-assessed health). Finally, Cramer's V was calculated to measure the correlation between dichotomous variables, as well as between dichotomous variables and ordinal variables. It is important to keep in mind, however, that Cramer's V varies only between 0 and 1, and therefore no conclusions about the direction of the correlation can be drawn (Agresti 1984). In order to understand the effect sizes of the correlation coefficients, Cohen's (1988, 1992) recommendations were applied: 0.1 represents a 'small' effect size, 0.3 represents a 'medium' effect size, and 0.5 represents a 'large' effect size. According to Cohen, a small effect is nontrivial, but requires careful study to be able to discern with the "naked eye," whereas as a large effect would be clearly discernible.

Three different tests of independence were applied to the correlations. First, given that the univariate analyses indicated that all interval variables violated the assumption of normality, the Kruskal–Wallis test was applied for non-parametric data to test independence between interval variables. This test assesses whether

Table 5.6 Overview of correlation measures and tests of independence

	Interval	Ordinal	Dichotomous
Interval	Pearson product moment correlation (r)/Kruskal–Wallis test	Spearman rank correlation coefficient (r_s)/Kruskal–Wallis test	Point biserial correlation (r_{pb})/t-test
Ordinal	–	Spearman rank correlation coefficient (r_s)/Kruskal–Wallis test[a]	Cramer's V/Chi-square (χ^2)
Dichotomous	–	–	Cramer's V/Chi-square (χ^2)

Adapted from Bortz and Döring (2006), Brzank (2012) and Rasch et al. (2010)

[a]Although the information for ordinal-ordinal is provided, no ordinal-ordinal correlations were necessary for the analysis

samples originate from the same distribution (Kruskal and Wallis 1952), and it was also applied to the correlations between ordinal and interval variables. Second, assessing the independence between dichotomous variables and interval variables, the independent samples *t*-test was applied. Finally, the chi-square (χ^2) test was used to test the independence between dichotomous variables and between dichotomous and ordinal variables. In order to determine whether the null hypothesis could be rejected for these tests of independence, a significance level of $p < 0.05$ and a confidence interval of 95 % were applied.

5.4.4 *Multivariate Analyses*

Building on the bivariate analyses, the next stage of analysis called for assessing the relationship between the dependent variables (i.e., IPV exposure, self-assessed health, mental health complaints) and independent variables. This was done using multiple regression models. A simple linear regression describes the relationship between one dependent variable and one independent variable using a straight line, whereas a multiple linear regression model incorporates multiple independent variables (Kohler and Kreuter 2009). In essence, the dependent variable is predicted on the basis of the independent variable(s) (Howell 2007). In this case, the regression coefficients represent the average change in the dependent variable, given a one-unit change in the independent variable. However, regression models predicting categorical, dichotomous, or count dependent variables require slightly different approaches. These approaches are explored in Sects. 5.4.4.1 and 5.4.4.2, arranged by research question.

5.4.4.1 Predicting Social Position's Impact on IPV Exposure

The first research question (RQ1) explored in this book asks to what extent social position impacts IPV exposure. This required fitting a multiple regression model separately for each data set predicting IPV exposure based on the independent variables of social position (i.e., income, education, employment) while correcting for the influence of the control variables (i.e., age, marital/partnership status, number of children, minority/migration background, alcohol consumption, other violence, health impairment) (see Chap. 7 for results). Given that the dependent variable of IPV exposure is a categorical measure, it was necessary to choose a non-linear regression model. Ordinal logistic regression models can be used with categorical dependent variables as long as it can be assumed that the relationship between every pair of outcome groups is the same (i.e., the proportional odds or parallel regression assumption) (UCLA: Statistical Consulting Group 2014a; Williams 2006). However, since this assumption could not be made for the categories of 'no IPV exposure,','minor IPV exposure', and 'severe IPV exposure,' a multinomial logit regression model was fitted instead, which does not assume any order in the categories. In this type of model, one is "essentially [simultaneously] estimating a separate binary logit for each pair of outcome categories," while imposing the necessary constraints on the coefficients (Long and Freese 2006, p. 223). In other words, the probability for every value of the dependent variable is predicted (Kohler and Kreuter 2009).

The coefficients in the multinomial model indicate the effect of the independent variables on each category of the dependent variable relative to the specified base category. Thus, 'no IPV exposure' was specified as the base category, so as to measure the effect of the independent variables on 'minor IPV exposure' in comparison to 'no IPV exposure', and 'severe IPV exposure' in comparison to 'no IPV exposure'. To measure the effect of 'minor IPV exposure' in comparison to 'severe IPV exposure,' an additional model was specified with 'minor IPV exposure' as the base category. Relative risk ratios were calculated to aid in the interpretation of the regression coefficients. These ratios represent "the probability of choosing one outcome category over the probability of choosing the baseline category" given a one-unit change in the independent variable (UCLA: Statistical Consulting Group 2014b).

Additionally, using a significance level of $p < 0.05$ and a confidence interval of 95 %, the null hypothesis that all coefficients related to each independent variable were simultaneously equal to zero was tested using the Wald statistic. In essence, the Wald statistic assessed the significance of the overall effects of each independent variable across the different categories of IPV exposure (Long and Freese 2006). A nonsignificant result would imply that removing the independent variable from the model would not alter the fit of the model. Moreover, using a significance level of $p < 0.05$ and a confidence interval of 95 %, the log likelihood ratio (LR) chi-squared test was used to compare the log likelihood of the full model to the intercept model. This "investigate[d] the hypothesis that the independent variables have no explanatory power or, equivalently, that all the coefficients other than the constant are all zero" (Kohler and Kreuter 2009, p. 268).

Finally, to illustrate results, predicted probabilities were calculated using the *margins* command and then graphed using the *marginsplot* command available in Stata 12. This provided the average predicted probabilities of either 'minor IPV exposure' or 'severe IPV exposure' as compared to 'no IPV exposure' for different values of the independent variables (i.e., income, education, employment) holding all other variables at their means (UCLA: Statistical Consulting Group 2014b). Graphically, the predicted probabilities of 'minor IPV exposure' and 'severe IPV exposure' were plotted against the independent variables of interest.

5.4.4.2 Predicting Social Position's Impact on Health: IPV Exposure as a Moderator

The second research question (RQ2) explored in this book is whether women with IPV exposure are more vulnerable to social position's impact on health outcomes. Another way of stating the same question is: does the impact of social position on health outcomes vary by level of IPV exposure? Statistically speaking, the question posed is one of the moderating effects of IPV exposure on the relationship between social position and health. "Questions involving moderators address 'when' or 'for whom' a variable most strongly predicts or causes an outcome variable" (Frazier et al. 2004, p. 116), so that the moderator alters the strength of the relationship between the independent and dependent variable (Baron and Kenny 1986). Moderating effects can be examined using multiple regression models that include interaction terms, where the effect of the independent variable (i.e., income, education, employment) on the dependent variable (i.e., self-assessed health, mental health complaints) is dependent upon the level of the moderating variable (i.e., 'no IPV exposure,' 'minor IPV exposure,' 'severe IPV exposure') (Jaccard 2001). Using the conceptual framework described in Chap. 3 as a theoretical guide, the aim was to test an "enhancing interaction" between social position and IPV exposure, where both social position and IPV exposure impact health outcomes in the same direction and "together have a stronger than additive effect" (Frazier et al. 2004, p. 117). The moderating effect of IPV exposure was tested for a dichotomous measure of self-assessed health and a count measure of mental health complaints, which necessitated two different types of regression models (see Chap. 8 for results).

For the dichotomous measure of self-assessed health, a logistic regression model was fit for each of the data sets, which allowed for the examination of how social position and IPV exposure affected the probability of a rating of poor self-assessed health. Given, the nonlinearity of logistic models, "the magnitude of the change in outcome probability that is associated with a given change in one of the independent variables depends on the levels of *all* of the independent variables" (Long and Freese 2006, p. 131, emphasis added). In other words, the coefficients in the logistic regression models indicate the logarithmic odds of poor self-assessed health given a one-unit increase in the social position or IPV exposure variables. Since this is challenging to understand in practical terms, odds ratios were calculated to aid in the interpretation of the regression coefficients. Odds ratios represent "the odds that an outcome will occur given a particular exposure, compared to the odds of the outcome occurring in the absence of that exposure" (Szumilas 2010, p. 227). Thus, the odds ratios indicate that for a unit change in social position or IPV exposure, the odds of poor self-assessed health are expected to change by a certain factor, while holding all other variables constant. The multiplicative nature of odds ratios is worth noting: positive effects are indicated by factors greater than one, while negative effects are indicated by factors between zero and one (Long and Freese 2006).

For the count variable of mental health complaints, a negative binomial regression model was fit for each data set. Although it is not uncommon to fit linear regression models for count variables (i.e., variables which count how many things there are, or how many times something has happened), this has the potential to lead to "inefficient, inconsistent, and biased estimates" (Long and Freese 2006, p. 349). Thus, Poisson regressions are often used as an alternative for modeling count outcomes, but in cases where the conditional variance of the outcome variable exceeds the conditional mean, the negative binomial regression is more appropriate because it includes a parameter which reflects the over-dispersion in the outcome variable (UCLA:

Statistical Consulting Group 2014c). As a result, the confidence intervals are narrower for the negative binomial regression as compared to those in a Poisson regression model. Analysis of the means and variance of the count of mental health complaints indicated that it was indeed overdispersed, thus leading to the decision to fit negative binomial regression models to predict mental health complaints.[13] The regression coefficients from these models indicate by how much the log count of mental health complaints is expected to change for each one-unit increase in the independent variable. In order to make the results easier to comprehend, incident rate ratios were calculated, which reflect the factor change in the expected count of mental health complaints given a one-unit change in the independent variable, while holding all other variables constant (Long and Freese 2006).

The first steps in building the regression models testing IPV exposure as a moderator involved centering the independent variables measured on an interval scale (i.e., income and education) and creating the interaction terms. The centering of interval variables has a number of advantages, especially when incorporating interaction terms in statistical models (Kohler and Kreuter 2009). Firstly, centering reduces the issue of multicollinearity caused by the high correlation of the independent and moderating variables with the interaction terms (Frazier et al. 2004). Secondly, centering simplifies the interpretation of the interactions between social position and IPV exposure. When interaction terms are included in regression models, the coefficients predicting the outcome according to the independent variables or the moderating variable are interpreted as conditional effects rather than main effects (Jaccard 2001). In other words, the coefficient represents the relationship when other variables in the model are held at zero. Thus, centering the interval variables involved in the interaction provides a meaningful zero point (e.g., the median of the interval variable) to aid in the interpretation. Finally, it also aids in the later comparison of results across the US, Germany, and Norway. These are the reasons for centering the variables for education and income. For education, this involved subtracting the number of years required to complete a high school education (for the US and Norway) or the median number of years of education completed (for Germany) from the number of years of education attained for each individual. In the same way, household income was also centered on the median.[14] Along with the dichotomous variable of employment, these centered independent variables were then each separately multiplied with the moderator of IPV exposure. Since IPV exposure consisted of three categorical levels, a total of six interaction terms were created: household income * minor IPV, household income * severe IPV, education * minor IPV, education * severe IPV, employment * minor IPV, employment * severe IPV.

Following the construction of the interaction terms, a series of nested regression models were fit for both health outcomes, separately for each data set. It is

[13]The over-dispersion, however, was not caused by an excess of zeros in the count of mental health complaints. If it would have been, then a zero-inflated model would have been more appropriate.

[14]Based on the results of the bivariate analyses (see Chap. 6), it was determined to eliminate personal income from the regression models and retain household income. Therefore, it is not included in the following explanations.

important to first add the independent and moderating variables into the model before the interaction terms, making sure that all variables contributing to the interaction terms are included, so as to avoid confounding the moderator effect with that of the independent and moderating variables (Frazier et al. 2004). Thus, the first three regression models fit were: a model with only social position as the independent variables (Model 1); a model adding IPV exposure as a categorical variable (Model 2); and a model incorporating the control variables (Model 3). The next step was to add the interaction terms, evaluating them individually with separate models.[15] This resulted in three additional models, including: the addition of the interactions between household income and IPV exposure (Model 4); a model replacing the previous interaction with the interactions between education and IPV exposure (Model 5); and a model replacing the previous interaction with the interactions between employment and IPV exposure (Model 6).

Given that the measure of IPV exposure was measured categorically, the overall contribution of all levels of IPV exposure to Models 2 and 3 was tested using the Wald statistic as an omnibus test with a significance level of $p < 0.05$. Furthermore, since at least two interactions were needed in Models 4–6 to represent IPV exposure as a categorical variable, the same omnibus test was also used to assess the overall contribution of the moderating effect.

Additionally, in order to compare the models against one another, several goodness of fit measures were considered using the Stata user-written post-estimation command *fitstat* (Long and Freese 2000). First was the LR chi-squared test described in Sect. 5.4.4.1. Second was McFadden's pseudo R-squared measure. Several different pseudo R-squared measures exist, none of which are equivalent to the R-squared calculated in linear regression models (Kohler and Kreuter 2009), and none of which can be compared across data sets or interpreted out of context (UCLA: Statistical Consulting Group 2014d). However, when comparing pseudo R-squareds of the same type, they are useful for looking at differences across models measuring the same outcome with the same data set. McFadden's R-squared is the most commonly used pseudo R-squared and is a comparison of the log likelihood of the intercept model to that of the full model, essentially measuring the improvement of the model using all parameters over that of the intercept model (Long and Freese 2006). When comparing McFadden's R-squared across models, a higher result indicates better model fit (Kohler and Kreuter 2009).

Finally, as another means of comparing nested models, the Bayesian information criterion (BIC') was applied, which is based on the LR chi-squared with degrees of freedom equal to the number of regressors (Long and Freese 2006; Raftery 1995). Essentially, the smaller or more negative the BIC' measure, the better the model fit.

[15] Ideally, when examining multiple moderating effects, all interactions should be added to the model at the same time and an omnibus F test should be used test the overall variance explained (Cohen et al. 2003; Frazier et al. 2004). This step was conducted for all regression models predicting health outcomes in all three data sets, but the omnibus tests were not significant. Therefore, it was decided to also test the interaction terms in separate models.

In assessing the strength of the evidence preferring one model over the other, the following suggested guidelines were applied: an absolute difference of 0–2 is 'weak', 2–6 is 'positive', 6–10 is 'strong', and greater than 10 is 'very strong' evidence (Raftery 1995). However, when using these goodness of fit measures, Long and Freese (2006) caution that "there is no convincing evidence that selecting a model that maximizes the value of a given measure of fit results in a model that is optimal in any sense other than the models having a larger value of that measure" (p. 154). In other words, these goodness of fit measures should be used as only one method of evaluation.

Finally, similar to the analysis of the previous research question, predicted probabilities were calculated and graphed for Model 3 and for any significant interaction effects found in Models 4–6. The graphs depict the average predicted probabilities of either poor self-assessed health or predicted count of mental health complaints at each level of IPV exposure for different values of social position, holding all other variables at their means.

5.4.5 *Cross-National Comparison*

The final step in the analysis was the cross-national comparison of the quantitative results in order to answer the questions of whether social position's impact on IPV exposure is reflective of policies enabling women to establish independent households (RQ3), and whether social position's impact on health among IPV survivors is reflective of policies addressing access to health care (RQ4). Given the differences in data collection and methodology present in the three national data sets, a direct statistical comparison would not be wise. Thus, in order to gain an understanding of the macro-level policy factors potentially influencing differential exposure to IPV and differential vulnerability to poor health, a structured examination of the distinct patterns present in the three sets of empirical results was undertaken. A comprehensive policy and literature review was the basis of the case descriptions presented in Chap. 4, detailing the national policy contexts which may potentially influence women's abilities to establish independent households and their access the health care. The review was informed by a number of different sources: governmental reports and documents, reports from NGOs, OECD and WHO data and reports, academic policy databases, as well as peer-reviewed academic research. In reflecting upon the different patterns revealed by the empirical results, these case descriptions serve as the foundation for a structured discussion of the potential policy entry points addressing the proposed mechanisms involved in the generation of health inequities. This discussion is found in Chap. 9.

References

Agresti, A. (1984). *Analysis of ordinal categorical data.* New York, NY: Wiley.

Ahnquist, J., Wamala, S. P., & Lindstrom, M. (2012). Social determinants of health—A question of social or economic capital? Interaction effects of socioeconomic factors on health outcomes. *Social Science and Medicine, 74*(6), 930–939. doi:10.1016/j.socscimed.2011.11.026

Au, N., & Johnston, D. W. (2014). Self-assessed health: What does it mean and what does it hide? *Social Science and Medicine, 121C*, 21–28. doi:10.1016/j.socscimed.2014.10.007

Bachman, R., & Saltzman, L. E. (1995). *Violence against women: Estimates from the redesigned survey.* Washington, DC: U.S. Department of Justice.

Band-Winterstein, T., & Eisikovits, Z. (2009). "Aging out" of violence: The multiple faces of intimate violence over the life span. *Qualitative Health Research, 19*(2), 164–180. doi:10.1177/1049732308329305

Baron, R. M., & Kenny, D. A. (1986). The moderator-mediator variable distinction in social psychological research: Conceptual, strategic, and statistical considerations. *Journal of Personality and Social Psychology, 51*(6), 1173–1182.

Bent-Goodley, T. B. (2007). Health disparities and violence against women: Why and how cultural and societal influences matter. *Trauma, Violence, and Abuse, 8*(2), 90–104. doi:10.1177/1524838007301160

Bhat, C. (1994). Imputing a continuous income variable from grouped and missing income observations. *Economics Letters, 46*(4), 311–319. doi:10.1016/0165-1765(94)90151-1

Bishara, A. J., & Hittner, J. B. (2012). Testing the significance of a correlation with nonnormal data: Comparison of Pearson, Spearman, transformation, and resampling approaches. *Psychological Methods, 17*(3), 399–417. doi:10.1037/a0028087

Black, M. C., Basile, K. C., Breiding, M. J., Smith, S. G., Walters, M. L., Merrick, M. T., et al. (2011). *The National Intimate Partner and Sexual Violence Survey (NISVS): 2010 summary report.* Atlanta, GA: CDC.

Bortz, J., & Döring, N. (2006). Hypothesenprüfende Untersuchungen [Hypotheses proving tests]. In *Forschungsmethoden und Evaluation: für Human- und Sozialwissenschaftler* (pp. 489–598). Berlin, Heidelberg: Springer. doi:10.1007/978-3-540-33306-7

Brzank, P. (2012). *Wege aus der Partnergewalt. Frauen auf der Suche nach Hilfe [Escaping partner violence: Women seeking help].* Wiesbaden: Springer VS.

Casey, E. A., & Nurius, P. S. (2005). Trauma exposure and sexual revictimization risk: Comparisons across single, multiple incident, and multiple perpetrator victimizations. *Violence Against Women, 11*(4), 505–530. doi:10.1177/1077801204274339

Chok, N. S. (2010). Pearson's versus Spearman's and Kendall's correlation coefficients for continuous data. http://d-scholarship.pitt.edu/8056/1/Chokns_etd2010.pdf. Accessed July 24, 2013.

Cohen, J. (1988). The analysis of variance. In *Statistical power for the social sciences* (2nd ed., pp. 273–406). Hillsdale, NJ: Lawrence Elbaum Associates.

Cohen, J. (1992). A power primer. *Psychological Bulletin, 112*(1), 155–159.

Cohen, J., Cohen, P., West, S. G., & Aiken, L. S. (2003). *Applied multiple regression/correlation analysis for the behavioral sciences* (3rd ed.). Mahwah, NJ: Erlbaum.

D'Agostino, R. B., Belanger, A., & D'Agostino, R. B, Jr. (1990). A suggestion for using powerful and informative tests of normality. *American Statistician, 44*(4), 316–321.

De Bruin, A., Picavet, H. S. J., & Nossikov, A. (1996). *Health interview surveys: Towards international harmonization of methods and instruments.* Copenhagen: World Health Organization.

DeMaris, A., Benson, M. L., Fox, G. L., Hill, T., & Van Wyk, J. (2003). Distal and proximal factors in domestic violence: A test of an integrated model. *Journal of Marriage and Family, 65*(3), 652–667. doi:10.1111/j.1741-3737.2003.00652.x

Derogatis, L. R., Lipman, R. S., Rickels, K., Uhlenhuth, E. H., & Covi, L. (1974). The Hopkins Symptom Checklist (HSCL): A self-report symptom inventory. *Behavioral Science, 19*, 1–15.

Dillon, G., Hussain, R., Loxton, D., & Rahman, S. (2013). Mental and physical health and intimate partner violence against women: A review of the literature. *International Journal of Family Medicine*, 1–15. doi:10.1155/2013/313909

European Central Bank. (2014). Euro foreign exchange reference rates. https://www.ecb.europa.eu/stats/exchange/eurofxref/html/eurofxref-graph-nok.en.html. Accessed July 19, 2014.

European Union Agency for Fundamental Rights [FRA]. (2014). *Violence against women: An EU-wide survey*. Luxembourg. http://fra.europa.eu/sites/default/files/fra-2014-vaw-survey-main-results_en.pdf. Accessed November 01, 2014.

Flåte, S. (2004). *Undersøkelse om trygghet i hverdagen: dokumentasjonsrapport [Survey of Everyday Safety: Documentation report]*. Oslo, Norway: Statistics Norway.

Follingstad, D. R. (2009). The impact of psychological aggression on women's mental health and behavior: The status of the field. *Trauma, Violence, and Abuse, 10*(3), 271–289. doi:10.1177/1524838009334453

Follingstad, D. R., Coker, A. L., Lee, E., Williams, C. M., Bush, H. M., & Mendiondo, M. M. (2015). Validity and psychometric properties of the measure of psychologically abusive behaviors among young women and women in distressed relationships. *Violence Against Women, 21*(7), 875–896. doi:10.1177/1077801215584070

Frazier, P. A., Tix, A. P., & Barron, K. E. (2004). Testing moderator and mediator effects in counseling psychology research. *Journal of Counseling Psychology, 51*(1), 115–134. doi:10.1037/0022-0167.51.1.115

Fredebeul, C., Gilberg, R., Hess, D., Kästner, G., Marwinski, K., & Prussog-Wagner, A. (2004). *Methodenbericht "Lebenssituation, Sicherheit und Gesundheit von Frauen in Deutschland" [Methods report "Health, Well-being and Personal Safety of Women in Germany"]*. Bonn: infas - Institut für angewandte Sozialwissenschaft GmbH.

Haaland, T., Clausen, S., & Schei, B. (2005). *Vold i parforhold - ulike perspektiver: resultater fra den første landsdekkende undersøkelsen i Norge [Violence in relationships - different perspectives: Results of the first nationwide survey in Norway]*. Oslo, Norway: Norwegian Institute of Urban and Regional Research.

Hamby, S. (2014). Intimate partner and sexual violence research: Scientific progress, scientific challenges, and gender. *Trauma, Violence, and Abuse, 15*(3), 149–158. doi:10.1177/1524838014520723

Hamby, S. (2015). A scientific answer to a scientific question: The gender debate on intimate partner violence. *Trauma, Violence, and Abuse, online first*. doi:10.1177/1524838015596963

Heise, L., & García-Moreno, C. (2012). Violence by intimate partners. In E. G. Krug, L. L. Dahlberg, J. A. Mercy, A. B. Zwi, & R. Lozano (Eds.), *World report on violence and health* (pp. 87–121). Geneva: World Health Organization.

Howell, D. (2007). Correlation and regression. In *Statistical methods for psychology* (7th ed., pp. 245–292). Belmont, CA: Cengage Wadsworth.

Idler, E. L., & Benyamini, Y. (1997). Self-rated health and mortality: A review of twenty-seven community studies. *Journal of Health and Social Behavior, 38*, 21–37.

Jaccard, J. (2001). *Interaction effects in logistic regressions*. Thousand Oaks, CA: Sage Publications.

Johnson, H., Ollus, N., & Nevala, S. (2008). *Violence against women: An international perspective*. New York, NY: Springer.

Jylhä, M. (2009). What is self-rated health and why does it predict mortality? Towards a unified conceptual model. *Social Science and Medicine, 69*(3), 307–316. doi:10.1016/j.socscimed.2009.05.013

Kaukinen, C. (2004). Status compatibility, physical violence, and emotional abuse in intimate relationships. *Journal of Marriage and Family, 66*(2), 452–471. doi:10.1111/j.1741-3737.2004.00031.x

Kohler, U., & Kreuter, F. (2009). *Data analysis using Stata* (2nd ed.). College Station, Texas: Stata Press.

Krantz, G., & Garcia-Moreno, C. (2005). Violence against women. *Journal of Epidemiology and Community Health, 59*, 818–821. doi:10.1136/jech.2004.022756

Kruskal, W. H., & Wallis, W. A. (1952). Use of ranks in one-criterion variance analysis. *Journal of the American Statistical Association, 47*(260), 583–621.

Landerman, L. R., Land, K. C., & Pieper, C. F. (1997). An empirical evaluation of the predictive mean matching method for imputing missing values. *Sociological Methods and Research, 26* (1), 3–33. doi:10.1177/0049124197026001001

Long, J. S., & Freese, J. (2000). sg145: Scalar measures of fit for regression models. *Stata Technical Bulletin, 56*, 34–40.

Long, J. S., & Freese, J. (2006). *Regression models for categorical dependent variables using Stata* (2nd ed.). College Station, Texas: Stata Press.

Loya, R. M. (2014). The role of sexual violence in creating and maintaining economic insecurity among asset-poor women of color. *Violence Against Women, 20*(11), 1299–1320. doi:10.1177/1077801214552912

Maiuro, R. D. (2001). Sticks and stones may break my bones, but names will also hurt me: Psychological abuse in domestically violent relationships. In K. D. O'Leary & R. D. Maiuro (Eds.), *Psychological abuse in violent domestic relations* (pp. ix–xx). New York, NY: Springer.

Manor, O., Matthews, S., & Power, C. (2000). Dichotomous or categorical response? Analysing self-rated health and lifetime social class. *International Journal of Epidemiology, 29*, 149–157. doi:10.1093/ije/29.1.149

Moxnes, K. (1991). *Kjernesprengning i familien? Familieforandring ved samlivsbrudd og dannelse av nye samliv [Destroying the core of the family? Family change during breakups and the formation of new relationships]*. Oslo, Norway: Universitetsforlaget.

Müller, U., & Schröttle, M. (2004). *Lebenssituation, Sicherheit und Gesundheit von Frauen in Deutschland: Eine repräsentative Untersuchung zu Gewalt gegen Frauen in Deutschland [Health, well-being and personal safety of women in Germany: A representative study of violence against women in Germany]*. Berlin: Bundesministerium für Familie, Senioren, Frauen und Jugend.

Müller, U., & Schröttle, M. (2005). *Lebenssituation, Sicherheit und Gesundheit von Frauen in Deutschland (Gewalt gegen Frauen - Zusatzbefragung) [Health, Well-being and Personal Safety of Women in Germany (Violence Against Women—Supplemental Survey)] (Version 1.0.0) [Data set]*. Cologne: GESIS Datenarchiv. doi:10.4232/1.4194

Nash, M., & McDermott, J. (2011). Mental health and long-term conditions 2: Managing depression. *Nursing Times, 107*, 21–23.

Nicolaidis, C., & Paranjape, A. (2009). Defining intimate partner violence: Controversies and implications. In C. Mitchell & D. Anglin (Eds.), *Intimate partner violence: A health-based perspective* (pp. 19–30). New York, NY: Oxford University Press.

OECD. (n.d.). *What are equivalence scales? Project on income distribution and poverty*. http://www.oecd.org/els/soc/OECD-Note-EquivalenceScales.pdf. Accessed December 05, 2011.

Park, H. M. (2008). *Univariate analysis and normality tests using SAS, Stata, and SPSS*. http://www.indiana.edu/~statmath/stat/all/normality/index.html. Accessed May 21, 2013.

Power, C., Manor, O., & Fox, A. J. (1991). *Health and class: The early years*. London: Chapman and Hall.

Raftery, A. E. (1995). Bayesian model selection in social research. *Sociological Methodology, 25*, 111–163.

Rasch, B., Hofmann, W., Friese, M., & Naumann, E. (2010). Merkmalszusammenhänge [Correlations]. In *Quantitative Methoden: Einführung in die Statistik für Psychologen und Sozialwissenschaftler* (pp. 119–171). Berlin, Heidelberg: Springer. doi:10.1007/978-3-642-05272-9

Schröttle, M., Martinez, M., Condon, S., Jaspard, M., Piispa, M., Westerstrand, J., et al. (2006). *Comparative reanalysis of prevalence of violence against women and health impact data in Europe—Obstacles and possible solutions. Testing a comparative approach on selected studies*. http://www.cahrv.uni-osnabrueck.de/reddot/D_20_Comparative_reanalysis_of_prevalence_of_violence_pub.pdf. Accessed November 11, 2010.

Scott-Storey, K. (2011). Cumulative abuse: Do things add up? An evaluation of the conceptualization, operationalization, and methodological approaches in the study of the phenomenon of cumulative abuse. *Trauma, Violence, and Abuse, 12*(3), 135–150. doi:10.1177/1524838011404253

Shapiro, S. S., & Francia, R. S. (1972). An approximate analysis of variance test for normality. *Journal of the American Statistical Association, 67*(337), 215–216.

Shapiro, S. S., & Wilk, M. B. (1965). An analysis of variance test for normality (complete samples). *Biometrika, 52*(3/4), 591–611.

SOEP Group. (2012). *SOEP 2011—Documentation of person-related status and generated variables in PGEN for SOEP v28* (No. 111). Berlin. http://panel.gsoep.de/soep-docs/surveypapers/diw_ssp0111.pdf. Accessed February 15, 2012.

Sokoloff, N. J., & Dupont, I. (2005). Domestic violence at the intersections of race, class, and gender: Challenges and contributions to understanding violence against marginalized women in diverse communities. *Violence Against Women, 11*(1), 38–64. doi:10.1177/1077801204271476

SSB. (2003). *Survey of everyday safety, 2003 (second NSD edition) [Data set]*. http://www.nsd.uib.no/. Accessed February 02, 2012.

SSCC. (2012a). *Multiple imputation in Stata: Creating imputation models*. http://www.ssc.wisc.edu/sscc/pubs/stata_mi_models.htm. Accessed May 12, 2012.

SSCC. (2012b). *Multiple imputation in Stata: Imputing*. http://www.ssc.wisc.edu/sscc/pubs/stata_mi_impute.htm. Accessed May 12, 2012.

StataCorp. (2011). *Stata statistical software: Release 12*. College Station, Texas: StataCorp LP.

Straus, M. A. (1979). Measuring intrafamily conflict and violence: The Conflict Tactics (CT) Scales. *Journal of Marriage and Family, 41*, 75–88.

Straus, M. A. (2001). *Scoring the CTS2 and CTSPC*. Durham, NH: University of New Hampshire, Family Research Laboratory.

Straus, M. A., Hamby, S. L., Boney-McCoy, S., & Sugarman, D. B. (1996). The Revised Conflict Tactics Scales (CTS2): Development and preliminary psychometric data. *Journal of Family Issues, 17*, 283–316. doi:10.1177/019251396017003001

Szumilas, M. (2010). Explaining odds ratios. *Journal of the Canadian Academy of Child and Adolescent Psychiatry, 19*(3), 227–229.

Tjaden, P., & Thoennes, N. (1999). *Violence and threats of violence against women and men in the United States, 1994–1996 (First ICPSR version) [Data set]*. doi:10.3886/ICPSR02566.v1

Tjaden, P., & Thoennes, N. (2000). *Extent, nature, and consequences of intimate partner violence: Findings from the National Violence Against Women Survey*. Washington, DC: U.S. Department of Justice.

Tolman, R. M., & Rosen, D. (2001). Domestic violence in the lives of women receiving welfare: Mental health, substance dependence, and economic well-being. *Violence Against Women, 7*(2), 141–158. doi:10.1177/10778012010070020003

UCLA: Statistical Consulting Group. (2014a). *Ordered logistic regression*. http://www.ats.ucla.edu/stat/stata/dae/ologit.htm. Accessed May 06, 2014.

UCLA: Statistical Consulting Group. (2014b). *Multinomial logistic regression*. http://www.ats.ucla.edu/stat/stata/dae/mlogit.htm. Accessed May 06, 2014.

UCLA: Statistical Consulting Group. (2014c). *Negative binomial regression*. http://www.ats.ucla.edu/stat/stata/dae/nbreg.htm. Accessed May 06, 2014.

UCLA: Statistical Consulting Group. (2014d). *What are pseudo R-squareds?* http://www.ats.ucla.edu/stat/mult_pkg/faq/general/Psuedo_RSquareds.htm. Accessed May 06, 2014.

Van Doorslaer, E., & Gerdtham, U. G. (2003). Does inequality in self-assessed health predict inequality in survival by income? Evidence from Swedish data. *Social Science and Medicine, 57*, 1621–1629. doi:10.1016/S0277-9536(02)00559-2

Ware, J. E., Snow, K. K., Kosinski, M., & Gandek, B. (1993). *SF-36® Health Survey manual and interpretation guide*. Boston: New England Medical Center, The Health Institute.

White, I. R., Royston, P., & Wood, A. M. (2011). Multiple imputation using chained equations: Issues and guidance for practice. *Statistics in Medicine, 30*(4), 377–399. doi:10.1002/sim.4067

WHO. (2001). *Putting women's safety first: Ethical and safety recommendations for research on domestic violence against women*. Geneva: World Health Organization.

WHO. (2005). *WHO multi-country study on women's health and domestic violence against women: Initial results on prevalence, health outcomes and women's responses*. Geneva: World Health Organization.

Williams, R. (2006). Generalized ordered logit/partial proportional odds models for ordinal dependent variables. *The Stata Journal, 6*(1), 58–82.

Winstok, Z. (2015). Critical review of Hamby's (2014) article titled "Intimate partner and sexual violence research, scientific progress, scientific challenges, and gender". *Trauma, Violence, and Abuse, online first.* doi:10.1177/1524838015596962

Zheng, H., & Thomas, P. A. (2013). Marital status, self-rated health, and mortality: Overestimation of health or diminishing protection of marriage? *Journal of Health and Social Behavior, 54*(1), 128–143. doi:10.1177/0022146512470564

Chapter 6
First Insights into the Relationships Between Social Position, IPV Exposure, and Health Outcomes

Abstract This chapter begins a series of three which present the quantitative analyses with the *National Violence Against Women Survey* (1995–96) in the US, the *Health, Well-being, and Safety of Women in Germany* survey (2003–04), and the *Survey of Everyday Safety* in Norway (2003–04). To begin, the chapter provides a descriptive overview of the US, German, and Norwegian samples based on the variables of interest. Following this are the results of the bivariate analyses determining the initial relationships and their significance between social position, IPV exposure, health outcomes, and the sociodemographic control variables. These analyses offer a clearer picture of the composition of each of the samples and provide the first clues toward answering this book's research questions. The chapter concludes with a brief summary of the key similarities and differences across countries and the remaining puzzles to be solved by the multiple regression analyses in Chaps. 7 and 8.

This chapter begins a series of three which present the quantitative analyses answering the first two research questions with the *National Violence Against Women Survey* in the US, the *Health, Well-being, and Safety of Women in Germany* survey, and the *Survey of Everyday Safety* in Norway. To begin, the chapter provides a descriptive overview of the US, German, and Norwegian samples based on the variables of interest. Following this are the results of the bivariate analyses determining the initial relationships between social position, IPV exposure, health outcomes, and the control variables. These analyses offer a clearer picture of the composition of each of the samples and provide the first clues toward answering the research questions. The chapter concludes with a brief summary of the key similarities and differences and the remaining puzzles to be solved by the multiple regression analyses in Chaps. 7 and 8.

© Springer International Publishing Switzerland 2016
M.M. Larsen, *Health Inequities Related to Intimate Partner Violence Against Women*, Social Disparities in Health and Health Care,
DOI 10.1007/978-3-319-29565-7_6

6.1 Study Samples

As mentioned in Chap. 5, the study samples were limited to women who had either not experienced IPV at all, or who had experienced it within the previous 5 years. This was to minimize the time between the respondents' social position at the time of the survey and the time of their last IPV incident, in order to decrease the chance of significant changes in social position due to other reasons. Moreover, in order to harmonize the data sets, all samples were further limited to women ages 20–56, which was the age span collected in the Norwegian survey. This resulted in a US sample of 4725 women, a German sample of 3724 women, and a Norwegian sample of 1575 women. A detailed description of the three country samples is broken down into the following sections: IPV exposure, health outcomes, social position, and control variables.

IPV exposure was measured overall as experiencing physical or sexual violence from a partner within the past five years, as well as specifically according to severity (see Table 6.1). In the US, a total of 9 % (n = 424) of the sample had experienced IPV. Of those, 43 % (n = 184) reported severe partner violence involving injury, while the remaining 57 % (n = 240) experienced minor IPV without injury. Approximately 12 % (n = 443) of the German sample had experienced IPV, with 65 % (n = 288) of those reporting severe IPV, and 35 % (n = 155) reporting minor IPV. Similarly, in Norway, 13 % (n = 212) of the sample had experienced physical or sexual violence from a partner within the past five years. Of those, 59 % (n = 125) of respondents reported severe IPV, while the remaining 41 % (n = 87) reported minor IPV.

To measure health outcomes, both self-assessed health and number of mental health complaints were chosen as indicators. In the US, nearly 10 % of respondents rated their health as poor (i.e., 'fair' or 'poor' on a five-point scale), and 10 % of the respondents in Germany also found this to be the case (i.e., a rating of 4, 5, or 6 on a scale of 1 'very good' to 6 'very poor') (see Table 6.2). Furthermore, in Norway, 16 % of respondents found their health to be poor (i.e., 'neither good nor poor,' 'poor,' or 'very poor' on a five-point scale). In terms of mental health complaints, the US respondents experienced an average of 2.4 in the past week either 'some' or 'most of the time.' In Germany, an average number of 3.5 mental health complaints were experienced either 'frequently' or 'occasionally' over the past 12 months.

Table 6.1 IPV prevalence for US, German, and Norwegian samples

Variables	US (N = 4725) (%)	Germany (N = 3724) (%)	Norway (N = 1575) (%)
No IPV	91 %	88 %	86 %
Minor IPV[a]	5 %	4 %	6 %
Severe IPV[a]	4 %	8 %	8 %

See Table 6.14 for complete information
[a]Within the past five years

Table 6.2 Health outcomes for US, German, and Norwegian samples

Variables	US (N = 4725) (%/mean)	Germany (N = 3724) (%/mean)	Norway (N = 1575) (%/mean)
Poor SAH	10 %	10 %	16 %
Mental health complaints	2.4	3.5	0.5

See Table 6.15 for complete information

Table 6.3 Social position for US, German, and Norwegian samples

Variables	US (N = 4725) (%/mean)	Germany (N = 3724) (%/mean)	Norway (N = 1575) (%/mean)
Annual household income (equivalent)	$24,615[a]	€16,667[b]	281,774 NOK[a]
Annual personal income (equivalent)	$14,080[a]	€7183[b]	132,383 NOK[a]
Education in years	14.8	13.0	14.2
Employed (FT/PT)	72 %	72 %	85 %

See Table 6.16 for complete information
[a]Before taxes and social contributions
[b]After taxes and social contributions

Finally, for Norway, an average of 0.5 mental health complaints found to be 'pretty much' or 'very much' bothersome in the past 14 days was reported.

Variables of social position relevant for the analyses included household income, personal income, education, and employment status (see Table 6.3). The annual household equivalent income in the US sample reported for 1995 before taxes was $24,615, of which the respondents themselves contributed an average of $14,080.[1] Meanwhile, the annual household equivalent income in the Norwegian sample reported for 2002 before taxes was 281,774 NOK, of which the respondents contributed an average of 132,383 NOK.[2] Finally, in contrast to the US and Norway, respondents in Germany were asked for information on household income for 2003 *after* taxes and social insurance contributions. The annual equivalent income amounted to €16,667, of which the respondents themselves contributed an average of €7183.[3] Moreover, respondents in the US sample had an average of 14.8 years of

[1]Approximately $38,415 and $21,973 before taxes, respectively, in 2015 currency (US Bureau of Labor Statistics n.d.).

[2]Approximately €45,812 and €21,523 before taxes, respectively, in 2015 currency (European Central Bank 2015).

[3]Approximately €20,858 and €8989 after taxes, respectively, in 2015 currency (European Central Bank 2015).

Table 6.4 Sociodemographic control variables for US, German, and Norwegian samples

Variables	US (N = 4725) (%/mean)	Germany (N = 3724) (%/mean)	Norway (N = 1575) (%/mean)
Age in years	37.3	39.3	37.9
Married/partnered	68 %	85 %	83 %
Number of children	1.2	0.8	1.1
Minority/migration	23 %[a]	12 %[b]	6 %[b]
Frequent alcohol	6 %	23 %	24 %
Other violence	25 %	28 %	28 %
Health impairment	10 %	9 %	7 %

See Table 6.17 for complete information
[a]Identification as a racial or ethnic minority
[b]Migration background

education (i.e., some post-secondary education), while the German respondents had an average of 13.0 years, and 14.2 years in Norway (i.e., some post-secondary education). Finally, 72 % of women in the US sample and 72 % of those in the Germany sample reported full- or part-time employment, while 85 % of women in the Norway sample did so.

The relevant control variables considered in the quantitative analyses included age, marital/partnership status, number of children under the age of 18, racial/ethnic identification or migration background, alcohol consumption, violence from a non-partner, and health impairment (see Table 6.4). The mean age of the US sample was 37.3, 39.3 years in Germany, and 37.9 years in Norway. While 68 % of the respondents in the US were married or cohabitating with a partner, this was the case for 85 % of women in the Germany sample, and 83 % in the Norway sample. In terms of the number of children in the household under the age of 18, women in the US reported an average of 1.2 children, while in Germany the average was 0.8, and 1.1 in Norway. Approximately 23 % of the US respondents identified themselves as being a racial or ethnic minority. A similar, but slightly different indicator regarding migration background was measured in Germany and Norway, where 12 and 6 % of respondents, respectively, reported a migration background.[4] In the US, about 6 % reported consuming alcohol at least a couple of times per week or more, while this was the case for 23 % of respondents in Germany and 24 % in Norway.[5] Of the US sample, 25 % indicated they had experienced physical or sexual violence as an

[4]It should be noted that results regarding migration background in Norway need to be interpreted with care due to the high nonresponse rate among nonnative Norwegians who received the survey (Flåte 2004; Sogn et al. 2006).

[5]Given the differences in time frames and amounts used to measure alcohol consumption across surveys (see Chap. 5), caution should be taken in ascribing too much meaning regarding differences in this indicator across countries.

adult from someone other than a partner (e.g., relative, co-worker, stranger), as was the case for 28 % of respondents since the age of 16 in Germany, and 28 % of respondents since the age of 15 in Norway. Finally, about 10 % of the US sample indicated that they had a chronic disease or health condition that prevented them from carrying out daily activities. This was the case for 9 % of the Germany sample and 7 % of the Norwegian sample.

6.2 Bivariate Findings

As an initial assessment of the relationships between the variables of interest, this section presents the results of the bivariate correlations and tests of independence for all three countries based on the applicable survey data.[6,7] Although direct statistical analysis across countries was not possible, this section does offer bivariate analyses of *within* country relationships. The first correlations presented are those relevant for the dependent variables of IPV exposure and then for health outcomes.[8] Due to space limitations, only statistically significant ($p < 0.05$) and meaningful correlations ($r/r_{pb}/r_s/V \geq 0.1$) are described.

6.2.1 IPV Exposure as the Dependent Variable

This section presents correlations of the independent variables with IPV exposure as the dependent variable. Results of tests of independence are also reported for those variables with meaningful correlations. These are arranged by country, starting with the US, followed by Germany and Norway.

Beginning with the correlations between social position and IPV exposure for the *US data*, household income was the only variable to have a significant and meaningful correlation with IPV exposure (see Tables 6.5 and 6.6). The negative correlation between household income and IPV exposure was small, but

---

[6]Based on tests of normality, it was determined that all interval variables (i.e., age, number of children, income levels, years of education, and number of mental health complaints) violated the assumption of normality. The statistical tests described here and in Chaps. 7 and 8 take this into account.

[7]A number of different correlation tests (i.e., Pearson's product moment correlation, point biserial correlations, Spearman's rank order, and Cramér's V) and independence tests (i.e., Kruskal–Wallis, Pearson chi-square, t tests) were utilized according to types of variables tested (e.g., interval, ordinal, dichotomous). Precise information on these tests, as well as explanations of the interpretation of the correlation coefficients, can be found in Chap. 5.

[8]Bivariate analyses of social position and control variables were also conducted and can be found in Tables 6.18, 6.19, and 6.20.

Table 6.5 Bivariate correlations with IPV exposure as dependent variable

Variables	IPV exposure correlation coefficients		
	US (N = 4725)	Germany (N = 3724)	Norway (N = 1575)
Social position			
Annual household income (equivalent)	−0.16***	−0.16***	−0.18***
Annual personal income (equivalent)	−.05***	0.06***	−0.03
Education in years	−0.06***	0.01	−0.05*
Employed (FT/PT)	0.03	0.04	0.14***
Controls			
Age in years	−0.14***	−0.13***	−0.17***
Married/partnered	0.20***	0.16***	0.22***
Number of children	0.09***	0.01	−0.01
Minority/migration	0.04*	0.07***	0.02
Frequent alcohol	0.02	0.04	0.07*
Other violence	0.10***	0.28***	0.36***
Health impairment	0.04*	0.03	0.14***

Significance levels for tests of independence: $^{*}p < 0.05$, $^{**}p < 0.01$, $^{***}p < 0.001$

Table 6.6 US: tests of independence for IPV exposure as a dependent variable

Variables	Significance	US IPV exposure (N = 4725) mean/%		
		No IPV	Minor IPV	Severe IPV
Social position				
Annual household income (equivalent) in USD	***	25,826	19,733	14,303
Annual personal income (equivalent) in USD	***	14,407	12,581	9896
Education in years	***	14.9	14.6	14.1
Employed (FT/PT)		72 %	73 %	65 %
Controls				
Age in years	***	37.7	33.1	33.1
Married/partnered	***	71 %	45 %	32 %
Number of children	***	1.1	1.4	1.6
Racial/ethnic minority	*	22 %	27 %	29 %
Frequent alcohol		6 %	8 %	5 %
Other violence	***	24 %	34 %	44 %
Health impairment	*	10 %	6 %	15 %

Significance levels for tests of independence: $^{*}p < 0.05$, $^{**}p < 0.01$, $^{***}p < 0.001$

demonstrated that those without a history of IPV have a higher household income than those who have experienced minor or severe IPV.

A few control variables were significantly related to IPV exposure in the US data, with the strongest correlation, though still classified as small, occurring with marital/partnership status (see Tables 6.5 and 6.6). Overall, more women without a history of IPV were married or in a partnership, as compared to women who had experienced minor IPV or severe IPV. IPV exposure was also correlated with having experienced violence from a non-partner, so that more women with histories of minor and severe IPV have experienced violence from a non-partner than women with no history of IPV. Finally, age had a small, negative correlation with IPV exposure, so that those without a history of IPV were on average older than those with such a history.

In testing the correlations between social position and IPV exposure in the *German data*, household income seems to have the strongest correlation with IPV, while the correlation with personal income is significant, but too small to be meaningful (see Tables 6.5 and 6.7). The negative correlation between household income and IPV exposure was small, but demonstrated that those without a history of IPV have higher household income than those with a history of minor or severe IPV.

Meanwhile, a few control variables were significantly and meaningfully related to IPV exposure in the German data (see Tables 6.5 and 6.7). The strongest correlation occurs between IPV exposure and having experienced violence from a

Table 6.7 Germany: tests of independence for IPV exposure as dependent variable

Variables	Significance	Germany IPV exposure (N = 3724) mean/%		
		No IPV	Minor IPV	Severe IPV
Social position				
Annual household income (equivalent) in EUR	***	17,116	15,081	12,412
Annual personal income (equivalent) in EUR	***	7093	8904	7289
Education in years		13.0	13.9	12.7
Employed (FT/PT)		73 %	69 %	67 %
Controls				
Age in years	***	39.7	35.9	35.7
Married/partnered	***	87 %	72 %	67 %
Number of children		0.83	0.89	0.83
Migration background	***	12 %	8 %	19 %
Frequent alcohol		22 %	30 %	25 %
Other violence	***	23 %	70 %	58 %
Health impairment		9 %	9 %	12 %

Significance levels for tests of independence: $^{*}p < 0.05$, $^{**}p < 0.01$, $^{***}p < 0.001$

non-partner. Overall, fewer women without a history of IPV had experienced violence from a non-partner than women who had experienced minor IPV or severe IPV. Marriage and partnership had a slightly smaller correlation with IPV exposure, so that fewer women with histories of minor and severe IPV are married or partnered when compared to women with no history of IPV. Finally, age had a small, negative correlation with exposure, so that those without a history of IPV were older than those who had experienced minor or severe IPV.

In terms of social position, household income and employment had the strongest correlations with IPV exposure in the *Norwegian data*, while the correlations with education and personal income were too small to be meaningful (see Tables 6.5 and 6.8). To begin, there was a small, negative correlation between annual household income and IPV exposure. Those who experienced minor or severe IPV had lower levels of household income on average than those without a history of IPV. Likewise, employment's correlation with IPV exposure was also small, but showed that a history of IPV was associated with unemployment.

A number of control variables were significantly related to IPV exposure in the Norwegian sample, with the strongest correlations occurring with violence from a non-partner, marital/partnership status, and age (see Tables 6.5 and 6.8). Having experienced violence from a non-partner was moderately correlated with IPV exposure. In fact, fewer women without IPV experience had experienced violence from a non-partner, as compared to women with minor IPV or severe IPV experience. Marriage/partnership had a small correlation with exposure, so that fewer

Table 6.8 Norway: tests of independence for IPV exposure as dependent variable

Variables	Significance	Norway IPV exposure (N = 1575) mean/%		
		No IPV	Minor IPV	Severe IPV
Social position				
Annual household income (equivalent) in NOK	***	290,357	247,354	212,141
Annual personal income (equivalent) in NOK		133,036	140,950	199,294
Education in years	*	14.3	14.7	13.3
Employed (FT/PT)	***	87 %	89 %	68 %
Controls				
Age in years	***	38.6	33.9	33.7
Married/partnered	***	86 %	68 %	58 %
Number of children		1.1	1.3	1.0
Migration background		6 %	7 %	5 %
Frequent alcohol	*	25 %	22 %	14 %
Other violence	***	22 %	54 %	76 %
Health impairment	***	5 %	9 %	18 %

Significance levels for tests of independence: $^{*}p < 0.05$, $^{**}p < 0.01$, $^{***}p < 0.001$

women with minor and severe IPV histories were married or partnered than those without any history of IPV. A smaller, negative correlation with IPV exposure occurred with age. In other words, women without histories of IPV tended to be older on average than those with histories of minor or severe IPV. Finally, IPV exposure was minimally correlated with health impairment of daily activities. These differences were significant, demonstrating more women with a history of minor IPV or severe IPV reported health impairment than those without IPV histories.

6.2.2 Health Outcomes as the Dependent Variables

This section presents correlations of independent variables with self-assessed health and mental health complaints as the dependent variables. Results of tests of independence are also reported for those variables with meaningful correlations. These are arranged by country, starting with the US, and followed by Germany and Norway.

Nearly all of the social position variables were significantly and meaningfully correlated with the measures of health in the *US data* (see Tables 6.9 and 6.10). A poor self-assessment of health had small, negative correlations with all of the

Table 6.9 Bivariate correlations with SAH as dependent variable

Variables	Poor SAH correlation coefficients		
	US (N = 4725)	Germany (N = 3724)	Norway (N = 1575)
Social position			
Annual household income (equivalent)	−0.17***	−0.06***	−0.14***
Annual personal income (equivalent)	−0.13***	−0.06***	−0.14***
Education in years	−0.18***	−0.08***	−0.14***
Employed (FT/PT)	−0.16***	−0.09***	−0.25***
IPV			
Exposure	0.08***	0.07***	0.18***
Controls			
Age in years	0.06***	0.09***	0.08**
Married/partnered	−0.05***	0.00	0.03
Number of children	0.00	−0.03	−0.05
Minority/migration	0.12**[a]	0.03[b]	0.07**[b]
Frequent alcohol	0.00	−0.02	0.04
Other violence	0.05***	0.05**	0.14***
Health impairment	0.31***	0.34***	0.50***

Significance levels for tests of independence: *$p < 0.05$, **$p < 0.01$, ***$p < 0.001$

[a]Identification as a racial or ethnic minority

[b]Migration background

Table 6.10 Bivariate correlations with mental health complaints as dependent variable

Variables	Mental health complaints correlation coefficients		
	US (N = 4725)	Germany (N = 3724)	Norway (N = 1575)
Social position			
Annual household income (equivalent)	−0.20***	−0.08***	−0.18***
Annual personal income (equivalent)	−0.12***	−0.01	−0.13***
Education in years	−0.14***	0.02	−0.08**
Employed (FT/PT)	−0.07***	−0.05**	−0.18***
IPV			
Exposure	0.12***	0.20***	0.25***
Controls			
Age in years	−0.05***	−0.06***	−0.10***
Married/partnered	−0.06***	−0.09***	−0.09***
Number of children	0.06	0.03*	−0.02
Minority/migration	0.06***[a]	−0.01[b]	0.03[b]
Frequent alcohol	0.02	0.07***	−0.05*
Other violence	0.12***	0.23***	0.26***
Health impairment	0.20***	0.17***	0.34***

Significance levels for tests of independence: *$p < 0.05$, **$p < 0.01$, ***$p < 0.001$
[a]Identification as a racial or ethnic minority
[b]Migration background

social position variables, so that it was associated with lower levels of household and personal income, lower levels of education, and being unemployed (see Table 6.11). Examining the number of mental health complaints, there were small, negative correlations with household and personal income, as well as with education. That is, higher levels of household and personal income as well as higher levels of education were associated with lower numbers of mental health complaints.

With regards to associations between IPV exposure and health in the US data, only a number of mental health complaints were both significantly and meaningfully correlated with IPV exposure (see Tables 6.9 and 6.10). There was a small, positive correlation between IPV exposure and the number of mental health complaints reported, showing that greater IPV exposure was associated with a greater number of mental health complaints. To illustrate, those without a history of IPV reported an average of 2.3 mental health complaints in the past week, while those with minor and severe IPV report an average of 3.0 and 3.1 complaints, respectively.

In terms of correlations between the control variables and health outcomes in the US data, meaningful correlations varied according to the health outcome itself (see Tables 6.9 and 6.10). For self-assessed health, there was a small, positive

Table 6.11 US: tests of independence for SAH as dependent variable

Variables	Significance	US SAH (N = 4725) mean/%	
		Good SAH	Poor SAH
Social position			
Annual household income (equivalent) in USD	***	25,948	16,138
Annual personal income (equivalent) in USD	***	14,693	8819
Education in years	***	14.9	13.6
Employed (FT/PT)	***	74 %	49 %
IPV			
Exposure	***		
No IPV		92 %	86 %
Minor		5 %	5 %
Severe		3 %	8 %
Controls			
Age in years	***	37.1	38.9
Married/partnered	***	69 %	61 %
Number of children		1.1	1.1
Racial/ethnic minority	**	21 %	38 %
Frequent alcohol		6 %	6 %
Other violence	***	24 %	32 %
Health impairment	***	7 %	38 %

Significance levels for tests of independence: $^{*}p < 0.05$, $^{**}p < 0.01$, $^{***}p < 0.001$

correlation with racial/ethnic minority identification and a moderate, positive correlation existed with health impairment. That is, racial or ethnic minorities more often rated their health as poor than as good. Likewise, a higher proportion of those impaired in daily activities also rated their health as poor than as good. Moreover, the number of mental health complaints had small, positive correlations with non-partner violence and health impairment. In other words, those having experienced violence from a non-partner had a greater number of mental health complaints on average than those who had not (2.7 vs. 2.3). Likewise, those impaired by health in daily activities had a higher average of mental health complaints than those without a health impairment (3.4 vs. 2.3).

While quite a number of the social position variables were significantly correlated with the measures of health for the *German data* (see Tables 6.9 and 6.10), there were no meaningful correlations. However, the largest among these were negative correlations between poor self-assessed health and education and employment (see Table 6.12), as well as between household income and mental health complaints.

Table 6.12 Germany: tests of independence for SAH as dependent variable

Variables	Significance	Germany SAH ($N = 3724$) mean/%	
		Good SAH	Poor SAH
Social position			
Annual household income (equivalent) in EUR	***	16,868	14,930
Annual personal income (equivalent) in EUR	***	7332	5891
Education in years	***	13.1	12.4
Employed (FT/PT)	***	74 %	60 %
IPV			
Exposure	***		
No IPV		89 %	84 %
Minor		4 %	3 %
Severe		7 %	13 %
Controls			
Age in years	***	38.9	41.8
Married/partnered		85 %	85 %
Number of children		0.85	0.75
Migration background		12 %	15 %
Frequent alcohol		23 %	20 %
Other violence	**	27 %	34 %
Health impairment	***	7 %	43 %

Significance levels for tests of independence: $^{*}p < 0.05$, $^{**}p < 0.01$, $^{***}p < 0.001$

Regarding associations between IPV exposure and health for the German data, only the number of mental health complaints was significantly and meaningfully correlated with IPV exposure (see Tables 6.9 and 6.10). This small, positive correlation between IPV exposure and the number of mental health complaints demonstrated that greater exposure of IPV was associated with a greater number of mental health complaints. To illustrate, those without a history of IPV reported an average of 3.2 mental health complaints in the past year, while those with minor and severe IPV reported an average of 4.4 and 5.6 complaints, respectively.

Regarding correlations between the control variables and health for the German data, violence from a non-partner and health impairment had the strongest relationships to health (see Tables 6.9 and 6.10). There was a small correlation between having experienced violence from a non-partner and the number of mental health complaints, so that a history of this kind of violence was associated with a greater number of mental health complaints than among those without this history (3.0 vs. 4.5). Likewise, there is a moderate, positive correlation between poor self-assessed health and health impairment and a small, positive correlation between mental health complaints and health impairment. In other words, those with a health

Table 6.13 Norway: tests of independence for SAH as dependent variable

Variables	Significance	Norway SAH (N = 1575) mean/%	
		Good SAH	Poor SAH
Social position			
Annual household income (equivalent) in NOK	***	288,978	244,654
Annual personal income (equivalent) in NOK	***	137,026	108,460
Education in years	***	14.4	13.4
Employed (FT/PT)	***	89 %	65 %
IPV			
Exposure	***		
No IPV		89 %	74 %
Minor		5 %	8 %
Severe		6 %	18 %
Controls			
Age in years	**	37.6	39.7
Married/partnered		83 %	80 %
Number of children		1.2	1.0
Migration background	**	6 %	10 %
Frequent alcohol		24 %	20 %
Other violence	***	25 %	42 %
Health impairment	***	1 %	35 %

Significance levels for tests of independence: $^{*}p < 0.05$, $^{**}p < 0.01$, $^{***}p < 0.001$

impairment rated their health as poor more often than good and reported more mental health complaints than those without such an impairment (3.3 vs. 5.1).

Nearly, all of the social position variables were significantly and meaningfully correlated with the measures of health in the *Norwegian data* (see Tables 6.9 and 6.10). Employment correlated the strongest with both health variables. Being employed either full- or part-time had a small, negative correlation with poor self-assessed health ratings. In other words, the employed more often reported their health as good than poor (see Table 6.13). There was also a small, negative correlation between employment and number of mental health complaints, so that the employed reported fewer bothersome mental health complaints on average than the non-employed (0.4 vs. 1.1). Additionally, there was a small, negative correlation between annual household income and reporting poor health. In other words, those who reported poor health had lower household incomes than those who reported good health. Additionally, annual household income showed a small, negative correlation with number of mental health complaints, where higher levels of household income were associated with lower numbers of bothersome mental health complaints. Personal income showed a very similar pattern of correlations with poor self-assessed health and mental health complaints. Lower levels of personal income were found among those reporting poor health than good health. Higher levels of personal income were also associated with fewer numbers of mental health complaints. For education, those reporting poor health had on average fewer years of education than those reporting good health.

It is also important to note that IPV exposure and health were significantly correlated for the Norwegian data (see Tables 6.9 and 6.10). The strongest of these was the small, positive correlation between IPV exposure and the number of mental health complaints reported, showing that those with minor or severe IPV reported a greater number of mental health complaints than those without a history of IPV. There was also a small relationship between exposure and having a poor self-assessment of health, so that greater IPV exposure was related to the tendency to report poor health. For example, those reporting minor or severe IPV more often reported poor health than good health.

In terms of correlations between the control variables and health, health impairment and violence from a non-partner had the strongest relationships to health in the Norwegian data (see Tables 6.9 and 6.10). To begin, there were strong and moderate positive correlations between health impairment and self-assessed health and mental health complaints. Unsurprisingly, this demonstrated that those impaired in daily activities rated their health as poor more often than as good, and reported higher numbers of mental health complaints on average than those without a health impairment (2.3 vs. 0.4). There were also small, positive correlations between having experienced violence from a non-partner and reporting poor health and the number of mental health complaints reported. In other words, those who had experienced violence from a non-partner more often reported poor health than good health and reported more bothersome mental health complaints than those without this history (1.1 vs. 0.3). Additionally, being older was associated with fewer numbers of mental health complaints.

6.3 Discussion

This chapter has provided an overview of the composition of each country's sample and offers some clues as to what could be especially important for predicting IPV exposure and health outcomes.

Based on the bivariate analyses, one gains an impression of what factors are particularly noteworthy in their relation to IPV exposure. In terms of social position, higher levels of household income were significantly associated with less IPV exposure for all three countries, as would be expected, while being employed was related to lower IPV exposure in Norway only. When focusing on control variables, being married or partnered was related to reduced IPV exposure in all three countries. Given that IPV was measured for the purposes of this book as violence experienced by a former or current partner within the past five years, it may be supposed that many respondents who had recently experienced minor or severe IPV had exited the abusive relationship and had not entered a new relationship within this time period. This may also hint at the possibility that the IPV reported in the surveys was more often related to former partnerships rather than current ones. Furthermore, it was clear across all three countries that IPV exposure was related to having also experienced violence from someone other than a partner. Although this is not specifically the subject of this book, it does highlight the complexity of measuring IPV and its overlaps with other forms of violence (Scott-Storey 2011). Finally, as has been found in previous studies, being younger was associated with IPV exposure in all three countries (e.g., Bachman and Saltzman 1995). These similarities in correlations, with the exception of employment in Norway, suggest that the three countries may share more commonalities regarding IPV exposure than differences. The multiple regression models predicting IPV exposure in Chap. 7 attempt to determine whether this holds true when all factors are taken into consideration at the same time.

When examining factors which could be predictive of health outcomes, there are fewer commonalities across the three countries. In terms of social position, lower levels of household and personal income were significantly and meaningfully correlated with both poor self-assessed health and more mental health complaints in the US and Norway. Likewise, lower levels of education were associated with poor self-assessed health for the US and Norway, and with more mental health complaints for the US. Similarly, unemployment was also associated with poor self-assessed health in the US and Norway samples, and with more mental health complaints in Norway. Contrary to what was expected, however, none of the social position variables were significantly and meaningfully correlated with health outcomes for Germany.

Focusing on IPV exposure's relationship to health outcomes, greater IPV exposure was significantly related to poor self-assessed health for Norway and with more mental health complaints for all three countries. Moreover, being a racial or ethnic minority was associated with poor self-assessed health in the US, but having a migration background was not related to health in Germany or Norway. Keeping in line with other research (e.g., Casey and Nurius 2005), having experienced violence from someone other than a partner was significantly and meaningfully related to poor self-assessed health for Norway, and with more mental health complaints for all three countries. Finally, unsurprisingly, having a chronic health impairment was also associated with both poor self-assessed health and more mental health complaints in each of the countries.

In sum, the correlations reveal somewhat different patterns across countries in the associations between social position, IPV exposure, and health outcomes. Employment distinguishes itself as a highly relevant factor for health in Norway, which may be related to the higher level of employment among women in the Norwegian sample than in the US or German samples. Why self-assessed health did not have a meaningful correlation with IPV exposure for the US and Germany despite proving to be statistically significant remains an open question. Furthermore, it was not clear based on the bivariate analyses why social position was not correlated with health for Germany. Thus, the analyses presented in Chap. 8 for the multiple regression models predicting health outcomes will fit these pieces together and examine these questions and relationships in more detail.

Appendix

Table 6.14 IPV prevalence for US, German, and Norwegian samples

Variables	US (*N* = 4725)		Germany (*N* = 3724)		Norway (*N* = 1575)	
	Mean (SD)	Min–max	Mean (SD)	Min–max	Mean (SD)	Min–max
Experienced IPV[a]	0.09 (0.29)	0–1	0.12 (0.32)	0–1	0.13 (0.34)	0–1
IPV exposure	0.13 (0.44)	0–2	0.20 (0.56)	0–2	0.21 (0.57)	0–2
No IPV	91 %		88 %		86 %	
Minor	5 %		4 %		6 %	
Severe	4 %		8 %		8 %	

Max maximum, *Min* minimum, *SD* standard deviation
[a]Within the past five years

Table 6.15 Health outcomes for US, German, and Norwegian samples

Variables	US (*N* = 4725)		Germany (*N* = 3724)		Norway (*N* = 1575)	
	Mean (SD)	Min–max	Mean (SD)	Min–max	Mean (SD)	Min–max
Poor SAH[a]	0.10 (0.29)	0–1	0.10 (0.30)	0–1	0.16 (0.37)	0–1
Mental health complaints[b]	2.4 (1.70)	0–8	3.5 (2.92)	0–14	0.5 (1.41)	0–8

Max maximum, *Min* minimum, *SD* standard deviation
[a]Specifically, 'fair' or 'poor' for the US; a rating of 4, 5, or 6 on a scale of 1 'very good' to 6 'very poor' for Germany; and 'neither good nor poor,' 'poor,' or 'very poor' for Norway
[b]Specifically, 'some' or 'most of the time' in the past week for the US; 'frequently' or 'occasionally' in the past 12 months for Germany; and 'pretty much' or 'very much' bothersome in the past 14 days for Norway

Table 6.16 Social position for US, German, and Norwegian samples

Variables	US (N = 4725)		Germany (N = 3724)		Norway (N = 1575)	
	Mean (SD)	Min–max	Mean (SD)	Min–max	Mean (SD)	Min–max
Household income[a]	24,615[b,c] (16,551)	0–100,000	16,667[d,e] (8801)	0–91,2000	281,774[b,f] (119,597)	204,124–900,000
Personal income[a]	14,080[b,c] (13,582)	0–100,000	7,183[d,e] (6846)	0–91,200	132,383[b,f] (76,550)	16,666–450,000
Education in years	14.8 (2.3)	0–19	13.0 (2.72)	0–18	14.2 (2.58)	0–20
Employed (FT/PT)	0.72 (0.45)	0–1	0.72 (0.45)	0–1	0.85 (0.36)	0–1

Max maximum, *Min* minimum, *SD* standard deviation
[a]Annual, equivalent income
[b]Before taxes and social contributions
[c]US dollars
[d]After taxes and social contributions
[e]Euros
[f]Norwegian Kroner

Table 6.17 Sociodemographic control variables for US, German, and Norwegian samples

Variables	US (N = 4725)		Germany (N = 3724)		Norway (N = 1575)	
	Mean (SD)	Min–max	Mean (SD)	Min–max	Mean (SD)	Min–max
Age in years	37.3 (9.71)	20–56	39.3 (9.47)	20–56	37.9 (9.45)	20–56
Married/partnered	0.68 (0.47)	0–1	0.85 (0.36)	0–1	0.83 (0.38)	0–1
Number of children	1.2 (1.24)	0–10	0.8 (0.99)	0–6	1.1 (1.13)	0–7
Minority/migration	0.23[a] (0.42)	0–1	0.12[b] (0.33)	0–1	0.06[b] (0.24)	0–1
Frequent alcohol	0.06 (0.24)	0–1	0.23 (0.42)	0–1	0.24 (0.43)	0–1
Other violence	0.25 (0.43)	0–1	0.28 (0.45)	0–1	0.28 (0.45)	0–1
Health impairment	0.10 (0.29)	0–1	0.09 (0.29)	0–1	0.07 (0.25)	0–1

Max maximum, *Min* minimum, *SD* standard deviation
[a]Identification as a racial or ethnic minority
[b]Migration background

Table 6.18 US: bivariate correlations between independent variables

Variables	US correlation coefficients ($N = 4725$)										
	Social position				Controls						
	1	2	3	4	5	6	7	8	9	10	11
Social position											
1. Household income	–	0.66^{***}	0.42^{***}	0.24^{***}	0.26^{***}	0.17^{***}	-0.30^{***}	-0.21^{***}	0.13^{***}	−0.02	$-.08^{***}$
2. Personal income		–	0.36^{***}	0.31^{***}	0.20^{***}	-0.04^{**}	-0.28^{***}	-0.09^{***}	0.12^{***}	0.01	-0.07^{***}
3. Education in years			–	0.21^{***}	0.03^{*}	0.01	-0.12^{***}	-0.17^{***}	0.10^{***}	−0.02	-0.10^{***}
4. Employed (FT/PT)				–	0.08^{***}	-0.03^{*}	-0.16^{***}	-0.07^{***}	0.02	−0.02	-0.10^{***}
Controls											
5. Age in years					–	0.22^{***}	-0.21^{***}	-0.13^{***}	0.10^{***}	-0.12^{***}	0.15^{***}
6. Married/partnered						–	0.15^{***}	-0.18^{***}	−0.01	-0.13^{***}	-0.03^{*}
7. Number of children							–	0.11^{***}	-0.05^{***}	0.03	-0.03^{*}
8. Racial/ethnic								–	-0.07^{***}	0.01	0.06^{***}
9. Frequent alcohol									–	0.03^{*}	−0.02
10. Other violence										–	0.03^{*}
11. Health impairment											–

Significance levels for tests of independence: $^{*}p < 0.05$, $^{**}p < 0.01$, $^{***}p < 0.001$

Table 6.19 Germany: bivariate correlations between independent variables

Variables	German correlation coefficients ($N = 3724$)										
	Social position				Controls						
	1	2	3	4	5	6	7	8	9	10	11
Social position											
1. Household income	–	0.48^{***}	0.28^{***}	0.24^{***}	0.20^{***}	0.15^{***}	-0.17^{***}	-0.16^{***}	0.16^{***}	-0.04^{*}	-0.02
2. Personal income		–	0.30^{***}	0.37^{***}	0.08^{***}	-0.24^{***}	-0.35^{***}	-0.16^{***}	0.11^{***}	0.05^{**}	-0.02
3. Education in years			–	0.15^{***}	-0.05^{***}	-0.01	-0.04^{*}	-0.08^{***}	0.14^{***}	0.08^{***}	-0.06^{**}
4. Employed (FT/PT)				–	0.05^{**}	0.04^{*}	-0.08^{***}	-0.10^{***}	0.05^{**}	-0.02	-0.10^{***}
Controls											
5. Age in years					–	0.09^{***}	-0.14^{***}	-0.06^{***}	0.10^{***}	-0.12^{***}	0.13^{***}
6. Married/partnered						–	0.17^{***}	0.03	-0.01	-0.06^{***}	-0.02
7. Number of children							–	0.08^{***}	-0.02	0.00	-0.07^{***}
8. Migration background								–	-0.09^{***}	0.00	-0.05^{**}
9. Frequent alcohol									–	0.06^{***}	-0.01
10. Other violence										–	0.04^{*}
11. Health impairment											–

Significance levels for tests of independence: $^{*}p < 0.05$, $^{**}p < 0.01$, $^{***}p < 0.001$

Table 6.20 Norway: bivariate correlations between independent variables

Variables	Norwegian correlation coefficients (N = 1575)										
	Social position				Controls						
	1	2	3	4	5	6	7	8	9	10	11
Social position											
1. Household income	–	0.66***	0.28***	0.29***	0.31***	0.43***	−0.25***	−0.04	0.23***	−0.10***	−0.11***
2. Personal income		–	0.34***	0.35***	0.18***	−0.23***	−0.34***	−0.02	0.19***	0.04	−0.11***
3. Education in years			–	0.17***	−0.10***	−0.02	0.04	0.10***	0.13***	−0.00	−0.09***
4. Employed (FT/PT)				–	0.04	0.06*	0.00	0.02	0.07*	0.06*	−0.23***
Controls											
5. Age in years					–	0.15***	−0.04	0.03	0.21***	−0.12***	0.10***
6. Married/partnered						–	0.20***	0.01	0.01	0.15***	−0.05
7. Number of children							–	0.01	−0.11***	−0.04	−0.04
8. Migration background								–	0.05	0.01	0.09***
9. Frequent alcohol									–	0.00	−0.02
10. Other violence										–	0.13***
11. Health impairment											–

Significance levels for tests of independence: $^{*}p < 0.05$, $^{**}p < 0.01$, $^{***}p < 0.001$

References

Bachman, R., & Saltzman, L. E. (1995). *Violence against women: Estimates from the redesigned survey*. Washington, DC: U.S. Department of Justice.

Casey, E. A., & Nurius, P. S. (2005). Trauma exposure and sexual revictimization risk: Comparisons across single, multiple incident, and multiple perpetrator victimizations. *Violence Against Women, 11*(4), 505–530. doi:10.1177/1077801204274339

European Central Bank. (2015). Euro foreign exchange reference rates. https://www.ecb.europa.eu/stats/exchange/eurofxref/html/eurofxref-graph-nok.en.html. Accessed July 22, 2015.

Flåte, S. (2004). *Undersøkelse om trygghet i hverdagen: dokumentasjonsrapport [Survey of everyday safety: Documentation report]*. Oslo: Statistics Norway.

Scott-Storey, K. (2011). Cumulative abuse: Do things add up? An evaluation of the conceptualization, operationalization, and methodological approaches in the study of the phenomenon of cumulative abuse. *Trauma, Violence, and Abuse, 12*(3), 135–150. doi:10.1177/1524838011404253

Sogn, H., Lorentzen, J., & Holter, Ø. G. (2006). *Research on violence in Norway*. Oslo, Norway.

US Bureau of Labor Statistics. (n.d.). CPI inflation calculator. http://www.bls.gov/data/inflation_calculator.htm. Accessed July 16, 2015.

Chapter 7
Findings on Differential Exposure to IPV

Abstract After the previous chapter's description of the country samples and the initial exploration of the data for the US, Germany, and Norway, this chapter presents findings regarding social position's impact on IPV exposure. According to the conceptual framework for understanding health inequities, a key initial mechanism leading to differences in health is *differential exposure* to health risks if those in lower social positions do not have the socioeconomic resources necessary to avoid exposure. Applying this mechanism to the context of IPV, it was therefore sought to examine whether women with lower social positions may be differentially exposed to IPV (RQ1), based on the literature linking socioeconomic resources to ending abusive relationships and establishing independent households. It was thus hypothesized that *higher levels of social position are related to lower levels of IPV exposure*. Even more specifically, social position was broken down into three different indicators: household income, education, and employment status. These formed three subhypotheses, where it was expected that higher levels of household income, education, and being employed are related to lower IPV exposure. After a detailed presentation of results country by country, the chapter concludes with a brief discussion of the results in the context of the conceptual framework, theory, and the empirical literature.

After the previous chapter's description of the country samples and the initial exploration of the data for the US, Germany, and Norway, this chapter presents findings regarding social position's impact on IPV exposure. According to the conceptual framework for understanding health inequities, a key initial mechanism leading to differences in health is *differential exposure* to health risks if those in lower social positions do not have the socioeconomic resources necessary to avoid exposure. Applying this mechanism to the context of IPV, it was therefore sought to examine whether women with lower social positions may be differentially exposed to IPV (RQ1), based on the literature linking socioeconomic resources to ending abusive relationships and establishing independent households. It was thus hypothesized that

© Springer International Publishing Switzerland 2016
M.M. Larsen, *Health Inequities Related to Intimate Partner Violence Against Women*, Social Disparities in Health and Health Care,
DOI 10.1007/978-3-319-29565-7_7

higher levels of social position are related to lower levels of IPV exposure.[1] Even more specifically, social position was broken down into three different indicators: household income, education, and employment status.[2] These formed three subhypotheses, where it was expected that higher levels of household income, education, and being employed are related to lower IPV exposure. After a detailed presentation of results country by country, the chapter concludes with a brief discussion of the results in the context of the conceptual framework, theory, and the empirical literature.

7.1 Social Position's Impact on IPV Exposure

To test the hypotheses related to RQ1, a multinomial logit regression model was fit for each country using IPV exposure as the categorical dependent variable. This involved using 'no IPV' as a base category to calculate separate dichotomous logits for 'minor IPV' and 'severe IPV'. As described in Chap. 5, the variable of IPV exposure is based on the understanding of partner violence as a series of escalating violent incidents over time (Mitchell and Vanya 2009). Thus, this analysis made the assumption that severe IPV involving injury is the result of longer and more intensive exposure to IPV than minor IPV without injury. The independent variables in the model included household income, education, and employment status as measures of social position. Age, marital/partnership status, number of children, racial/ethnic minority status or migration background, alcohol consumption, and violence from a nonpartner were also included in the model as control variables in order to account for their potential impact on IPV exposure. The results of the regression models are presented in terms of relative risk ratios (RRR). Additionally, in order to offer a somewhat clearer visualization of the significant findings, the predicted probabilities of minor and severe IPV were calculated at each level of the relevant social position measure, while holding all other variables in the models at their means.

Based on the regression model that was fit for the *US data*, results revealed that household income and education were related to IPV exposure (see Table 7.1). For every $1000-increment increase in household income, the relative risk of experiencing minor IPV as compared to no IPV was slightly smaller, as was the relative risk of severe IPV as compared to no IPV. Additionally, the level of education predicted the severity of IPV, so that for every year increase in education, the

---

[1]It is worth emphasizing that the same hypotheses were tested for each country, and due to the methodological considerations described in Chap. 5, the countries were not statistically compared against one another. Whether differences across countries could be attributable to differences in the policy context will be explored in Chap. 9.

[2]Readers should note that annual personal income was eliminated as a variable of social position for all regression models in Chaps. 7 and 8. Given the strong correlation between household and personal income in each of the countries (see Tables 6.18–6.20), household income was retained for its ability to capture valuable information regarding household resources, while individual-level resources were captured with education and employment.

Table 7.1 US: relative risk ratios of social position predicting IPV exposure

Predictors	US: IPV exposure (N = 4725) RRR (SE)		
	No IPV	Minor IPV	Severe IPV
Social position			
Household income[a]	Base	0.99 (0.01)*	0.97 (0.01)***
Education in years[b]	Base	0.97 (0.03)	0.92 (0.04)*
Employed (FT/PT)[c]	Base	1.25 (0.20)	1.03 (0.18)
Controls			
Age in years	Base	1.24 (0.08)***	1.27 (0.09)**
Married/partnered	Base	0.35 (0.05)***	0.21 (0.04)***
Number children	Base	1.15 (0.07)*	1.17 (0.08)*
Racial/ethnic minority	Base	0.83 (0.13)*	0.68 (0.13)*
Frequent alcohol	Base	1.75 (0.44)*	1.11 (0.39)
Other violence	Base	1.31 (0.19)	1.92 (0.31)***
Constant	Base	0.00 (0.00)***	0.00 (0.00)***
Likelihood ratio test	357.72***		
McFadden's r^2	0.10		

95 % confidence intervals. Standard errors in parentheses

*$p < 0.05$; **$p < 0.01$; ***$p < 0.001$

[a]Annual, equivalized household income *before* taxes and centered on the median in increments of $1000

[b]Centered on a high school education

[c]'Not employed' is base category

relative risk of severe IPV was reduced as compared to no IPV at all. Employment, however, did not impact IPV exposure.[3]

While holding all other variables at their means, the predicted probabilities of minor and severe IPV exposure given household income (see Fig. 7.1), as well as the predicted probabilities of severe IPV exposure given education (see Fig. 7.2), offer a visualization of the results. The probability of minor IPV decreased from 5 % at the lowest levels of household income to 1 % at the highest levels of household income. This decrease was slightly more pronounced for predicted probability of severe IPV exposure, with the lowest levels of household income having a probability of 5 %, while the highest levels approached zero. Similarly, when predicting the probabilities of severe IPV according to education, the probability decreased from 7 % at the lowest levels of education to less than 2 % at the highest levels of education.

Finally, Wald tests indicated that the effect of household income on minor and severe IPV exposure was strong enough to have a significant overall effect on IPV exposure as a whole ($\chi^2(2)$ = 21.18, p < 0.001), but this is not the case for

[3]The results also revealed that the relative risk of severe IPV as compared to minor IPV did not vary significantly by social position.

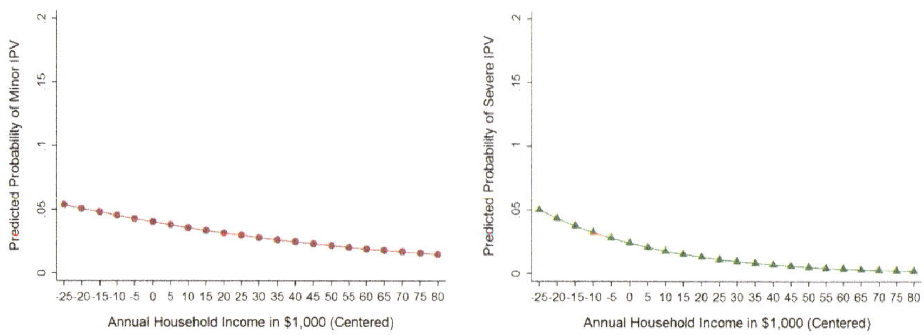

Fig. 7.1 US: predicted probabilities of IPV exposure by household income, only significant levels of IPV exposure shown

Fig. 7.2 US: predicted probabilities of IPV exposure by education, only significant levels of IPV exposure shown

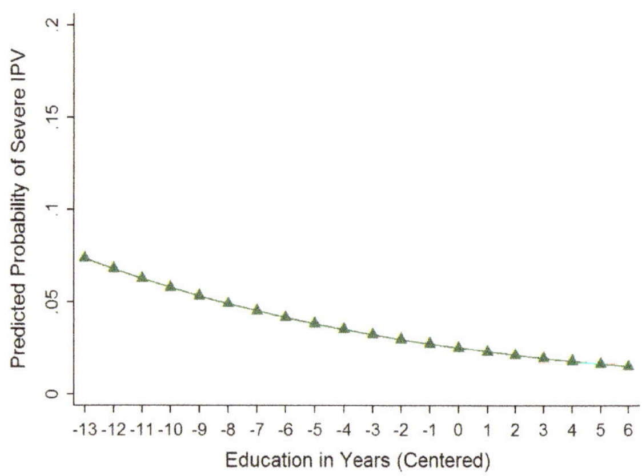

education, although it did approach significance ($\chi^2(2) = 5.28$, $p = 0.07$). In summary, evidence confirmed that higher levels of household income are related to decreased levels of IPV exposure in the US data. The data partially confirmed that higher levels of education are related to decreased levels of IPV exposure, but this only applies to severe IPV exposure. However, the evidence did not show that employment has any impact on IPV exposure in the US data.

The results predicting IPV exposure for the *German data* were somewhat less straightforward. The model revealed that household income predicted both minor and severe IPV exposure as compared to no IPV, while education predicted only minor IPV as compared to no IPV (see Table 7.2). For every €1000 increase in the equivalized annual household income, the relative risk of having experienced minor IPV as compared to none at all decreased by a factor of 0.97, while the risk of severe IPV decreased by a factor of 0.93. Surprisingly, however, for every year increase in the number of years of education, the relative risk of minor IPV exposure as compared to none at all would be expected to increase by a factor of 1.10. In other words, yearly increases in education increased the risk of minor IPV exposure. Employment status, however, was not related to IPV exposure.

Table 7.2 Germany: relative risk ratios of social position predicting IPV exposure

Predictors	Germany: IPV exposure (N = 3724) RRR (SE)		
	No IPV	Minor IPV	Severe IPV
Social position			
Household income[a]	Base	0.97 (0.01)*	0.93 (0.01)***
Education in years[b]	Base	1.10 (0.03)**	0.96 (0.03)
Employed (FT/PT)[c]	Base	0.90 (0.18)	1.14 (0.17)
Controls			
Age in years	Base	1.07 (0.09)	1.09 (0.07)
Married/partnered	Base	0.44 (0.09)***	0.40 (0.06)***
Number children	Base	1.08 (0.11)	0.91 (0.07)
Migration background	Base	0.65 (0.20)	1.48 (0.26)*
Frequent alcohol	Base	1.40 (0.27)	1.36 (0.21)*
Other violence	Base	6.73 (1.23)***	4.25 (0.56)***
Constant	Base	0.02 (0.03)**	0.03 (0.04)**
Likelihood ratio test	466.22***		
McFadden's r^2	0.14		

95 % confidence intervals. Standard errors are shown in parentheses

$^{*}p < 0.05$; $^{**}p < 0.01$; $^{***}p < 0.001$

[a]Annual, equivalized household income *after* taxes and centered on the median in increments of €1000

[b]Centered on median of number of years of education

[c]'Not employed' is base category

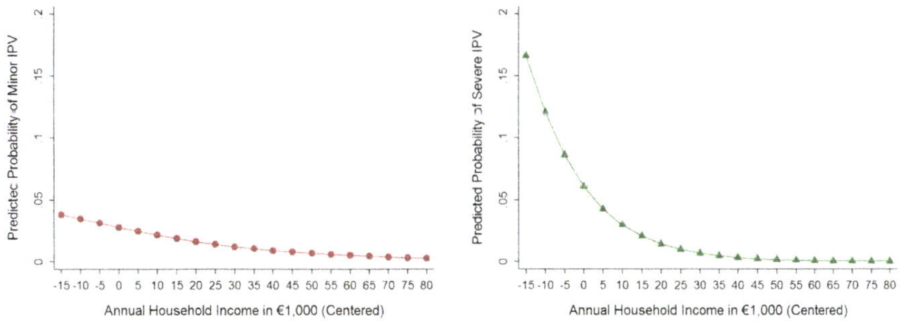

Fig. 7.3 Germany: predicted probabilities of IPV exposure by household income, only significant levels of IPV exposure shown

Estimating predicted probabilities of minor and severe IPV given household income (see Fig. 7.3), as well as minor IPV given education (see Fig. 7.4) illustrates the regression results. The probability of minor IPV decreased from 4 % at the lowest levels of household income and approached zero at the highest levels of household income. This is even more pronounced when looking at the predicted probabilities of severe IPV exposure, with the lowest levels of household income

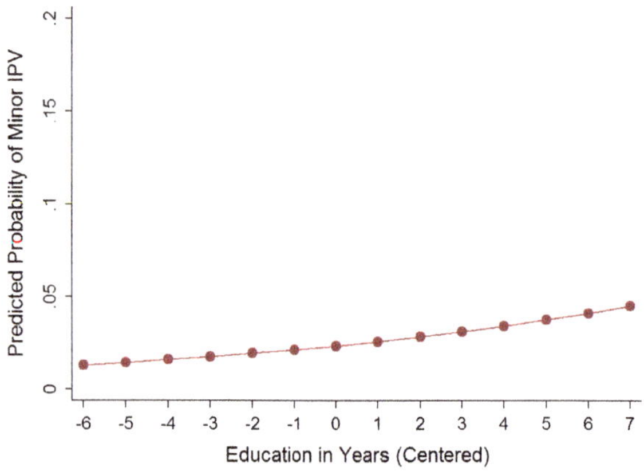

Fig. 7.4 Germany: predicted probabilities of IPV exposure by education, only significant levels of IPV exposure shown

having a probability of 17 %, while the probability at the highest levels of income approached zero. The opposite occurred with education and minor IPV exposure, however. As the number of years of education increased, the probability of minor IPV increased from 1 % at the lowest level of education to nearly 5 % at the highest level of education.

According to the Wald statistics, the effects of both household income ($\chi^2(2) = 44.50$, $p < 0.001$) and education ($\chi^2(2) = 12.03$, $p < 0.01$) were also strong enough to have a significant overall effect on the IPV exposure variable as a whole. Taken together, the analysis confirmed that higher levels of household income are related to decreased levels of IPV exposure in the German data. However, evidence only partially confirmed education's effect on IPV exposure. While it proved to be a significant predictor of minor IPV exposure and had a strong enough effect to impact IPV exposure overall, its effect moved in the opposite direction as predicted. Finally, that employment is related to decreased levels of IPV exposure could not be confirmed for the German data.

Moving on to the *Norwegian data*, the regression model revealed that education and employment status were associated with severe IPV exposure as compared to no IPV (see Table 7.3). For every year increase in education, the relative risk of severe IPV exposure as compared to no IPV decreased by a factor of 0.85. Similarly, if a respondent was employed part- or full-time, the relative risk of severe IPV exposure as compared to no IPV decreased by a factor of 0.53. In other words, being employed halved the relative risk of severe IPV exposure. Household income, however, did not influence severe IPV exposure. Additionally, social position did not influence minor IPV as compared to no IPV.

While holding all other variables at their means, the predicted probabilities of severe IPV exposure given education (see Fig. 7.5), as well as the predicted probabilities of severe IPV exposure given employment (see Fig. 7.6), offer a visualization of the results. As the number of years of education increased, the probability of severe IPV exposure decreased from 10 % at the lowest levels of education to 1 % at the highest levels of education. Likewise, the probability of

Table 7.3 Norway: relative risk ratios of social position predicting IPV exposure

Predictors	Norway: IPV exposure (N = 1575) RRR (SE)		
	None	Minor IPV	Severe IPV
Social position			
Household income[a]	Base	0.99 (0.01)	0.98 (0.01)
Education in years[b]	Base	1.04 (0.05)	0.85 (0.04)**
Employed (FT/PT)[c]	Base	1.41 (0.52)	0.53 (0.13)*
Controls			
Age in years	Base	1.17 (0.16)	1.17 (0.12)
Married/partnered	Base	0.44 (0.14)*	0.40 (0.11)**
Number children	Base	1.16 (0.16)	0.86 (0.11)
Migration background	Base	1.06 (0.48)	0.86 (0.41)
Frequent alcohol	Base	1.04 (0.29)	0.69 (0.20)
Other violence	Base	3.77 (0.87)***	9.27 (2.09)***
Constant	Base	0.01 (0.02)*	0.01 (0.03)*
Likelihood ratio test	288.65***		
McFadden's r^2	0.19		

95 % confidence intervals. Standard errors shown in parentheses

$^{*}p < 0.05$; $^{**}p < 0.01$; $^{***}p < 0.001$

[a]Annual, equivalized household income *before* taxes centered on the median in increments of 10,000 NOK

[b]Centered on a high school education

[c]'Not employed' is base category

Fig. 7.5 Norway: predicted probabilities of IPV exposure by education, only significant levels of IPV exposure shown

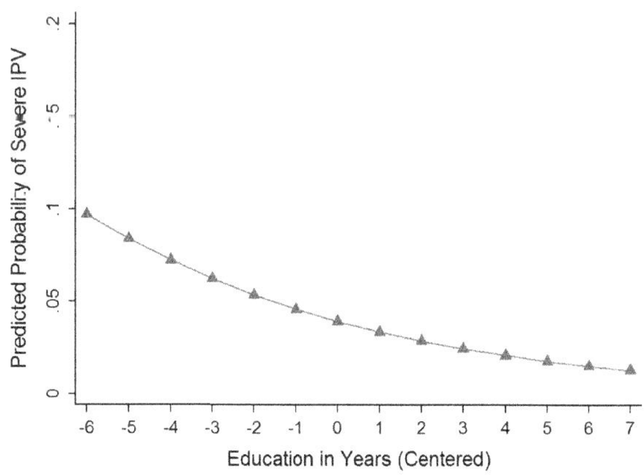

severe IPV exposure decreased from 6 to 3 % if the respondent was not employed as opposed to being employed full- or part-time.

Finally, Wald tests indicated that while none of the social position variables specifically predicted minor IPV exposure as opposed to no IPV, the effects of education ($\chi^2(2) = 12.54$, $p < 0.001$) and employment ($\chi^2(2) = 8.06$, $p < 0.05$) were

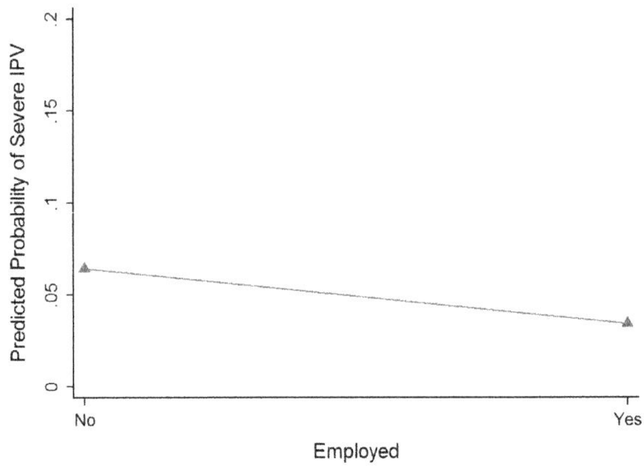

Fig. 7.6 Norway: predicted probabilities of IPV exposure by employment, only significant levels of IPV exposure shown

strong enough to have a significant overall effect on the variable of IPV exposure. Overall, this analysis confirmed that higher levels of education and employment were related to decreased levels of severe IPV exposure in the Norway data. At the same time, the results did not support the hypothesis that higher levels of household income are related to decreased levels IPV exposure.

7.2 Discussion

The primary goal of this chapter was to examine whether women with lower social positions experienced greater levels of IPV exposure. The analyses presented were based on the conceptual framework suggesting that women with lower levels of social position are *differentially exposed* to IPV due to limited socioeconomic resources limiting their ability to end abusive relationships and establish independent households. This required fitting multinomial regression models predicting IPV exposure based on social position, while accounting for other important factors. Overall, the evidence presented in this chapter confirmed the hypothesis that higher levels of social position are generally related to lower IPV exposure in the US, Germany, and Norway. However, the results also clearly demonstrate distinctive patterns across the countries (see Table 7.4, H1a-c), which generated three key findings that are discussed in the following paragraphs.

The first major finding is that higher levels of household income predicted lower levels of exposure (H1a) for the US and Germany. In both countries, the relationship between household income and IPV exposure was strongest when examining severe IPV. More specifically, those women with household incomes below the median had increasing probabilities of experiencing severe IPV, while those at the very high ends of household income had probabilities that approached zero. Given that household income in Germany was measured after taxes and social contributions, which may be expected to level out the social gradient, it is particularly noteworthy that the relationship between household income and IPV

Table 7.4 Evaluation of hypotheses: social position's impact on IPV exposure (RQ1)

Country	Hypotheses	Indicators	Confirmation		
			Significant predictor	Expected direction	Improves model fit
US	H1: higher social position is related to less exposure to IPV				
	1a	Income	✓	✓	✓
	1b	Education	✓	✓	x
	1c	Employment	x	–	x
Germany	H1: higher social position is related to less exposure to IPV				
	1a	Income	✓	✓	✓
	1b	Education	✓	x	✓
	1c	Employment	x	–	x
Norway	H1: higher social position is related to less exposure to IPV				
	1a	Income	x	–	x
	1b	Education	✓	✓	✓
	1c	Employment	✓	✓	✓

✓ confirmed, x not confirmed, – not applicable

exposure remained significant. These findings are in line with previous studies demonstrating the relationship between household income and abuse, where income sometimes showed it itself to be the strongest factor related to IPV (Bachman and Saltzman 1995; Cunradi et al. 2002; Tolman and Rosen 2001; Vest et al. 2002). In the case that household income represented women's financial resources *during* a violent relationship, these results could indicate that minimal household financial resources may have made it difficult for women to end an abusive relationship and may have exposed them to severe IPV. Alternatively, following family conflict theory, the social structural stress associated with low-income households may have been the trigger for severe IPV. In the case that household income represented women's economic resources *after* an abusive relationship, these results could be indicative of the diminished resources available to women after establishing autonomous households. Overall, these results fall in line with studies showing that concerns regarding the financial consequences of relationship dissolution negatively impact the decision to end the abusive relationship, and consequently result in longer exposure to IPV (Anderson and Saunders 2003; Kim and Gray 2008; Meyer 2012).

The second major finding is related to the rather distinctive pattern found in the Norwegian data. Employment was the strongest predictor of IPV exposure for the Norwegian sample, but did not play a role in either the US or Germany. Specifically, not being actively employed predicted higher risk of severe IPV than active employment (H1c). Given the overall high levels of employment and the negative correlation found between severe IPV exposure and employment in the Norwegian data (see Chap. 6), it was already clear that employment may play a deciding factor in exposure. Other studies have shown that employment status is one of the strongest predictors of women's decision to leave or stay in an abusive relationship (for a review, see Anderson and Saunders 2003). Thus, in the case that employment status measured at the time of the survey was during a relationship, lack of part- or full-time employment may have made it difficult for women to end an abusive relationship and may have exposed them to severe IPV. Likewise, for women coping with the aftermath of an abusive relationship, their opportunities and abilities to work may have been hindered by previous severe IPV (e.g., through injuries or harassment at the workplace by the abusive [ex-] partner) (Bell 2003; Browne et al. 1999; Moe and Bell 2004).

The third major finding is related to the effect of education on IPV exposure. As opposed to household income and employment, education was related to IPV exposure (H1b) in all three countries. Women in the US and Norwegian samples with fewer years of education, especially those with less than a high school education, had an increased risk of severe IPV exposure. Education is an individual resource that women carry with them throughout their adult lives, affording them the economic opportunities necessary to exit relationships before violence escalates. Thus, lack of education may increase women's economic dependence on their partners and place them at higher risk of IPV exposure (Farmer and Tiefenthaler 1997; Golden et al. 2013; Shobe and Dienemann 2008). In the German sample, however, increasing levels of education predicted increasing levels of risk of minor IPV exposure. Following the relative resource theory of IPV, one possible explanation may be that risk of IPV increases when women have access to a greater level of resources (e.g., education) than their partner. Thus, given that education represents women's own stable resources in these analyses, an imbalance of relative resources may potentially be the source of the higher level of risk of minor IPV in the German sample. It is also noteworthy that the increased risk was for minor IPV exposure, indicating that the violence had not yet escalated to violence causing injury. Despite the increased risk according to an imbalance in resources, perhaps education still served as a protector against more severe forms of IPV. Unfortunately, it was not possible to test this idea with the current data. Even so, it is remains clear that education is a significant factor for IPV exposure risk for the US, Germany, and Norway.

Although these three findings offer valuable contributions to the literature, there are critical issues which should be considered. It was not possible in all data sets to differentiate whether the violence reported occurred in the current relationship or a previous relationship. Significantly fewer women reporting IPV within the past five years were married or partnered in all three countries (see Chap. 6), so it may be reasonable to infer that measures of social position in the data represented resources after exiting an abusive relationship for the majority of survivors. Even so, no causal directionality could be established between social position and IPV exposure with the cross-sectional data. Although this book's conceptual framework suggests a causal link leading from social position to IPV exposure, the overview of the literature presented in Chap. 2 instead suggests that the relationship may move in both directions. In other words, lower social position may increase risk of IPV exposure, but increased IPV exposure may also decrease social position. I argue, however, that both possibilities are relevant for understanding differential exposure. Finally, employment was measured using a dichotomous variable, combining part-time and full-time employment together, and not differentiating between the unemployed actively seeking work and those unemployed by choice. This was done to combat the problem of small case numbers in such a detailed categorization, but may have led to a decreased effect of the variable overall.

Despite these issues, the analyses presented in this chapter provide a rare look at the relationship between social position and IPV exposure in a variety of national settings. The commonalities in the results for the US, Germany, and Norway stress the importance of considering women's socioeconomic resources within the context of IPV, implying that increased resources generally serve as a protection against IPV exposure. Education, specifically, proved to be an important factor for all three countries, with household income also impacting IPV exposure in the US and Germany, and employment playing the strongest role for Norway. The puzzle remains, however, why the patterns of social position's impact on IPV exposure vary across these national settings. The link between these results and the national policy contexts will be explored in detail in Chap. 9. But first, analyses of the link between IPV and women's health outcomes are presented in the following chapter.

References

Anderson, D. K., & Saunders, D. G. (2003). Leaving an abusive partner: An empirical review of predictors, the process of leaving, and psychological well-being. *Trauma, Violence, and Abuse, 4*(2), 163–191. doi:10.1177/1524838002250769

Bachman, R., & Saltzman, L. E. (1995). *Violence against women: Estimates from the redesigned survey*. Washington, DC: U.S. Department of Justice.

Bell, H. (2003). Cycles within cycles. *Violence Against Women, 9*(10), 1245–1262. doi:10.1177/1077801203255865

Browne, A., Salomon, A., & Bassuk, S. S. (1999). The impact of recent partner violence on poor women's capacity to maintain work. *Violence Against Women, 5*(4), 393–426. doi:10.1177/10778019922181284

Cunradi, C. B., Caetano, R., & Schafer, J. (2002). Socioeconomic predictors of intimate partner violence among white, black, and Hispanic couples in the United States. *Journal of Family Violence, 17*(4), 377–389. doi:0885-7482/02/1200-0377/0

Farmer, A., & Tiefenthaler, J. (1997). An economic analysis of domestic violence. *Review of Social Economy, 55*(3), 337–358. doi:10.1080/00346769700000004

Golden, S. D., Perreira, K. M., & Durrance, C. P. (2013). Troubled times, troubled relationships: How economic resources, gender beliefs, and neighborhood disadvantage influence intimate partner violence. *Journal of Interpersonal Violence, 28*, 2134–2155. doi:10.1177/0886260512471083

Kim, J., & Gray, K. A. (2008). Leave or stay? Battered women's decision after intimate partner violence. *Journal of Interpersonal Violence, 23*(10), 1465–1482. doi:10.1177/0886260508314307

Meyer, S. (2012). Why women stay: A theoretical examination of rational choice and moral reasoning in the context of intimate partner violence. *Australian and New Zealand Journal of Criminology, 45*(2), 179–193. doi:10.1177/0004865812443677

Mitchell, C., & Vanya, M. (2009). Explanatory frameworks of intimate partner violence. In C. Mitchell & D. Anglin (Eds.), *Intimate partner violence: A health-based perspective* (pp. 39–52). New York, NY: Oxford University Press.

Moe, A. M., & Bell, M. P. (2004). Abject economics. *Violence Against Women, 10*(1), 29–55. doi:10.1177/1077801203256016

Shobe, M. A., & Dienemann, J. (2008). Intimate partner violence in the United States: An ecological approach to prevention and treatment. *Social Policy and Society, 7*(2), 185–195. doi: http://dx.doi.org/10.1017/S1474746407004137

Tolman, R. M., & Rosen, D. (2001). Domestic violence in the lives of women receiving welfare: Mental health, substance dependence, and economic well-being. *Violence Against Women, 7* (2), 141–158. doi:10.1177/10778012010070020003

Vest, J. R., Catlin, T. K., Chen, J. J., & Brownson, R. C. (2002). Multistate analysis of factors associated with intimate partner violence. *American Journal of Preventive Medicine, 22*(3), 156–164.

Chapter 8
Findings on Differential Vulnerability to Poor Health

Abstract This chapter addresses whether women with IPV exposure are more vulnerable to social position's impact on health outcomes than women without IPV exposure. According to the conceptual framework, for IPV survivors in lower social positions, *differential vulnerability* to poor health is a further mechanism contributing to health inequities, particularly if women do not have the resources necessary to adequately access health care. Therefore, for the US, Germany, and Norway, it was first hypothesized that *higher social position is related to better health*. Second, it was hypothesized that *IPV exposure negatively contributes to health outcomes*. The final hypothesis is that *social position's negative impact on health increases with IPV exposure*. The present chapter is split into two primary sections. Section 8.1 presents the results related to the impact of IPV exposure on health, beyond what can be attributed to social position. Building on these results, Sect. 8.2 specifically addresses the moderating effect of IPV on the relationship between social position and health. The chapter concludes with an overview of the results for each country and a discussion of the key findings in the context of the conceptual framework and the empirical literature.

After investigating the differential exposure of women to IPV according to social position in Chap. 7, this chapter addresses the second research question (RQ2) posed in this book: whether women with IPV exposure are more vulnerable to social position's impact on health outcomes than women without IPV exposure. According to the conceptual framework, for IPV survivors in lower social positions, *differential vulnerability* to poor health is a further mechanism contributing to health inequities, particularly if women do not have the resources necessary to adequately access health care. From a statistical standpoint, the question posed is one of the moderating effects of IPV exposure on the relationship between social position and health. This is best tested using a series of nested models, first establishing whether social position affects health, and then whether IPV contributes to health outcomes, before finally testing the interaction between social position and IPV exposure.

© Springer International Publishing Switzerland 2016

M.M. Larsen, *Health Inequities Related to Intimate Partner Violence Against Women*, Social Disparities in Health and Health Care,
DOI 10.1007/978-3-319-29565-7_8

Therefore, for all three countries, it was first hypothesized that *higher social position is related to better health.*[1] Even more specifically, a series of sub-hypotheses were created by breaking down social position and health outcomes, so that higher household income, education, and employment were hypothesized to result in better self-assessed health and fewer mental health complaints. Second, it was hypothesized that *IPV exposure negatively contributes to health outcomes.* Again creating sub-hypotheses, health was broken down into self-assessed health and mental health complaints. The final hypothesis is that *social position's negative impact on health increases with IPV exposure.* Specifically, it was hypothesized that household income's, education's, and employment's impact on poor self-assessed health increases with IPV exposure. The same was hypothesized for their impact on number of mental health complaints.

The present chapter is split into two primary sections. Section 8.1 presents the results related to the impact of IPV exposure on health, beyond what can be attributed to social position. Building on these results, Sect. 8.2 specifically addresses the moderating effect of IPV on the relationship between social position and health. The chapter concludes with three tables presenting an overview of the results for each country and a discussion of the key findings related to RQ2 in the context of the conceptual framework and the empirical literature.

8.1 IPV Exposure's Impact on Health

To begin, logit regression models were fit for self-assessed health as a dichotomous-dependent variable, and negative binomial regression models for mental health complaints as a count-dependent variable. Initially, three nested models were fit for each health outcome: a model with only social position as the independent variable (Model 1); a model adding IPV exposure as a categorical moderating variable (Model 2); and an additional model incorporating the control variables (Model 3). The results of the logit regression models are presented in terms of odds ratios (OR) and the results of the negative binomial regression models are presented in terms of incident rate ratios (IRR). Furthermore, calculations of predicted probabilities of poor self-assessed health and predicted counts of mental health complaints, taking into account IPV exposure and social position, are presented for the purposes of further illustrating the findings. In order to inform decision-making about the successive, nested models, information on the improvement of model fit is also presented. The findings from Model 3 were used to confirm the hypotheses.

[1]It is worth emphasizing that the same hypotheses were tested for each country, and due to the methodological considerations described in Chap. 5, the countries were not statistically compared against one another. Whether differences across countries could be attributable to differences in the policy context will be explored in Chap. 9.

8.1.1 Impact of IPV Exposure on Self-assessed Health

This section begins with the results from the *US data* testing whether social position alone has an impact on respondents' self-assessment of health. Annual household income, education, and employment were found to predict whether a respondent rated her health as poor, so that increases in income, education, and employment resulted in lower odds of a poor health rating (see Table 8.1, Model 1). For every $1000 increase in the equivalized annual household income, the odds of rating health as poor were 0.97 smaller. Likewise, for every additional year of education, the odds of a poor health rating were 0.84 smaller. Finally, the odds of a poor health rating were more than halved for those who were employed full- or part-time as compared to those who were not.

Table 8.1 US: odds ratios predicting poor SAH

Predictors	US: poor SAH (N = 4725) OR (SE)		
	Model 1	Model 2	Model 3
Social position			
Household income[a]	0.97 (0.00)***	0.98 (0.00)***	0.97 (0.00)***
Education in years[b]	0.84 (0.02)***	0.84 (0.02)***	0.87 (0.02)***
Employed (FT/PT)[c]	0.48 (0.05)***	0.48 (0.05)***	0.49 (0.06)***
IPV exposure			
No IPV	–	Base	Base
Minor	–	0.91 (0.21)	1.11 (0.27)
Severe	–	1.89 (0.37)***	1.93 (0.41)**
Controls			
Age in years	–	–	1.07 (0.05)
Married/partnered	–	–	0.97 (0.12)
Number of children	–	–	0.88 (0.04)**
Racial/ethnic minority	–	–	1.67 (0.20)***
Frequent alcohol	–	–	1.36 (0.31)
Other violence	–	–	1.46 (0.18)**
Health impairment	–	–	6.14 (0.77)***
Constant	0.21 (0.02)***	0.20 (0.02)***	0.02 (0.02)***
Likelihood ratio test	265.14***	275.01***	565.52***
McFadden's r^2	0.09	0.09	0.19
Wald test	–	10.82**	294.21***
BIC'	−239.78	−232.71	−455.53

95 % confidence intervals. Standard errors are shown in parentheses

$*p < 0.05$, $**p < 0.01$, $***p < 0.001$

[a]Annual, equivalized household income before taxes and centered on the median in increments of $1000

[b]Centered on a high school education

[c]'Not employed' is base category

When IPV exposure was added to create Model 2, the odds of a poor health rating were 1.89 times larger for those reporting severe IPV exposure as compared to no IPV, even when controlling for the effects of social position. However, the experience of minor IPV did not significantly impact the odds of a poor health rating. The impact of household income, education, and employment on self-assessed health held steady. When comparing Models 1 and 2, adding the measure of IPV exposure improved the prediction of poor health ($\chi^2(2) = 10.82$, $p < 0.01$), despite the fact that minor IPV was not significant. While the pseudo R-squared stayed the same, the BIC' measures for these models indicated strong support for Model 1 over Model 2.

Even so, given the significance of severe IPV in Model 2 and the contribution of IPV exposure overall to predicting poor health in the US data, IPV exposure was kept in Model 3 as the control variables were added. When accounting for the newly added control variables, severe IPV continued to increase the odds of poor self-assessed health, and the overall measure of IPV exposure continued to contribute to the model's prediction of poor self-assessed health. At the same time, the effects of household income, education, and employment on poor self-assessed health remained stable. Finally, including the control variables improved the pseudo R-squared and the BIC' measures indicated very strong support for including control variables.

As a means of illustrating the results for Model 3 for the US data, predicted probabilities were calculated of poor self-assessed health at different levels of social position, according to IPV exposure (see Fig. 8.1). For instance, at the lowest levels of household income, the predicted probability of poor health was 12 % for those with no IPV, and 13 % for those with minor IPV, as compared to 21 % for those with severe IPV exposure. These probabilities of poor self-assessed health decreased for respondents as household income increased, with the predicted probabilities at the highest levels of income ranging from 1 to 2 % and barely differentiating from one another.

The predicted probabilities of poor self-assessed health according to education and IPV exposure presented a similar pattern. At the lowest levels of education, the predicted probability of poor health was 33 % for those with no IPV, and 37 % for those with minor IPV, as compared to 49 % for those with severe IPV exposure. Given that the lowest level of education was absolutely no education at all, the extremity of these predicted probabilities is perhaps not surprising. A less extreme example of lower levels of education would be those without a high school education. For these women, the predicted probability of poor health was 13 % for those with no IPV, and 14 % for those with minor IPV, as compared to 22 % for those with severe IPV exposure. These probabilities decreased as education levels increased, so that at the highest levels of education, the predicted probabilities of poor health according to IPV exposure were 4, 4, and 7 %, respectively.

Furthermore, for the unemployed, the predicted probability of poor self-assessed health was 10 % for those with no IPV, and 11 % for those who have experienced minor IPV, as compared to 24 % for those with severe IPV exposure. The same pattern prevailed for the employed, with the predicted probability of poor health

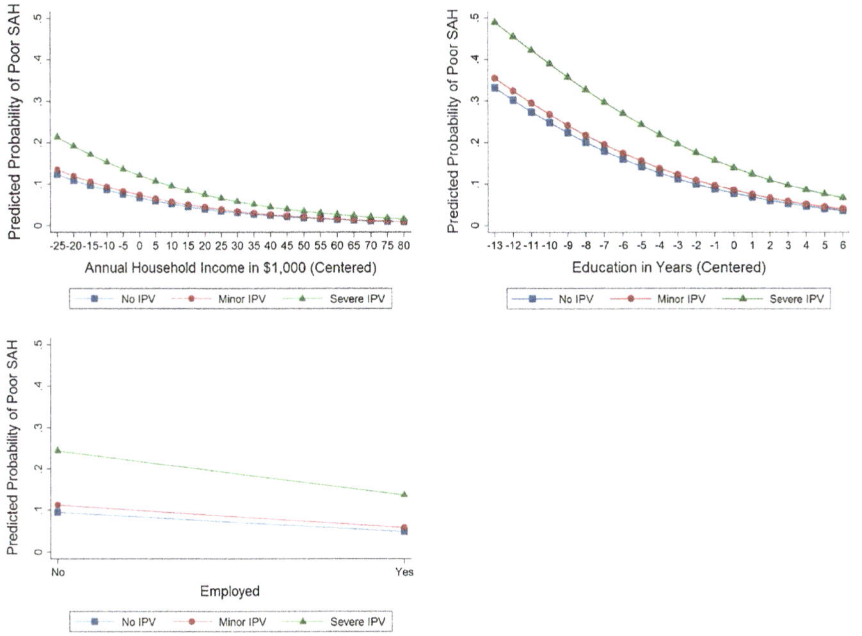

Fig. 8.1 US: predictive probabilities of poor SAH by social position according to IPV exposure (Model 3), only significant variables presented

being 5, 6, and 11 %, respectively. In sum, Fig. 8.1 illustrates that severe IPV increases the probability of poor self-assessed health in the US data, in addition to the impact of social position on poor self-assessed health. Additionally, given that the lines representing IPV exposure tend toward overlapping, the graphs hint at a possible interaction between IPV exposure and household income, as well as between IPV exposure and education.

Altogether, these results provide evidence confirming that increases in household income, education, and employment contribute to better self-assessed health in the US data. Moreover, the results confirm the hypothesis that IPV exposure contributes to poor self-assessed health, beyond what can be explained by social position alone.

Moving on to the *German data*, first it was tested whether social position alone had an impact on respondents' self-assessment of health. For Germany, education and employment predicted whether a respondent rated her health as poor, so that increases in education and employment resulted in lower odds of poor self-assessed health (see Table 8.2, Model 1). For every additional year of education, the odds of a poor health rating were 0.92 smaller. Likewise, the odds of a poor health rating were 0.61 smaller for those who were employed full- or part-time as compared to those who were not employed. The effect of household income on poor self-assessed health was not significant, although it did approach significance.

Table 8.2 Germany: odds ratios predicting poor SAH

Predictors	Germany: poor SAH (N = 3724) OR (SE)		
	Model 1	Model 2	Model 3
Social position			
Household income[a]	0.98 (0.01)	0.99 (0.01)	0.98 (0.01)*
Education in years[b]	0.92 (0.02)***	0.93 (0.02)***	0.95 (0.02)*
Employed (FT/PT)[c]	0.61 (0.07)***	0.60 (0.07)***	0.73 (0.09)*
IPV exposure			
No IPV	–	Base	Base
Minor	–	0.71 (0.23)	0.68 (0.23)
Severe	–	1.78 (0.30)***	1.76 (0.34)**
Controls			
Age in years	–	–	1.01 (0.06)
Married/partnered	–	–	1.27 (0.22)
Number of children	–	–	0.97 (0.07)
Migration background	–	–	1.31 (0.22)
Frequent alcohol	–	–	0.91 (0.13)
Other violence	–	–	1.37 (0.18)*
Health impairment	–	–	8.51 (1.15)***
Constant	0.18 (0.02)***	0.17 (0.02)***	0.04 (0.04)***
Likelihood ratio test	52.73***	65.02***	349.64***
McFadden's r^2	0.02	0.03	0.14
Wald test	–	13.18***	300.30***
BIC'	−28.06	−23.91	−242.74

95 % confidence intervals. Standard errors are shown in parentheses

*p < 0.05, **p < 0.01, ***p < 0.001

[a]Annual, equivalized household income after taxes and centered on the median in increments of €1000

[b]Centered on median number of years of education

[c]'Not employed' is base category

When adding IPV exposure as a variable to fit Model 2, the odds of a poor self-assessed health rating were 1.78 times larger for those reporting severe IPV as compared to no IPV, even when controlling for the effects of social position. However, minor IPV did not significantly impact the odds of a poor health rating in Model 2. The impact of education and employment on self-assessed health remained steady. When comparing Models 1 and 2, adding the measure of IPV exposure improved the prediction of poor self-assessed health ($\chi^2(2) = 13.18, p < 0.01$), despite the fact that minor IPV was not significant. However, while the pseudo R-squared was minimally better for Model 2, the BIC' measures indicated positive support for Model 1 without IPV exposure over Model 2 with IPV exposure.

However, given the significance of severe IPV in Model 2 and the contribution of IPV exposure overall to predicting poor self-assessed health, IPV exposure was kept in Model 3 as the control variables were added. With the addition of these variables, the effect of severe IPV remained constant and minor IPV remained nonsignificant in its prediction of self-assessed health. Furthermore, the overall measure of IPV exposure still contributed to the model's prediction of poor self-assessment of health ($\chi^2(2) = 10.80$, $p < 0.01$). At the same time, the effects of social position on health changed slightly, with household income becoming significant, education remaining relatively stable, and employment becoming slightly weaker. Finally, including the control variables dramatically improved Model 3's pseudo R-squared and the BIC' measures indicated very strong support for including control variables.

As a means of illustrating the results for Model 3 for the Germany data, predicted probabilities were calculated of poor self-assessed health at different levels of social position, according to IPV exposure (see Fig. 8.2). For instance, at the lowest levels of household income, the predicted probability of poor self-assessed health was 11 % for those with no IPV and 8 % for those with minor IPV, as compared to 18 % for those with severe IPV exposure. These probabilities decreased as household income increased, so that at the highest levels of income, the predicted probabilities of poor health ranged from 2 % for no IPV, 1 % for minor IPV, to 3 % for severe IPV exposure. Similarly, at the lowest levels of education, the predicted probability of poor self-assessed health was 11 % for no IPV and 8 % for minor IPV, as compared to 17 % for severe IPV exposure. These probabilities also

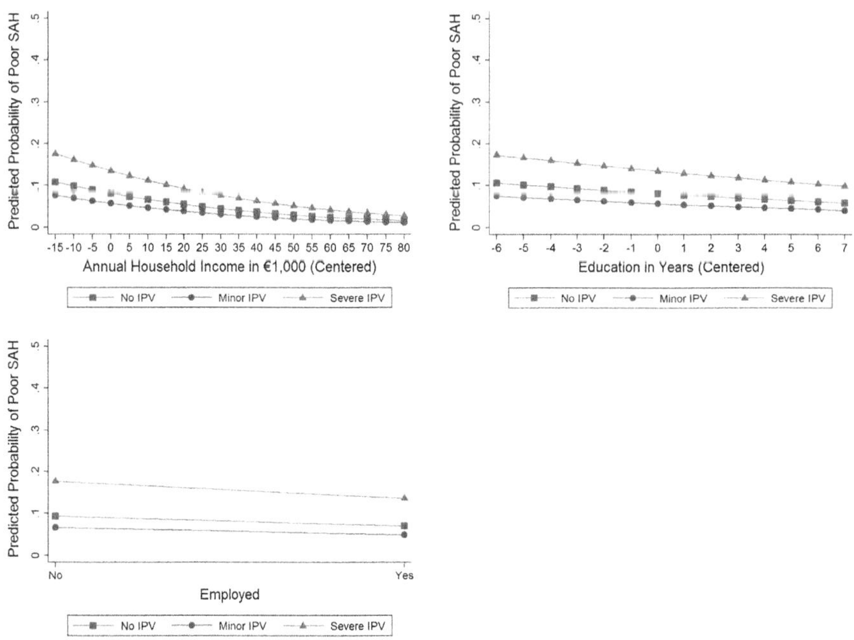

Fig. 8.2 Germany: predictive probabilities of poor SAH by social position according to IPV exposure (Model 3), only significant variables presented

decreased as education levels increased, with the highest levels of education showing probabilities of 6, 4, and 10 %, respectively. Finally, for the unemployed, the predicted probability of poor self-assessed health was 10 % for no IPV and 7 % for minor IPV, as compared to 18 % for severe IPV exposure. These probabilities were lower for the employed respondents, with predicted probabilities of 7, 5, and 14 % for no IPV, minor IPV, and severe IPV, respectively. In sum, Fig. 8.2 illustrates that severe IPV increased the probability of poor self-assessed health in the German data, in addition to the impact of social position on poor self-assessed health. Minor IPV exposure, however, appeared to have an effect closer to that of no IPV exposure. Additionally, given that the lines representing IPV exposure tend toward overlapping for household income, the graph hints at a possible interaction between IPV exposure and household income.

These results provide evidence confirming that increases in household income, education, and employment contribute to better self-assessed health in the German data. Moreover, the results confirm the hypothesis that IPV exposure contributes to poor self-assessed health, beyond what can be explained by social position alone.

Finally, for the *Norwegian data*, lower social position was also found to be related to poor self-assessed health. Specifically, annual household income, education, and employment predicted whether a respondent rated her health as poor, so that increases in income, education, and employment resulted in lower odds of a poor health rating (see Table 8.3, Model 1). For every 10,000 NOK[2]-increment increase in the equivalized annual household income, the odds of rating health as poor were 0.99 smaller. Likewise, for every additional year of education, the odds of a poor health rating were 0.90 smaller. Finally, for those employed full- or part-time, the odds of a poor health rating were 0.28 smaller as compared to those who were not.

When creating Model 2 by adding IPV exposure as a variable, the odds of a poor health rating were 2.17 times larger for those reporting minor IPV, and 2.63 times larger for those reporting severe IPV as compared to no IPV, even when controlling for the effects of social position. The impact of education and employment on self-assessed health remained steady, but the effect of household income was no longer significant. When comparing Models 1 and 2, adding the measure of IPV significantly improved the prediction of self-assessed health ($\chi^2(2) = 25.20$, $p < 0.001$). Additionally, the pseudo R-squared improved for Model 2 and the BIC' measures indicated very strong support for Model 2 over Model 1.

Based on the significance of IPV exposure in Model 2 and its contribution to the prediction of self-assessed health in the Norway data, IPV exposure was kept in Model 3 as the control variables were added. With the addition of these variables, the effects of minor and severe IPV on self-assessed health remained significant. Additionally, the overall measure of IPV exposure continued to contribute to the model's prediction of poor self-assessment of health ($\chi^2(2) = 11.53$, $p < 0.01$). At the same time, the effects of social position changed slightly, so that household

[2]Which was equal to approximately €1376 in 2003 (European Central Bank 2014).

Table 8.3 Norway: odds ratios predicting poor SAH

Predictors	Norway: poor SAH (N = 1575) OR (SE)		
	Model 1	Model 2	Model 3
Social position			
Household income[a]	0.99 (0.01)*	0.99 (0.01)	0.97 (0.01)*
Education in years[b]	0.90 (0.03)***	0.90 (0.03)***	0.93 (0.03)*
Employed (FT/PT)[c]	0.28 (0.05)***	0.29 (0.05)***	0.41 (0.09)***
IPV exposure			
No IPV	–	Base	Base
Minor	–	2.17 (0.59)**	2.13 (0.68)*
Severe	–	2.63 (0.57)***	2.19 (0.60)**
Controls			
Age in years	–	–	1.08 (0.09)
Married/partnered	–	–	1.76 (0.47)*
Number of children	–	–	0.82 (0.08)*
Migration background	–	–	1.55 (0.48)
Frequent alcohol	–	–	0.85 (0.18)
Other violence	–	–	1.53 (0.29)*
Health impairment	–	–	29.3 (8.94)***
Constant	0.51 (0.08)***	0.44 (0.07)***	0.02 (0.03)*
Likelihood ratio test	102.35***	126.07***	357.54***
McFadden's r^2	0.07	0.09	0.26
Wald test	–	25.20***	155.29***
BIC'	−80.26	−89.26	−261.83

95 % confidence intervals. Standard errors are shown in parentheses

*$p < 0.05$, **$p < 0.01$, ***$p < 0.001$

[a]Annual, equivalized household income before taxes centered on the median in increments of 10,000 NOK

[b]Centered on a high school education

[c]'Not employed' is base category

income became significant, employment weakened slightly, and education remained stable. Furthermore, including the control variables dramatically improved Model 3's pseudo R-squared and the BIC' measures indicated very strong support for including control variables.

Predicted probabilities of poor self-assessed health at different levels of social position according to IPV exposure illustrate the results from Model 3 for the Norway data (see Fig. 8.3). For example, at the lowest levels of household income, the predicted probability of poor health was 20 % for no IPV, as compared to 34 % for minor IPV, and 35 % for severe IPV. These probabilities decreased for respondents as household income increased, and the pattern according to IPV exposure remained the same, so that the probability of poor self-assessed health for those at the highest levels of household income were 3, 6, and 6 %, respectively.

Likewise, at the lowest levels of education, the predicted probability of poor health was 18 % for no IPV, as compared to 32 % for minor IPV and 32 % for severe IPV exposure. These probabilities also decreased as education increased, so that at the highest levels of education, the predicted probabilities of poor self-assessed health were 8, 15, and 16 %, respectively. For the unemployed in the Norway data, the predicted probability of poor self-assessed health was 22 % for no IPV, as compared to 37 and 47 % for minor and severe IPV exposure. These probabilities were lower for the employed respondents, so that the predicted probability of poor self-assessed health was 12 % for no IPV, as compared to 23 % for minor IPV, and 32 % for severe IPV exposure. In conclusion, Fig. 8.3 illustrates that minor and severe IPV increased the probability of poor self-assessed health in the Norwegian data to a similar degree, in addition to the impact of social position on poor self-assessed health. Additionally, given that the lines representing IPV exposure tended toward overlapping for household income, the graph hints at a possible interaction between IPV exposure and household income.

Taken together, these results provide evidence confirming that increases in household income, education, and employment contributed to better self-assessed health in the Norwegian data. Moreover, the results confirm the hypothesis that IPV exposure contributes to poor self-assessed health, beyond what can be explained by social position alone.

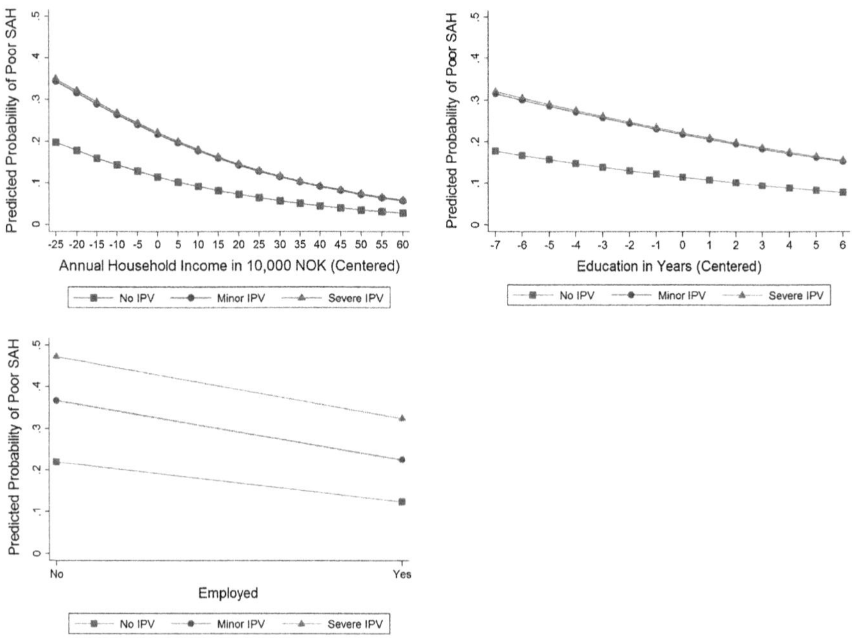

Fig. 8.3 Norway: predictive probabilities of poor SAH by social position according to IPV exposure (Model 3), only significant social position variables presented

After examining self-assessed health, the next set of results for the US, Germany, and Norway examine the impact of IPV exposure on mental health complaints.

8.1.2 Impact of IPV Exposure on Mental Health Complaints

Similar to the previous section, the first model with the *US data* predicting number of mental health complaints first tested whether social position alone had an impact. Annual household income and education predicted the number of mental health complaints experienced by respondents in the week prior to the survey, so that increases in income and education resulted in fewer mental health complaints in the US data (see Table 8.4, Model 1). For every $1000 increase in the equivalized annual household income, the number of mental health complaints decreased by a factor of 0.99. Likewise, for every additional year of education, the number of mental health complaints decreased by a factor of 0.98. Employment status, on the other hand, did not significantly predict mental health complaints.

When creating Model 2 by adding IPV exposure, the number of mental health complaints increased by a factor of 1.24 for minor IPV and by a factor of 1.23 for severe IPV exposure, as compared to no IPV, even when controlling for the effects of social position. The effects of household income and education on the number of mental health complaints remained steady. When comparing Models 1 and 2, adding the measure of IPV exposure improved the prediction of the number of mental health complaints in the past week ($\chi^2(2) = 43.15$, $p < 0.001$). Moreover, the BIC' measures for these models indicated very strong support for Model 2 with IPV exposure over Model 1 without it.

Given these results, IPV exposure remained in Model 3 as the control variables were added. When accounting for these newly added variables, the effects of minor and severe IPV on mental health complaints remained relatively stable, so that IPV exposure increased the number of mental health complaints. Importantly, in Model 3, the overall measure of IPV exposure continued to significantly contribute to the model's prediction of mental health complaints, even after accounting for the newly added control variables ($\chi^2(2) = 41.97$, $p < 0.001$). The effects of household income and education on the number of mental health complaints also remained stable, and the effect of employment remained nonsignificant. Finally, including the control variables improved Model 3's pseudo *R*-squared and the BIC' measures indicated very strong support for including the control variables.

The predicted counts of mental health complaints at different levels of social position according to IPV exposure illustrate the results for Model 3 of the US data (see Fig. 8.4). For example, at the lowest levels of household income data, the predicted count of mental health complaints was 2.8 for no IPV, 3.4 for minor IPV, and 3.3 for severe IPV exposure. These predicted counts decreased as household

Table 8.4 US: incident rate ratios predicting mental health complaints

Predictors	US: number of mental health complaints (N = 4725) IRR (SE)		
	Model 1	Model 2	Model 3
Social position			
Household income[a]	0.99 (0.00)***	0.99 (0.00)***	0.99 (0.00)***
Education in years[b]	0.98 (0.00)***	0.98 (0.00)***	0.98 (0.00)***
Employed (FT/PT)[c]	0.99 (0.02)	0.98 (0.02)	1.00 (0.02)
IPV exposure			
No IPV	–	Base	Base
Minor	–	1.24 (0.05)***	1.23 (0.05)***
Severe	–	1.23 (0.06)**	1.17 (0.05)**
Controls			
Age in years	–	–	1.02 (0.01)*
Married/partnered	–	–	1.01 (0.02)
Number of children	–	–	0.99 (0.01)
Racial/ethnic minority	–	–	1.00 (0.02)
Frequent alcohol	–	–	1.14 (0.05)**
Other violence	–	–	1.16 (0.03)***
Health impairment	–	–	1.44 (0.04)***
Constant	2.56 (0.05)***	2.50 (0.05)***	1.68 (0.25)**
Likelihood ratio test	216.75***	258.11***	461.68***
McFadden's r^2	0.01	0.02	0.03
Wald test	–	43.15***	221.41***
BIC'	−191.37	−215.81	−351.70

95 % confidence intervals. Standard errors are shown in parentheses
*p < 0.05, **p < 0.01, ***p < 0.001
[a]Annual, equivalized household income before taxes and centered on the median in increments of $1000
[b]Centered on high school education
[c]'Not employed' is base category

income increased, so that at the highest levels of income, the predicted count of mental health complaints was 1.4 for no IPV, 1.7 for minor IPV, and 1.6 for severe IPV exposure. A similar pattern was seen for the predicted counts of mental health complaints according to education and IPV exposure. At the lowest levels of education, the predicted count of mental health complaints was 3.2 for no IPV, as opposed to 3.9 for minor IPV and 3.7 for severe IPV exposure. These predicted counts decreased as education levels increased, so that the predicted counts of mental health complaints were 2.1, 2.6, and 2.5 for no IPV, minor IPV, and severe IPV exposure, respectively. In sum, Fig. 8.4 illustrates the overall similar impact of both minor and severe IPV on mental health complaints, in addition to the impact of social position on mental health complaints.

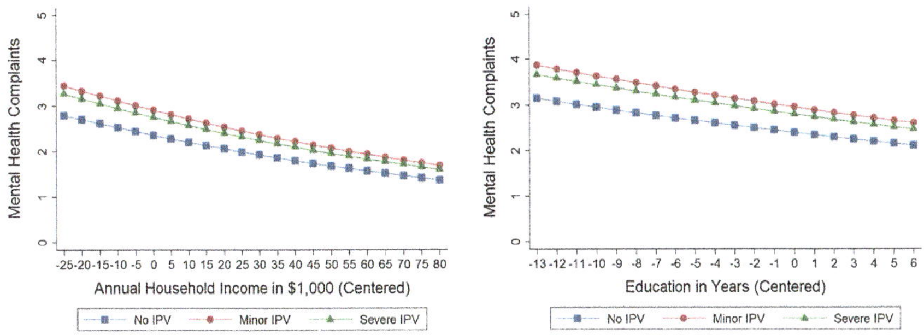

Fig. 8.4 US: predicted count of mental health complaints by social position according to IPV exposure (Model 3), only significant social position variables presented

Hence, these results provide evidence confirming the hypotheses that increases in household income and education contributed to fewer mental health complaints in the US data. However, evidence could not confirm this for employment. The results also confirmed the hypothesis that IPV exposure contributed to mental health complaints, beyond what could be explained by social position alone.

The first model in the *German data* predicting the number of mental health complaints experienced by respondents in the 12 months prior tested whether social position alone had an impact. Annual household income, education, and employment predicted mental health complaints (see Table 8.5, Model 1). For every $1000-increment increase in the equivalized annual household income, the number of mental health complaints decreased by a factor of 0.99. Likewise, the number of mental health complaints decreased by a factor of 0.93 for the employed. Yet surprisingly, for every year increase in education, the number of mental health complaints increased slightly by a factor of 1.01.

When creating Model 2 by adding IPV exposure, the number of mental health complaints increased by factors of 1.33 for minor IPV and 1.72 for severe IPV exposure, as opposed to no IPV. The effects of household income, education, and employment on the number of mental health complaints remained steady. When comparing Models 1 and 2, adding the measure of IPV exposure improved the model's explanatory power ($\chi^2(2)$ = 122.01, $p < 0.001$). Moreover, the BIC' measures for these models indicated very strong support for Model 2 with IPV exposure over Model 1 without.

Given both the significance of minor and severe IPV, as well as IPV exposure's improvement of the explanatory power of the model, IPV exposure was kept in Model 3 as the control variables were added. When accounting for these newly added variables, the effect of minor IPV lost significance, and the effect of severe IPV decreased slightly but remained significant. Even so, the overall measure of IPV exposure continued to contribute to the model's prediction of mental health complaints ($\chi^2(2)$ = 64.43, $p < 0.001$). The effect of education and household income on the number of mental health complaints remained stable, but the effect of employment became nonsignificant. Including the control variables improved

Table 8.5 Germany: incident rate ratios predicting mental health complaints

Predictors	Germany: number of mental health complaints (N = 3724) IRR (SE)			
	Model 1	Model 2	Model 3	Model 3a
Social position				
Household income[a]	0.99 (0.00)***	0.99 (0.00)*	0.99 (0.00)*	1.00 (0.00)
Education in years[b]	1.01 (0.01)**	1.01 (0.01)*	1.01 (0.01)*	1.01 (0.01)*
Employed (FT/PT)[c]	0.93 (0.03)*	0.93 (0.03)*	0.97 (0.03)	0.96 (0.03)
hh income*education	–	–	–	0.99 (0.00)*
IPV exposure				
No IPV	–	Base	Base	Base
Minor	–	1.33 (0.09)***	1.13 (0.08)	1.13 (0.08)
Severe	–	1.72 (0.09)***	1.51 (0.08)***	1.52 (0.08)***
Controls				
Age in years	–	–	0.99 (0.01)	0.99 (0.01)
Married/partnered	–	–	0.91 (0.04)*	0.90 (0.04)*
Number of children	–	–	1.05 (0.02)**	1.06 (0.02)**
Migration background	–	–	0.93 (0.04)	0.94 (0.04)
Frequent alcohol	–	–	1.13 (0.04)***	1.14 (0.04)***
Other violence	–	–	1.36 (0.04)***	1.36 (0.04)***
Health impairment	–	–	1.54 (0.07)***	1.54 (0.07)***
Constant	3.65 (0.11)***	3.39 (0.10)***	3.99 (0.98)***	3.97 (0.98)***
Likelihood ratio test	30.48***	155.89***	363.30***	368.04***
McFadden's r^2	0.00	0.01	0.02	0.02
Wald test	–	122.01***	209.16***	4.74*
BIC'	−5.81	−114.78	−256.40	−252.92

95 % confidence intervals. Standard errors are shown in parentheses
*$p < 0.05$, **$p < 0.01$, ***$p < 0.001$
[a]Annual, equivalized household income after taxes and centered on the median in increments of €1000
[b]Centered on median number of years of education
[c]'Not employed' is base category

Model 3's pseudo R-squared and the BIC' measures indicated very strong support for including the control variables as compared to without these variables.

To illustrate the results of the Germany data for Model 3, predicted counts of mental health complaints are presented at different levels of household income and education according to IPV exposure (see Fig. 8.5). For instance, at the lowest levels of household income, the predicted count of mental health complaints was 3.4 for those with no IPV, 3.9 for minor IPV, and 5.2 for severe IPV exposure. For all levels of IPV exposure, these predicted counts decreased as household income increased. This is evident when examining the highest levels of household income, where the predicted count of mental health complaints was 2.4 for no IPV and 2.7 for minor IPV, as compared to 3.6 for severe IPV exposure.

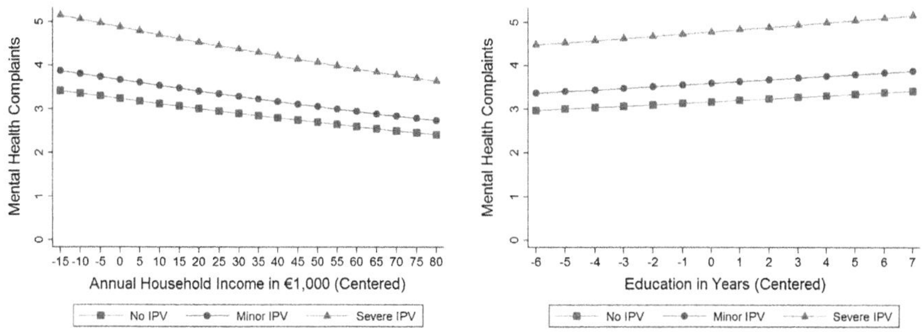

Fig. 8.5 Germany: predicted count of mental health complaints by social position according to IPV exposure (Model 3), only significant social position variables presented

The picture, however, for education in predicting mental health complaints was quite different. The predicted count of mental health complaints for those at the lowest levels of education was 3.0 for no IPV, 3.4 for minor IPV, and 4.5 for severe IPV exposure. These predicted counts increased as education increased for all levels of IPV exposure. For example, at the highest levels of education, the predicted count of mental health complaints was 3.4, 3.9, and 5.2 for no IPV, minor IPV, and severe IPV exposure, respectively. In sum, Fig. 8.5 illustrates that severe IPV had the greatest impact on mental health complaints, in addition to the impact of social position on mental health. Moreover, it highlights that household income and education impacted IPV exposure in opposite directions.

Since the effect of education on mental health complaints moved in the opposite direction as hypothesized, follow-up negative binomial regression models were fit interacting social position variables to assess whether variation across these variables may account for this result. The findings revealed a significant interaction between household income and education (see Table 8.5, Model 3a).[3] The interaction demonstrates that when household income was held at the median, the incident rate ratio of mental health complaints increased by a factor of 1.01 for every additional year of education. Likewise, if education was held at the median, then household income did not have a significant impact on mental health complaints. Furthermore, in Model 3a the overall measure of IPV exposure continued to contribute to the prediction of mental health complaints ($\chi^2(2) = 66.29$, $p < 0.001$). However, including the interaction between household income and education did not improve Model 3a's pseudo R-squared as compared to Model 3. Moreover, the BIC' measures indicated positive (but not strong) support for the model without the interaction term. Still, it is important to note that the interaction term did contribute significantly to the explanatory power of the model ($\chi^2(1) = 4.74$, $p < 0.05$). Based

[3]The models interacting household income and employment, and education and employment were not significant and are, therefore, not discussed in the text. For full tables of these results, please contact the author.

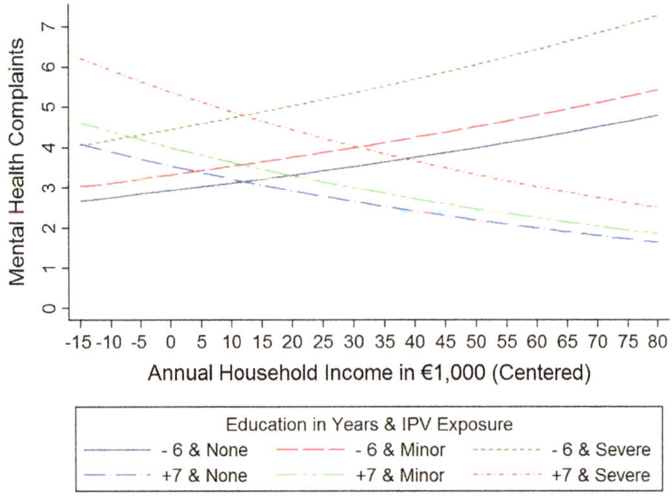

Fig. 8.6 Germany: predicted count of mental health complaints according to IPV exposure, interacting household income and education (Model 3a)

on these results, one may cautiously attribute the positive effect of increasing education on increasing mental health complaints to this interaction.

As an aid to understanding the interaction between household income and education in the German data, the results are presented here in terms of predicted count of mental health complaints according to IPV exposure (see Fig. 8.6). For those with both the lowest level of household income and the lowest level of education, the predicted count of mental health complaints ranged from 2.7 for no IPV to 4.1 for severe IPV exposure. This is in contrast to those at the lowest level of household income but the highest level of education, where the predicted count of mental health complaints ranged from 4.1 for no IPV to 6.2 for severe IPV exposure. However, at the other end of the income spectrum, the picture looks very different. For those with the highest level of household income but the lowest education level, the predicted count of mental health complaints ranged from 4.8 for no IPV to 7.3 for severe IPV exposure. On the other hand, for those with both the highest level of household income and the highest level of education, the predicted count of mental health complaints ranged from 1.6 for no IPV to 2.5 for severe IPV exposure. In other words, the two groups with the highest predicted count of mental health complaints were those with severe IPV exposure and an apparent inconsistency in levels of household income and education: first those with the highest level of household income but the lowest education level, and then those with the highest level of education but lowest household income. In sum, Fig. 8.6 continues to illustrate that severe IPV had the greatest impact on mental health complaints, in addition to the interaction of household income and education on mental health.

Altogether, these results provide evidence confirming the hypotheses that increases in household income contributed to fewer mental health complaints in the

German data. While the effect of education on mental health was clear, it was not in the direction predicted. However, the results could not confirm the effect of employment on mental health complaints. Finally, results confirmed the hypothesis that IPV exposure contributed to mental health complaints, beyond what could be explained by social position alone.

For the *Norwegian data*, to begin predicting the number of mental health complaints found bothersome by the respondents in the two weeks prior to the survey, it was first tested whether social position alone had an impact. Annual household income and employment predicted the number of mental health complaints in the Norway data (see Table 8.6, Model 1). For every 10,000 NOK[4] increase in the equivalized annual household income, the number of mental health complaints decreased by a factor of 0.97. Additionally, the number of mental health complaints decreased by a factor of 0.48 for those who were employed full- or part-time as compared to those who were not. Education, however, did not predict mental health complaints in the Norway data.

IPV exposure was added to create Model 2. When this was done, the number of mental health complaints increased by a factor of 2.42 for minor IPV and by 3.45 for severe IPV, as opposed to no IPV, even when controlling for the effects of social position. The effects of household income and employment on the number of mental health complaints remained steady. When comparing Models 1 and 2, adding the measure of IPV exposure significantly improved the prediction of mental health complaints ($\chi^2(2) = 31.29, p < 0.001$). Moreover, the BIC' measures for these models indicated very strong support for Model 2 with IPV exposure over Model 1 without.

Given the significance of minor and severe IPV, as well as IPV exposure's improvement of the explanatory power of the model and the improvement in model fit, IPV exposure was kept in Model 3 as the control variables were added. When accounting for these newly added variables, the effect of severe IPV decreased, but remained significant. However, the effect of minor IPV on mental health complaints became nonsignificant, although the p value did border on significance. Even so, the overall contribution of IPV exposure to the model's prediction of mental health complaints continued to be significant ($\chi^2(2) = 8.11, p < 0.05$). Furthermore, the effect of household income remained stable, but the effect of employment became nonsignificant. Finally, including the control variables improved Model 3's pseudo *R*-squared and the BIC' measures indicated very strong support for including the control variables compared to Model 2 without.

To illustrate the Norway results for Model 3, the predicted count of mental health complaints at different levels of household income and IPV exposure are presented (see Fig. 8.7). At the lowest levels of household income, the predicted count of mental health complaints reported as bothersome was 0.60 for no IPV, as compared to 1.01 for minor IPV, and 1.08 for severe IPV exposure. These counts of mental health complaints decreased for respondents as household income increased. For instance, at the highest levels of income, the predicted counts of mental health

[4]Which was equal to approximately €1376 in 2003 (European Central Bank 2014).

Table 8.6 Norway: incident rate ratios predicting mental health complaints

Predictors	Norway: number of mental health complaints (N = 1575) IRR (SE)		
	Model 1	Model 2	Model 3
Social position			
Household income[a]	0.97 (0.01)***	0.97 (0.01)***	0.97 (0.01)**
Education in years[b]	0.98 (0.03)	0.99 (0.03)	0.99 (0.03)
Employed (FT/PT)[c]	0.48 (0.10)***	0.55 (0.11)**	0.82 (0.16)
IPV exposure			
No IPV	–	Base	Base
Minor	–	2.42 (0.72)**	1.68 (0.47)
Severe	–	3.45 (0.86)***	1.80 (0.44)*
Controls			
Age in years	–	–	0.99 (0.07)
Married/partnered	–	–	1.31 (0.29)
Number of children	–	–	0.92 (0.08)
Migration background	–	–	1.42 (0.39)
Frequent alcohol	–	–	1.12 (0.21)
Other violence	–	–	2.67 (0.41)***
Health impairment	–	–	4.13 (1.03)***
Constant	0.82 (0.15)***	0.58 (0.11)**	0.34 (0.44)
Likelihood ratio test	55.96***	90.59***	183.62***
McFadden's r^2	0.02	0.04	0.07
Wald test	–	31.29***	81.79***
BIC'	−33.88	−53.78	−87.91

95 % confidence intervals. Standard errors are shown in parentheses
* $p < 0.05$, ** $p < 0.01$, *** $p < 0.001$
[a]Annual, equivalized household income before taxes centered on the median in increments of 10,000 NOK
[b]Centered on a high school education
[c]'Not employed' is base category

complaints approached zero and were barely distinguishable across levels of exposure (i.e., 0.08 for no IPV, 0.10 for minor IPV, and 0.11 for severe IPV exposure). In sum, Fig. 8.7 illustrates the overall similar impact of both minor and severe IPV on predicting mental health complaints. With this in mind, it should be taken into consideration that minor IPV's nonsignificant impact on mental health complaints may have been at least partially due to small sample sizes, rather than truly having no impact. Additionally, given that the lines representing IPV exposure tended toward overlapping for household income, the graph hints at a possible interaction between IPV exposure and household income.

Altogether, these results provide evidence confirming the hypotheses that increases in household income contributed to fewer mental health complaints in the Norway data. However, evidence could not confirm this for education or

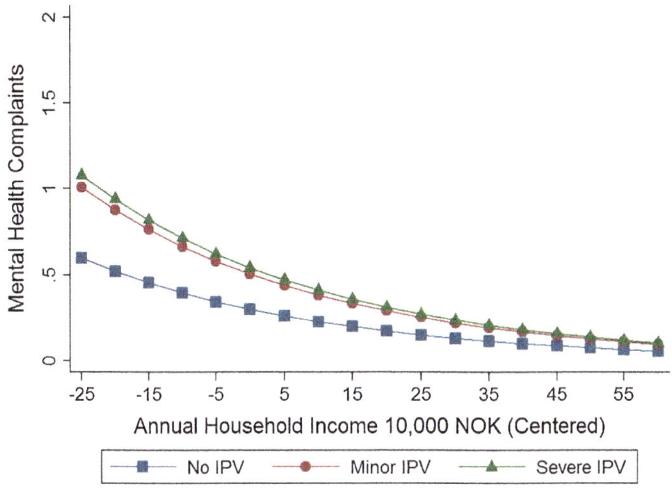

Fig. 8.7 Norway: predicted count of mental health complaints by social position according to IPV exposure (Model 3), only significant social position variables presented

employment. The results also confirmed the hypothesis that IPV exposure contributed to mental health complaints, beyond what could be explained by social position alone.

8.2 Social Position's Impact on Health: IPV Exposure as a Moderator

This section describes the last set of analyses for RQ2 as to whether women with IPV exposure are more vulnerable to social position's impact on health outcomes than women without IPV exposure. Building on the previous nested models, it was first tested whether social position's negative impact on health increases with IPV exposure. Some of the graphs presented in Sect. 8.1 hinted at possible interactions between social position and IPV exposure (i.e., Figs. 8.1, 8.2, 8.3, and 8.7), so to test this statistically, interactions of social position and IPV exposure were added to Model 3 for each health outcome and country. This resulted in the following models: one adding the interaction between household income and IPV exposure (Model 4); a model replacing the previous interaction with one between education and IPV exposure (Model 5); and a model replacing the previous interaction with one between employment and IPV exposure (Model 6).[5] As in Sect. 8.1, the results

[5]Models including all three interaction terms together were first tested, but omnibus tests of significance indicated that the three interaction terms together did not significantly impact the results. Thus, models with the individual interaction terms were also tested (Frazier et al. 2004).

are organized by health outcome and presented in terms of odds ratios and incident rate ratios, predicted probabilities and counts, and goodness-of-fit measures.

8.2.1 Impact on Self-assessed Health: IPV Exposure as a Moderator

When separately including variables interacting social position and IPV exposure for the *US data*, the interaction between household income and severe IPV significantly predicted self-assessed health (see Table 8.7, Model 4). The conditional effects of the model demonstrated that when there is no IPV exposure, household income has a negative impact on the odds of poor self-assessed health. In other words, when there is no IPV, the odds of poor health decrease by a factor of 0.97 for every $1000 increase in the equivalized annual household income. It also revealed that when household income is held at the median, severe IPV exposure no longer significantly predicted poor self-assessed health. Adding the interaction term of household income and overall IPV exposure to create Model 4 resulted in an improvement over Model 3 which approached significance ($\chi^2(2) = 5.39$, $p = 0.067$). While the pseudo R-squareds did not vary between Models 3 and 4, comparing measures of BIC' suggested strong support for Model 3 over Model 4.

The predicted probability of poor self-assessed health according to household income and IPV exposure provides an illustration of the results of Model 4 (see Fig. 8.8). For no IPV, the predicted probability of poor health was 12 % for the lowest levels of income, as compared to 1 % for the highest income levels. Similarly, for minor IPV, the predicted probability of poor health was 12 % for the lowest levels of income, as compared to 1 % for the highest levels of income. However, for those with severe IPV exposure, the predicted probability of poor health was 41 % for the lowest levels of income, as compared to nearly 0 % for the highest levels of income. In other words, Fig. 8.8 illustrates that household income's impact on self-assessed health was strongest for severe IPV exposure as compared to minor IPV exposure or no exposure.

Although Fig. 8.1 from Sect. 8.1.1 revealed a tendency towards overlap for the lines representing IPV exposure according to education, the interaction between IPV exposure and education was not significant for the US data (see Table 8.7, Model 5). Likewise, the interaction between IPV exposure and employment was also not significant (Model 6). Given their nonsignificance, adding these interactions did not result in statistically significant improvements to the models, and the BIC' measures indicated positive support for Model 4 over Models 5 and 6, and very strong support for Model 3 without any interactions.

Altogether, the significance of the interaction between household income and severe IPV exposure in Model 4, along with a Wald statistic approaching significance for the overall interaction between income and overall IPV exposure, partially confirmed for the US data that household income's impact on self-assessed

Table 8.7 US: odds ratios predicting poor SAH with interactions

Predictors	US: poor SAH (N = 4725) OR (SE)		
	Model 4	Model 5	Model 6
Social position			
Household income[a]	0.97 (0.00)***	0.97 (0.00)***	0.97 (0.01)***
Education in years[b]	0.87 (0.02)***	0.87 (0.02)***	0.87 (0.02)***
Employed (FT/PT)[c]	0.50 (0.06)***	0.49 (0.06)***	0.52 (0.21)
IPV exposure			
No IPV	Base	Base	Base
Minor	1.15 (0.31)	1.05 (0.29)	1.48 (0.52)
Severe	0.89 (0.39)	2.00 (0.45)**	1.90 (0.60)*
Controls			
Age in years	1.07 (0.05)	1.08 (0.05)	1.08 (0.05)
Married/partnered	0.98 (0.12)	0.97 (0.12)	0.97 (0.12)
Number of children	0.87 (0.04)**	0.88 (0.04)**	0.87 (0.04)**
Racial/ethnic minority	1.69 (0.21)***	1.68 (0.21)***	1.66 (0.20)***
Frequent alcohol	1.36 (0.31)	1.36 (0.31)	1.37 (0.31)
Other violence	1.47 (0.18)**	1.46 (0.18)**	1.46 (0.18)**
Health impairment	6.19 (0.78)***	6.15 (0.78)***	6.14 (0.78)***
*Social position *IPV*			
Income[a] *exposure:			
No IPV	Base	–	–
Minor	1.00 (0.02)	–	–
Severe	0.93 (0.03)*	–	–
Education[b] *exposure:			
No IPV	–	Base	–
Minor	–	1.05 (0.12)	–
Severe	–	0.95 (0.11)	–
Employed*exposure:			
No IPV	–	–	0.97 (0.40)
Minor	–	–	0.57 (0.35)
Severe	–	–	1.0 (omitted)[d]
Constant	0.02 (0.02)***	0.02 (0.02)***	0.02 (0.02)***
Likelihood ratio test	572.29***	565.93***	566.74***
McFadden's r^2	0.19	0.19	0.19
Wald test	5.39[e]	0.41	0.83
BIC'	−445.39	−439.02	−439.83

95 % confidence intervals. Standard errors are shown in parentheses

$*p < 0.05$, $**p < 0.01$, $***p < 0.001$

[a]Annual, equivalized household income before taxes centered on the median in increments of $1000

[b]Centered on a high school education

[c]'Not employed' is base category

[d]Due to the collinearity of severe IPV*employed

[e]Marginal significance at $p = 0.067$

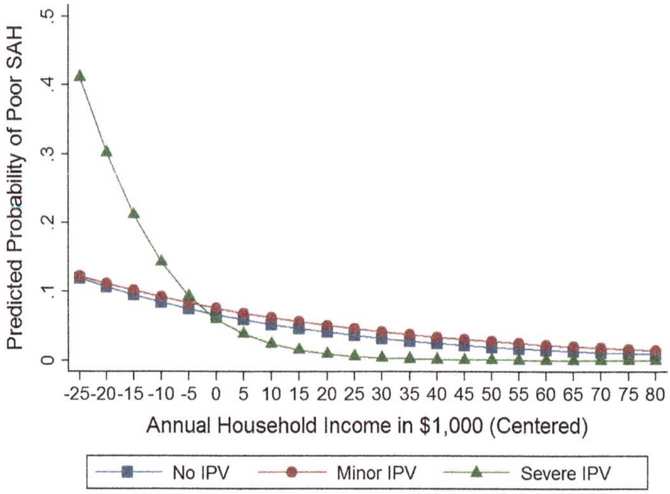

Fig. 8.8 US: predictive probabilities of poor SAH, interacting household income and IPV exposure (Model 4)

health should vary according to IPV exposure. However, hypotheses of an interaction between IPV exposure and education and employment could not be confirmed.

When separately including variables interacting social position and IPV exposure for the *German data*, none of the interactions had a significant impact on poor self-assessment of health.[6] This was the case even though Fig. 8.2 revealed a tendency towards overlap for the lines representing IPV exposure according to household income, which may have led one to expect at least one potential interaction. Moreover, adding the interaction terms did not result in statistically significant improvements to the models. Finally, while the pseudo R-squareds did not vary between Model 3 (r^2 = 0.14) as compared to Models 4 (r^2 = 0.14), 5 (r^2 = 0.14), and 6 (r^2 = 0.14), comparing measures of BIC' suggested very strong support for Model 3 (BIC'_3 = −242.74) without interactions over Models 4 (BIC'_4 = −229.51), 5 (BIC'_5 = −226.69), and 6 (BIC'_6 = −229.05).[7]

Likewise, including interaction variables for social position and IPV exposure for the *Norwegian data* did not result in any significant impacts on poor self-assessment of health.[8] Also for Norway, Fig. 8.3 had indicated a tendency

[6]Income * minor IPV: OR = 0.92 (0.06), income * severe IPV: 1.03 (0.03), education * minor IPV: 0.94 (0.11), education * severe IPV: 1.02 (0.07), employed * no IPV: 1.08 (0.40), employed * minor IPV: 0.34 (0.27).

[7]For full tables of these results, please contact the author.

[8]Income * minor IPV: OR = 1.03 (0.03), income * severe IPV: 0.98 (0.02), education * minor IPV: 0.99 (0.12), education * severe IPV: 0.93 (0.11), employed * no IPV: 1.05 (0.56), employed * minor IPV: 0.83 (0.77).

towards overlap between IPV exposure and household income, but this did not hold statistically. None of the interaction terms resulted in statistically significant improvements to the models. Similar to Germany, the pseudo *R*-squareds did not vary between Model 3 (r^2 = 0.26) when compared to Models 4 (r^2 = 0.26), 5 (r^2 = 0.26), and 6 (r^2 = 0.26). However, comparing BIC' suggested very strong support for Model 3 (BIC'_3 = −261.83) without interactions over Models 4 (BIC'_4 = −248.91), 5 (BIC'_5 = −247.52), and 6 (BIC'_6 = −247.19) (see Footnote 7). Altogether, this evidence did not confirm for the German or Norwegian data that the impact of household income, education, and employment on poor self-assessed health, respectively, should vary according to IPV exposure.

8.2.2 *Impact on Mental Health Complaints: IPV Exposure as a Moderator*

When separately including variables interacting social position and IPV exposure for the *US data*, *German data*, and *Norwegian data* none of the interactions had a significant impact on the number of mental health complaints.[9, 10, 11] At least for Norway, Fig. 8.7 in the previous section hinted at a potential interaction between household income and IPV exposure. However, this did not hold up statistically. Moreover, adding the interaction terms did not result in statistically significant improvements to Models 4–6 in any of the countries. Finally, for all three countries, the pseudo *R*-squareds did not vary between Models 3 (US: r^2 = 0.03, Germany: r^2 = 0.02, Norway: r^2 = 0.07) when compared to Models 4 (US: r^2 = 0.03, Germany: r^2 = 0.02, Norway: r^2 = 0.07), 5 (US: r^2 = 0.03, Germany: r^2 = 0.02, Norway: r^2 = 0.07), and 6 (US: r^2 = 0.03, Germany: r^2 = 0.02, Norway: r^2 = 0.07). Additionally, comparing measures of BIC' suggested very strong support for Model 3 (US: BIC'_3 = −351.70, Germany: BIC'_3 = −252.92, Norway: BIC'_3 = −87.91) without interactions over Models 4 (US: BIC'_4 = −335.52, Germany: BIC'_4 = −248.91, Norway: BIC'_4 = −73.46), 5 (US: BIC'_5 = −338.32, Germany: BIC'_5 = −247.52, Norway: BIC'_5 = −74.25), and 6 (US: BIC'_6 = −335.38, Germany: BIC'_6 = −247.19, Norway: BIC'_6 = −74.68) for all three countries (see Footnote 7). Thus, taken together, this evidence did not confirm for the US, Germany, or Norway that the impact of household income, education, and

---

[9] US: income * minor IPV: OR = 0.99 (0.00), income * severe IPV: 0.99 (0.00), education * minor IPV: 1.03 (0.02), education * severe IPV: 1.02 (0.02), employed * no IPV: 1.07 (0.20), employed * minor IPV: 1.07 (0.13).

[10] Germany: income * minor IPV: OR = 0.99 (0.01), income * severe IPV: 0.99 (0.01), education * minor IPV: 0.98 (0.02), education * severe IPV: 0.98 (0.02), employed * no IPV: 0.93 (0.10), employed * minor IPV: 0.99 (0.17).

[11] Norway: income * minor IPV: OR = 1.01 (0.02), income * severe IPV: 1.01 (0.02), education * minor IPV: 0.96 (0.10), education * severe IPV: 0.90 (0.10), employed * no IPV: 1.41 (0.67), employed * minor IPV: 0.62 (0.55).

employment on mental health complaints, respectively, should vary according to IPV exposure.

8.2.3 Discussion

The primary aim of this chapter was to examine whether women with histories of IPV are more vulnerable to social position's impact on health outcomes. The analyses presented were based on a conceptual framework that argues that women in lower social positions with IPV exposure experience *differential vulnerability* to poor health. Statistically, this required testing IPV exposure's moderating effect on the relationship between social position and health. This necessitated first examining: (1) social position's impact on health, and then (2) whether IPV contributed to health outcomes, even after accounting for the effect of social position. Only after these issues were examined could it be tested whether (3) social position's impact on health varied by IPV exposure. These analyses generated three important findings, which are described in the following paragraphs.

First, the results replicated what has been repeatedly shown in the literature: social gradients in health exist across a wide variety of national settings (e.g., Mackenbach et al. 2008). Even in societies with relatively low levels of social inequality, socioeconomic status serves as a "fundamental cause" of ill health, so that those with access to resources are able to avoid health risks and reduce the costs of poor health (Link and Phelan 1995). Results in this chapter demonstrated that not being employed, as well as lower levels of household income and education, were related to increased odds of poor self-assessed health for all three countries (see Table 8.8, Hypotheses $2a_{1-6}$).[12] Moreover, lower household income predicted more mental health complaints in both the US and Norway, as did fewer years of education in the US. In contrast, the data from Germany revealed an interaction between household income and education, so that the greatest levels of mental health complaints were reported among those with high household income but low levels of education, and those with high levels of education but low household income. According to the literature, such status inconsistency may be related to poorer mental health outcomes, whether it be individual status inconsistency or status inconsistency between individuals in a partnership (Dressler 1988; Gal et al. 2008; Hornung 1977). It is argued that departure from expected societal norms which dictate that financial rewards should be proportionate to education levels may lead to conflicting role expectations and uncertainty, resulting in psychological distress (Lenski 1954; Stehr 1968; Vernon and Buffler 1988). This may serve as a partial explanation for why women in Germany living with household incomes

[12]As mentioned in Chap. 7, it is important to note that the measure of household income in the German data was after taxes and social contributions. It would be expected that this would level out the social gradient to a certain extent. In this sense, it is particularly interesting that the relationship remained between household income and both health outcome variables.

Table 8.8 Evaluation of hypotheses: social position's impact on health (RQ2)

Hypotheses	Outcomes	Indicators	Confirmation		
			US	Germany	Norway
H2a: higher social position is related to better health					
	Self-assessed health				
$2a_1$		Household income	✓	✓	✓
$2a_2$		Education	✓	✓	✓
$2a_3$		Employment	✓	✓	✓
	Mental health complaints				
$2a_4$		Household income	✓	/	✓
$2a_5$		Education	✓	/	x
$2a_6$		Employment	x	x	x

✓ confirmed, x not confirmed, / not in predicted direction

inconsistent with their education reported a higher number of mental health complaints than women with more consistent income and education levels.[13] In sum, corresponding to previous research, social gradients were found for women's physical and mental health outcomes in all three countries.

Second, the results provided evidence that IPV exposure within the past five years negatively contributed to health outcomes beyond what was attributable to social position (see Table 8.9, Hypotheses $2b_{1-2}$). Specifically, in the US and Germany, severe IPV exposure nearly doubled the odds of poor self-assessed health, while in Norway, those with either minor or severe IPV exposure had odds of poor self-assessed health that were more than twice as high as for women without exposure. Likewise, the findings demonstrated that the incident rate for mental health complaints was one-and-a-half to two times greater for those women in Germany and Norway with severe IPV exposure. Meanwhile, in the US, both minor and severe IPV exposure lead to higher incident rates of mental health complaints.

By examining the effect of IPV exposure using harmonized data for three different countries, these results make a valuable contribution to an abundance of previous research examining the negative health consequences of IPV (for a recent review, see Dillon et al. 2013). In particular, the results confirm previous studies by demonstrating that increased severity of IPV exposure is associated with increased negative health consequences in all three countries studied (Dutton et al. 2005; Hegarty et al. 2013; Straus et al. 2009; Wuest et al. 2010). In my analyses, severe IPV was operationalized as exposure with injury, while minor IPV was operationalized as exposure without injury. Thus, based on these results, injuries resulting from IPV can clearly be conceptualized as having both acute and

[13]Although the correlation between education and household income in Norway was in the same moderately low range as in Germany (see Chap. 6), no interaction was found in the Norwegian data. In contrast, a moderately strong correlation between education and household income was found in the US data, which may explain a reduced tendency toward status inconsistency.

Table 8.9 Evaluation of hypotheses: IPV exposure's impact on health (RQ2)

Country	Hypotheses	Outcomes	Confirmation			
			Significant predictor	Expected direction	Improved model fit	Goodness of fit
US	H2b: IPV negatively contributes to health outcomes					
	$2b_1$	Self-assessed health	✓	✓	✓	✓
	$2b_2$	Mental health complaints	✓	✓	✓	✓
Germany	H2b: IPV negatively contributes to health outcomes					
	$2b_1$	Self-assessed health	✓	✓	✓	✓
	$2b_2$	Mental health complaints	✓	✓	✓	✓
Norway	H2b: IPV negatively contributes to health outcomes					
	$2b_1$	Self-assessed health	✓	✓	✓	✓
	$2b_2$	Mental health complaints	✓	✓	✓	✓

✓ confirmed, x not confirmed, – not applicable

"long-term, residual consequences" leading to poorer self-assessment of health and more mental health symptoms (Weaver and Resnick 2004, p. 1344). Moreover, the contribution of minor IPV highlights that even without injury, IPV is capable of negatively impacting health. This supports the argument that IPV also influences health through the psychological stress caused by constant fear of violence (Coker et al. 2000; Wong et al. 2014). Furthermore, given that IPV exposure was operationalized as violence from a current or former partner within the past five years, the prolonged effect of IPV on health several years after women exit an abusive relationship was also evident in these results (Alsaker et al. 2007; Campbell and Lewandowski 1997; Ford-Gilboe et al. 2009; Rivara et al. 2007).

Most importantly, the impact of IPV exposure went beyond what could be explained by the social gradient in both physical and mental health outcomes in all three countries. This provides support for those who argue that we cannot fully understand how IPV affects health without also acknowledging the socioeconomic context in which it occurs (Humphreys 2007; Purvin 2007). Given that lower social positions co-occurred with IPV exposure in all three countries, it was also critical to further examine whether they produced susceptibilities to one another. Investigating the interactions between social position and IPV exposure indeed led to the final major finding of this chapter.

Third, and most to the point of this chapter, the results demonstrated that social position's impact on health increased with IPV exposure for the US data (see Table 8.10, Hypotheses $2c_{1-6}$). Specifically, the US data revealed that the effect of household income on poor self-assessed health was strongest for those with severe

Table 8.10 Evaluation of hypotheses: IPV exposure as a moderator (RQ2)

Country	Hypotheses	Outcomes and indicators	Confirmation			
			Significant predictor	Expected direction	Improved model fit	Goodness of fit
US	2c: social position's impact on health increases with IPV exposure					
		Self-assessed health				
	$2c_1$	Income	✓	✓	✓[a]	x
	$2c_2$	Education	x, T	–	x	x
	$2c_3$	Employment	x	–	x	x
		Mental health complaints				
	$2c_4$	Income	x	–	x	x
	$2c_5$	Education	x	–	x	x
	$2c_6$	Employment	x	–	x	x
Germany	2c: social position's impact on health increases with IPV exposure					
		Self-assessed health				
	$2c_1$	Income	x, T	–	x	x
	$2c_2$	Education	x	–	x	x
	$2c_3$	Employment	x	–	x	x
		Mental health complaints				
	$2b_4$	Income	x	–	x	x
	$2c_5$	Education	x	–	x	x
	$2c_6$	Employment	x	–	x	x
Norway	2c: social position's impact on health increases with IPV severity					
		Self-assessed health				
	$2c_1$	Income	x, T	–	x	x
	$2c_2$	Education	x	–	x	x
	$2c_3$	Employment	x	–	x	x
		Mental health complaints				
	$2c_4$	Income	x, T	–	x	x
	$2c_5$	Education	x	–	x	x
	$2c_6$	Employment	x	–	x	x

✓ confirmed, x not confirmed, – not applicable, T trending towards overlap in graphs of predicted probabilities
[a]Marginal significance at the $p = 0.065$ level

IPV exposure. Women in the US at the lowest household income levels with severe IPV exposure were the most vulnerable to poor self-assessed health, being more than twice as likely as women with a history of minor or no IPV exposure to report poor self-assessed health. Conversely, as income increased, the differences in the probabilities of poor self-assessed health based on women's IPV exposure decreased, and the probabilities of poor self-assessed health at the higher ends of household income began to approach zero for all levels of IPV exposure. This significant interaction should be interpreted cautiously since the interaction term contributed to the explanatory power of the model at a level of marginal significance. Even so, these findings imply that in the US sample, the lack of financial resources represented a serious risk for poor self-assessed health among women with severe IPV exposure. These findings also suggest that greater household income leveled out risk of poor self-assessed health regardless of IPV exposure. However, the impact of social position on mental health complaints did not vary by IPV exposure in the US data. Neither did such interactions prove to be significant in either Germany or Norway, despite the fact that both social position and IPV exposure predicted physical and mental health outcomes in these countries, and despite tendencies toward interactions revealed in Sect. 8.1. In other words, the results show that respondents in the Germany and Norway samples with IPV exposure were not more vulnerable to social position's impact on health than the respondents without IPV exposure.

The literature investigating the intersections between women's social position, IPV, and health outcomes is limited, but generally makes the argument that the social gradient in health is magnified by IPV exposure. This is indeed what was found with the significant interaction between household income and severe IPV exposure for the US data. A small community-based study in the US found a similar negative trend in the relationship between severity of IPV exposure and physical health symptoms for all household income levels, while also noting that IPV was more strongly associated with more symptoms among low-income women (Sutherland et al. 2001). Furthermore, given that this interaction was not found for either Germany or Norway, the intersections between household income, IPV exposure, and self-assessed health may potentially be dependent upon macro-level factors that differ across countries. This is explored in greater detail in Chap. 9. Contrary to what the literature would suggest (Ford-Gilboe et al. 2009; Goodman et al. 2009), however, the results in this chapter did not reveal any significant interactions for the impact on mental health complaints for any of the countries. This suggests either similarities at the macro-level, or potential measurement issues with the mental health outcome variable, which is explored in the following paragraphs.

The findings presented in this chapter expand upon the previous limited research examining how social position and IPV exposure interact to affect health outcomes. First, most previous studies have analyzed smaller community-based samples (Weaver and Resnick 2004). Using larger, nationally representative data sets, these analyses captured a much wider spectrum of social position, partner violence experience, and health outcomes that are typically not represented in smaller samples. Another important contribution of the current work is that it examines three different national settings, as opposed to the single-country or North American focus that is typical in the literature. Allowing a look at where similarities and differences may be apparent is vital to understanding whether there are certain "universal truths" regarding IPV's impact on health, and whether additional macro-level factors may indeed be involved.

Although these results offer a significant contribution to the limited amount of research examining the health inequities experienced by IPV survivors, there are some methodological issues to consider.[14] First, the same population-based survey data that offers so many advantages is commonly understood to be more sensitive to situational couple violence than to intimate partner terrorism.[15] Additionally, the household income item used here as a proxy of social position may also be more apt at capturing situational couple violence caused by structural stress, as argued by family conflict researchers. Even so, the similarity of the interaction between household income and IPV found by Sutherland et al. (2001) using a community-based sample focusing on IPV survivors in the US, and the interaction found in the present analyses using nationally representative data, lends some support to the notion that the present study has captured both types of IPV to a certain degree using a measure of severity.

Second, the data used were cross-sectional and included both women whose abusive relationships were either ongoing or in the recent past. In this sense, claims cannot be made about the causality of the relationship between social position, IPV exposure, and health. It remains plausible that poor health negatively impacted women's social position, particularly their ability to be engaged in employment or contribute to household income. Likewise, it is also possible that women with poor health were more susceptible to IPV exposure. Studies using longitudinal data are necessary to examine these relationships in further detail. Third, although psychological violence has a salient and important effect on the physical and mental health of IPV survivors (Nicolaidis and Paranjape 2009), its inconsistent measurement in the three surveys presented analytical difficulties and it was therefore not included in the operationalization of IPV exposure. This may have led to significant underestimation of IPV's impact on health in the results, and may also be part of the explanation for why no significant interaction between social position and IPV was found for mental health complaints as an outcome variable. Fourth, it is important to consider the possibility that a lack of significant interactions, especially where the graphs demonstrated a tendency toward overlap, may have been related to uneven sample sizes across groups of IPV exposure. This could have had the effect of decreasing the power of the models to a level which could not detect a significant interaction (Frazier et al. 2004).

Additionally, there are two issues specific to the health outcome variables themselves. First, although information on self-assessed health was collected in the three surveys along a scale, the analyses operationalized it as a dichotomous variable of poor and good self-assessed health. This was done to address the heavy skew toward positive responses, which precluded both a linear regression approach and an ordinal regression approach. An outcome variable with dichotomous response options may not have been able to reveal the interactions and may have resulted in a loss of power (Russell and Bobko 1992), thus potentially contributing

[14]See also Sect. 7.2 for issues specific to the relationship between social position and IPV exposure.

[15]The reader is referred to Chap. 2 for a more comprehensive discussion of the controversy regarding types of IPV and their measurement.

to nonsignificant interaction terms for self-assessed health for Germany and Norway. The same loss of power also applies when summing responses to scale items, as was done for the mental health complaints variable, because the span of the scale (i.e., four points for all three countries), rather than the number of items (i.e., ranging from 8 in the US to 12 in Germany), represents total response options. This may offer an additional explanation for the nonsignificant interaction terms for mental health complaints for all three countries. Ideally, the outcome measure should "have as many response options as the product of the response options of the predictor and moderator variables" (Frazier et al. 2004, p. 119). However, this is difficult to achieve and is thus a common and sometimes unavoidable issue when testing moderating effects.

Despite these issues, these analyses fill a meaningful gap in IPV research and reveal intriguing intersections between social position, IPV, and health which have previously not been directly investigated using multiple countries and nationally representative survey data. The results demonstrated that IPV exposure negatively contributed to physical and mental health outcomes in the US, Germany, and Norway data, beyond what the existing social gradients in health could explain. Only in the US, however, was there evidence that IPV survivors in lower social positions experience *differential vulnerability* to poor health, specifically when looking at household income and self-assessed health. In this context, the double burden of severe IPV and limited financial resources presents itself as an access issue requiring broader attention in the US. The connections between these results and the policy contexts of the US, Germany, and Norway, will be presented in Chap. 9.

References

Alsaker, K., Moen, B. E., & Kristoffersen, K. (2007). Health-related quality of life among abused women one year after leaving a violent partner. *Social Indicators Research, 86*(3), 497–509. doi:10.1007/s11205-007-9182-7

Campbell, J. C., & Lewandowski, L. A. (1997). Mental and physical health effects of intimate partner violence on women and children. *The Psychiatric Clinics of North America, 20*(2), 353–374. doi:10.1016/S0193-953X(05)70317-8

Coker, A. L., Smith, P. H., Bethea, L., King, M. R., & McKeown, R. E. (2000). Physical health consequences of physical and psychological intimate partner violence. *Archives of Family Medicine, 9*, 451–457.

Dillon, G., Hussain, R., Loxton, D., & Rahman, S. (2013). Mental and physical health and intimate partner violence against women: A review of the literature. *International Journal of Family Medicine*, 1–15. doi:10.1155/2013/313909

Dressler, W. W. (1988). Social consistency and psychological distress. *Journal of Health and Social Behavior, 29*(1), 79–91.

Dutton, M., Kaltman, S., Goodman, L. A., Weinfurt, K., & Vankos, N. (2005). Patterns of intimate partner violence: Correlates and outcomes. *Violence and Victims, 20*, 483–497. doi:10.1891/0886-6708.2005.20.5.483

European Central Bank. (2014). Euro foreign exchange reference rates. Retrieved from https://www.ecb.europa.eu/stats/exchange/eurofxref/html/eurofxref-graph-nok.en.html. Accessed on November 09, 2014.

Ford-Gilboe, M., Wuest, J., Varcoe, C., Davies, L., Merritt-Gray, M., Campbell, J. C., et al. (2009). Modelling the effects of intimate partner violence and access to resources on women's health in the early years after leaving an abusive partner. *Social Science and Medicine, 68*, 1021–1029. doi:10.1016/j.socscimed.2009.01.003

Frazier, P. A., Tix, A. P., & Barron, K. E. (2004). Testing moderator and mediator effects in counseling psychology research. *Journal of Counseling Psychology, 51*(1), 115–134.

Gal, G., Kaplan, G., Gross, R., & Levav, I. (2008). Status inconsistency and common mental disorders in the Israel-based world mental health survey. *Social Psychiatry and Psychiatric Epidemiology, 43*(12), 999–1003. doi:10.1007/s00127-008-0393-2

Goodman, L. A., Smyth, K. F., Borges, A. M., & Singer, R. (2009). When crises collide: How intimate partner violence and poverty intersect to shape women's mental health and coping? *Trauma, Violence, and Abuse, 10*, 306–329. doi:10.1177/1524838009339754

Hegarty, K. L., O'Doherty, L. J., Chondros, P., Valpied, J., Taft, A. J., Astbury, J., et al. (2013). Effect of type and severity of intimate partner violence on women's health and service use: Findings from a primary care trial of women afraid of their partners. *Journal of Interpersonal Violence, 28*(2), 273–294. doi:10.1177/0886260512454722

Hornung, C. A. (1977). Social status, status inconsistency and psychological stress. *American Sociological Review, 42*(4), 623–638.

Humphreys, C. (2007). A health inequalities perspective on violence against women. *Health and Social Care in the Community, 15*(2), 120–127.

Lenski, G. E. (1954). Status crystallization: A non-vertical dimension of social status. *American Sociological Review, 19*(4), 405–413.

Link, B. G., & Phelan, J. (1995). Social conditions as fundamental causes of disease. *Journal of Health and Social Behavior, 35*(Extra Issue), 80–94.

Mackenbach, J. P., Stirbu, I., Roskam, A. R., Schaap, M. M., Menvielle, G., Leinsalu, M., & Kunst, A. E. (2008). Socioeconomic inequalities in health in 22 European countries. *The New England Journal of Medicine, 358*, 2468–2481. doi:10.1056/NEJMsa0707519

Nicolaidis, C., & Paranjape, A. (2009). Defining intimate partner violence: Controversies and implications. In C. Mitchell & D. Anglin (Eds.), *Intimate partner violence: A health-based perspective* (pp. 19–30). New York, NY: Oxford University Press.

Purvin, D. M. (2007). At the crossroads and in the crosshairs: Social welfare policy and low-income women's vulnerability to domestic violence. *Social Problems, 54*(2), 188–210. doi:10.1525/sp.2007.54.2.188

Rivara, F. P., Anderson, M. L., Fishman, P., Bonomi, A. E., Reid, R. J., Carrell, D., et al. (2007). Healthcare utilization and costs for women with a history of intimate partner violence. *American Journal of Preventative Medicine, 32*, 89–96. doi:10.1016/j.amepre.2006.10.001

Russell, C. J., & Bobko, P. (1992). Moderated regression analysis and Likert scales: Too coarse for comfort. *Journal of Applied Psychology, 77*, 336–342.

Stehr, N. (1968). Status consistency: The theoretical concept and its empirical referent. *The Pacific Sociological Review, 11*(2), 95–99. doi:10.2307/1388323

Straus, H., Cerulli, C., McNutt, L. A., Rhodes, K. V., Conner, K. R., Kemball, R. S., et al. (2009). Intimate partner violence and functional health status: Associations with severity, danger, and self-advocacy behaviors. *Journal of Women's Health, 18*(5), 625–631.

Sutherland, C. A., Sullivan, C. M., & Bybee, D. I. (2001). Effects of intimate partner violence versus poverty on women's health. *Violence Against Women, 7*, 1122–1143. doi:10.1177/10778010122183775

Vernon, S. W., & Buffler, P. A. (1988). The status of status inconsistency. *Epidemiologic Reviews, 10*, 65–86.

Weaver, T. L., & Resnick, H. (2004). Toward developing complex multivariate models for examining the intimate partner violence-physical health relationship. *Journal of Interpersonal Violence, 19*(11), 1342–1349. doi:10.1177/0886260504269692

Wong, J. Y.-H., Fong, D. Y.-T., Lai, V., & Tiwari, A. (2014). Bridging intimate partner violence and the human brain: A literature review. *Trauma, Violence, and Abuse*, *15*(1), 22–33. doi:10.1177/1524838013496333

Wuest, J., Ford-Gilboe, M., Merritt-Gray, M., Wilk, P., Campbell, J. C., Lent, B., et al. (2010). Pathways of chronic pain in survivors of intimate partner violence. *Journal of Women's Health*, *19*(9), 1665–1674. doi:10.1089/jwh.2009.1856

Chapter 9
Comparing Policy Contexts: IPV Exposure and Health

Abstract This book's comparison of the US, Germany, and Norway enables a discussion of whether patterns in differential exposure and vulnerability vary across welfare state contexts, and whether institutional arrangements may contribute to health inequities for IPV survivors. Thus, based on the results of the empirical analyses, it is the aim of the present chapter to explore the macro-level policy context with the following research questions. Is social position's impact on IPV exposure reflective of national policies supporting women to establish independent households? And are the vulnerabilities to social position's impact on health among IPV survivors reflective of national policies regarding access to health care? The specific cross-national hypotheses addressing the effect of institutional arrangements are informed primarily by the detailed case descriptions presented in Chap. 4, which explored the gender, safety net, family, and health policy arrangements for each country. This chapter brings together the evidence from the social policy contexts relevant to the national survey data (i.e., mid-1990s for the US, early 2000s for Germany and Norway) and the empirical findings to assess the cross-national hypotheses. The chapter concludes with the acknowledgement of additional contextual factors and a brief discussion.

The previous chapters have examined the social determinants of IPV exposure and health outcomes at the individual level, but the macro-level social and policy context in which women live cannot be ignored (Whitaker 2014). A core notion of sociology is that institutional arrangements impact individual life chances, and it has been argued that protecting vulnerable citizens is a vital task of the welfare state (Esping-Andersen 1990). Even more to the point, the welfare state influences women's position in society (e.g., Orloff 1996). These ideas are at the center of the conceptual framework used in this book: exploring the pathways from the social and policy context to health inequities by focusing on IPV survivors as a group sensitive to welfare policy (for a review of the framework, see Fig. 9.1). By selecting countries with varying approaches to social stratification, this book has indirectly investigated the first mechanism proposed in the framework, which argues that the social and policy context shapes the overall social position of

© Springer International Publishing Switzerland 2016
M.M. Larsen, *Health Inequities Related to Intimate Partner Violence Against Women*, Social Disparities in Health and Health Care,
DOI 10.1007/978-3-319-29565-7_9

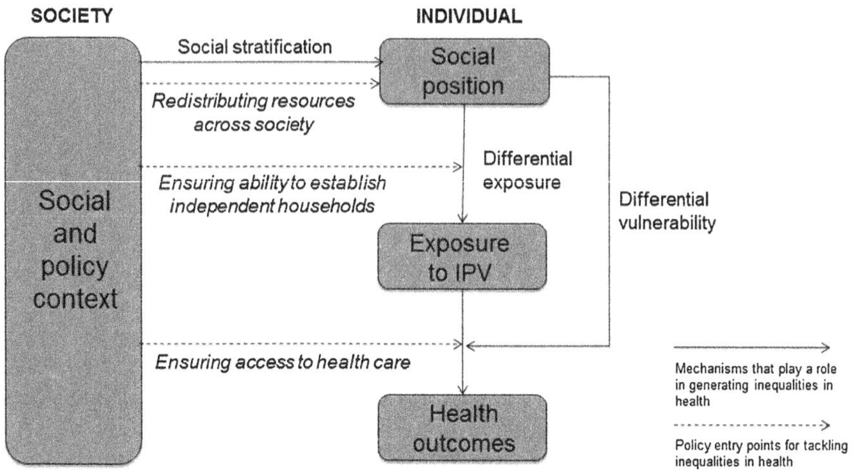

Fig. 9.1 Review of conceptual framework, adapted from Diderichsen et al. (2001)

women. More directly, this book has tested two further mechanisms at the individual level: whether women in lower social positions may be *differentially exposed* to IPV (Chap. 7), and whether women in lower social positions who have experienced IPV may be *differentially vulnerable* to poor health outcomes (Chap. 8).

Still unexplored, however, are the corresponding policy entry points where macro-level institutional arrangements may influence health inequities for survivors of IPV. To begin, the conceptual framework suggests that welfare policy emphasizing a more equal redistribution of resources across society may serve to impact the overall stratification of women. What interests me most, however, are the following two policy entry points. First, the suggestion that policies affecting defamilization or women's *ability to establish independent households* will also influence their IPV exposure. Second, that policy may affect vulnerability to poor health outcomes for IPV survivors with lower social positions by ensuring *access to health care.* If the conceptual framework holds true, then these policy entry points are potential means of intervening in the development of health inequities for survivors of IPV.

This book's comparison of the US, Germany, and Norway enables a discussion of whether patterns in differential exposure and vulnerability vary across welfare state contexts, and whether institutional arrangements may contribute to health inequities for IPV survivors. Thus, based on the results of the empirical analyses, it is the aim of the present chapter to explore the macro-level policy context with the following research questions. Is social position's impact on IPV exposure reflective of national policies supporting women to establish independent households (RQ3)? And are the vulnerabilities to social position's impact on health among IPV survivors reflective of national policies regarding access to health care (RQ4)? The specific cross-national hypotheses addressing the effect of institutional arrangements are informed primarily by the detailed case descriptions presented in Chap. 4, which explored the gender, safety net, family, and health policy arrangements for each country. This chapter brings together the evidence from the social policy contexts relevant to the national survey data (i.e., mid-1990s for the US, early 2000s for Germany and Norway) and the empirical findings to assess the cross-national hypotheses. The chapter concludes with the acknowledgement of additional contextual factors and a brief discussion.

9.1 Policy Context and Its Effect on IPV Exposure

Chapter 7 examined the effect of social position on IPV exposure at the individual level in the US, Germany, and Norway. Specifically investigated were the effects of household income, education, and employment on the dependent variable of IPV exposure. The current section briefly describes the macro-level, cross-national hypothesis regarding IPV exposure,[1] draws upon the policy context of each case, and highlights the individual-level empirical evidence necessary for assessing this hypothesis.

Based on substantial differences in institutional arrangements affecting women's abilities to establish independent households, I expected that social position's impact on IPV exposure would vary considerably across the countries (Table 9.1). Given the extensiveness of Norway's dual-earner family policies, as compared to a lack of support in the US, and family policies in Germany which presuppose a male breadwinner/female part-time carer norm, it was hypothesized that *social position's impact on IPV exposure would be generally smaller in Norway, and greater in the US and Germany* (H3). Overall, the empirical results did not specifically confirm this hypothesis. Instead, there was evidence of distinctive patterns in the social gradient of IPV exposure for the three countries. For example, although higher household income was correlated with less IPV exposure in all three countries, it only played a significant role in predicting IPV exposure in the US and German data. In contrast, being employed was a significant predictor of reduced IPV exposure in the Norwegian data, but not in the other two countries. Finally, education predicted IPV exposure for all three countries, but not always in the same direction. How these patterns reflect the institutional arrangements regarding women's abilities to establish independent household in each of the case countries is explored in the following paragraphs.

To begin, the findings show that in the US, lower levels of household income and fewer years of education predicted IPV exposure, even after accounting for a number of other related factors. Moreover, the data showed that women with IPV exposure in the past 5 years were less likely to be currently married or partnered, and had more children under the age of 18 in the household than women without IPV exposure. However, as described in Chap. 4, today as in the mid-1990s, the US

[1]See Sect. 4.5 for a comprehensive description of all cross-national hypotheses.

Table 9.1 Evaluation of cross-national hypotheses: IPV exposure (RQ3)

Hypotheses	Outcomes	Indicators	Confirmation
3a: Social position's effect on IPV exposure is smaller in Norway, and greater in Germany and the US			
	Minor IPV		
$3a_1$		Household income	✓
$3a_2$		Education	x
$3a_3$		Employment	x
	Severe IPV		
$3a_4$		Household income	✓
$3a_5$		Education	x
$3a_6$		employment	x

✓ confirmed, x not confirmed

provides little to no institutional support for women's economic independence, particularly in their role as caregivers. Nonexistent federal parental leave, high costs of market-based childcare, and minimal regulation of working hours lead some US women in current relationships to sever ties to the labor market and instead become economically dependent on partners (Gornick et al. 1998; Korpi et al. 2013). Those not in partnerships may also face financial strains while establishing independent, single-parent households. These include organizing childcare, and perhaps the necessity of part-time work, which often brings with it lower wages, minimal to no employment benefits or protections, and often no health insurance (Gornick and Meyers 2009; Ray et al. 2010). The empirical evidence presented in Chap. 7 for the US suggests that minimal household financial resources make it difficult to end *current abusive relationships* or, alternatively, reflect women's diminished resources when establishing an independent household *after an abusive relationship*. In both cases, the lack of institutional supports affects women's exposure to IPV by weakening their abilities to maintain economic independence and avoid poverty. Likewise, when women have fewer years of education, they may be particularly limited in the choices available to them.

Similar to the US, lower levels of household income predicted greater IPV exposure in Germany. This fits with the understanding of Germany's welfare state as a social insurance model which primarily benefits the employed middle classes (Leisering 2001) and perpetuates the prevailing occupational and class stratification (Beckfield and Krieger 2009). Particularly in combination with the male breadwinner/female part-time carer family policies that were in place in the early 2000s (e.g., extensive parental leave without income replacement, part-time childcare for children older than three, a joint tax system penalizing women's incomes in partnerships), women who became single parents when establishing an independent household did not fit the typical mold for benefits from the welfare state (i.e., neither full-time breadwinners nor full-time carers) (Hobson 1994). Cross-national comparative studies have confirmed that these institutional arrangements are related to greater financial losses among females after relationship dissolution than males, and to a greater degree in Germany than in countries with dual-earner family policies (Andreß et al. 2006; van Damme et al. 2009; Hansen et al. 2006). The empirical findings presented in this book additionally suggest that women establishing autonomous households in the early 2000s may have instead needed to rely on means-tested income assistance if they were not already plugged into the labor market.

Education also plays a central role in the empirical findings for Germany, although not in the expected direction, with more years of education increasing the likelihood of exposure to minor IPV (i.e., IPV without injury). As discussed in Sect. 7.2, this may partially be explained by an imbalance in resources, and therefore status, between partners. If women have higher levels of education than their partner, research suggests that this may be perceived as a threat if the male partner holds a more traditional male breadwinner gender ideology (Atkinson et al. 2005). Reflecting back on the family policies described in Chap. 4, the institutional arrangements in place in Germany in the early 2000s assumed that men are the primary breadwinners, while women are the secondary breadwinners and the primary caregivers. According to Pfau-Effinger (1998, 2012), these institutional arrangements (i.e., the *gender order*) are interconnected with a society's values and beliefs systems (i.e., the *gender culture*), and create the social practice within households of the division of labor (i.e., the *gender arrangement*). In other words, policies and culture interact to create the division of labor within households (Budig et al. 2012). Thus, I argue that Germany's family and welfare policies interacted with societal norms assuming male breadwinner/female part-time carer households, and therefore may have contributed to minor levels of IPV exposure when male partners with traditional gendered ideologies felt threatened by their female partner's education levels. In sum, Germany's family policies in the early 2000s, and perhaps also the overall social insurance welfare model which reinforced existing stratification, played an important role in women's exposure to IPV.

For the Norwegian sample, the empirical findings provide evidence of a social gradient in severe IPV exposure related to both employment status and education. As can be seen by the overall high levels of employment among women in the Norwegian sample (85 % vs. 72 % in the US and German samples), labor market involvement is central to women's lives (Skevik and Hatland 2008). Reflecting the interplay between Norway's *gender order* and *gender culture*, many institutional arrangements ensure women's ties to the labor market. For example, Norwegian family policy, today as well as in the early 2000s, emphasizes employment for both men and women as the best strategy to improve living standards, and simultaneously discourages long gaps between employment (Kjeldstad 2000). Having dual-earner families is made possible by daylong care for children after the age of one, flexible working hours for parents, and parental leave with high-income replacement up until children are eligible to attend childcare. Moreover, assistance for single parents with children over the age of one requires at least part-time employment, education enrollment, or actively seeking employment (Kjeldstad 2000; Strand 2012; Syltevik 1999).[2]

However, the great value placed on employment may serve as a double-edged sword. While employment offers women greater opportunities for establishing independent households, my findings suggest that the minority of women who are not employed may "fall between the cracks" of Norway's institutional arrangements, opening them up to specific vulnerabilities to IPV exposure. For women in a *current partnership*, not being employed in a predominantly dual-earner family culture may represent real economic dependence within a relationship and may indeed present a barrier to ending an abusive relationship (Anderson and Saunders 2003; Moe and Bell 2004). For women *after ending a relationship*, the connection between nonemployment and severe IPV may provide evidence that the consequences of violence hindered labor market involvement (Moe and Bell 2004; Swanberg and Logan 2007). Moreover, given the significant positive correlation found between employment and education, it is important to consider that fewer years of education also predicted severe IPV in Norway. Despite the comprehensive dual-earner institutional arrangements in Norway supporting women in establishing an independent household, women without employment and with fewer years of education remain vulnerable to severe IPV.

Importantly, household income was not predictive of severe IPV exposure in the Norway sample, although more women with IPV exposure were unmarried or unpartnered at the time of the survey than women without IPV exposure. This reflects to some degree the institutional supports available for women in Norway, which have been shown to help offset financial losses due to relationship dissolution (van Damme et al. 2009; Hansen et al. 2006; Misra et al. 2007; Strand 2012). For example, in the early 2000s, single parents with small children in Norway were eligible for a three-year-long allowance to help transition into single parenthood and balance work and family responsibilities. Likewise, family allowances and cash-for-care benefits are universally available benefits (as opposed to means-tested) which help maintain household income at a minimal standard, although they are often criticized by Scandinavian researchers as promoting a reduction in women's employment (Knudsen and Waerness 2001). A qualitative study of partnership dissolution in Norway found that these forms of financial support from the state were vital for IPV survivors' ability to end abusive relationships (Moxnes 1991). Thus, these aspects of the Norwegian institutional arrangement may play an important role in enabling women to establish independent households without entering into poverty.

In sum, comparing the social gradient in IPV exposure across the policy contexts of the three countries revealed interesting insights into the role of welfare policy in affecting women's IPV exposure. Different patterns of family policy reflect different patterns in the ability to prevent or exit abusive relationships. Policies which enable

[2]This focus on employment for single parents is balanced with both a transitional allowance and a good deal of assistance with childcare arrangements.

women's ties to the labor market and decrease economic dependence on partners, such as paid parental leave, subsidized childcare, and flexible working arrangements, appear to support women's opportunities to prevent, or end abusive relationships. Moreover, policies aimed at preventing poverty during the transition period after relationship dissolution appear to increase women's abilities to establish autonomous households.

9.2 Policy Context and Its Effect on Vulnerability to Poor Health

Chapter 8 examined whether IPV exposure affects the relationship between social position and health at the individual level in the US, Germany, and Norway. In order to examine this, it was necessary to test a series of hypotheses building upon one another. To begin, it was investigated whether social position (i.e., household income, education, and employment) has an impact on self-assessed health and mental health complaints. Following this, the effects of IPV exposure on these health outcomes was measured, beyond what could be attributed to social position. Finally, it was examined whether the impact of social position on health outcomes varied with IPV exposure. The current section reviews the cross-national hypotheses related to vulnerability to poor health for women who have experienced IPV, draws upon the relevant policy context of each country, and highlights the individual-level empirical evidence necessary for assessing these hypotheses.

Based on the understanding of socioeconomic status as a resource enabling good health and the avoidance of health risks (Link and Phelan 1995), the empirical results are in accordance with the hypothesis that *all countries would show evidence of a social gradient in health* (H4a) (see Table 9.2). The data from the US, Germany, and Norway revealed that higher household income ($H4a_1$), more years of education ($H4a_2$), and being employed ($H4a_3$) were associated with good self assessed health, despite the substantial differences in welfare policy in each of these case countries. These results support previous research demonstrating that social position continues to impact health, even in countries with universal access to health care. For example, although US health care is heavily linked to employment and ability to pay, whereas Iceland offers universal access, Olafsdottir (2007) found similar social gradients in health related to education, employment, and relative poverty. She argued that, "while the safety net provided by the Icelandic welfare state may result in fewer individuals living in poverty, once individuals are poor the effects are similar across institutional contexts" (Olafsdottir 2007, p. 249). Moreover, while absolute inequalities seem to decrease, the relative inequalities remain because those with more socioeconomic resources are able to take better advantage of universal health systems and therefore reap better health outcomes (Bergqvist et al. 2013; Deaton 2002). The empirical results showing social

Table 9.2 Evaluation of cross-national hypotheses: vulnerability to poor health (RQ4)

Hypotheses	Outcomes	Indicators	Confirmation
H4a: Social gradient in health in all countries			
	Self-assessed health		
$4a_1$		Household income	✓
$4a_2$		Education	✓
$4a_3$		Employment	✓
	Mental health complaints		
$4a_4$		Household income	✓, /
$4a_5$		Education	✓, /
$4a_6$		Employment	x
H4b: IPV impacts health, beyond social position in all countries			
$4b_1$	Self-assessed health		✓
$4b_2$	Mental health complaints		✓
H4c: Social position's impact on health for IPV survivors will be smallest in Norway and Germany, greatest in US			
$4c_1$	Self-assessed health		✓
$4c_2$	Mental health complaints		x

✓ confirmed, x not confirmed, / not in predicted direction

inequalities in self-assessed health for all three countries, even in Germany and Norway with their strong safety nets, confirm these observations from the literature.

While following a similar pattern as the results for self-assessed health, there were slight differences in the social gradient of mental health complaints, particularly for the German sample. Higher levels of household income were predictive of fewer mental health complaints in the US and Norway ($H4a_4$), as were more years of education ($H4a_5$) in the US sample. In Germany, however, having 'inconsistent' levels of household income and education (e.g., high household income and low education, or low household income and high education) was linked to a greater number of mental health complaints. As described in Sect. 8.3, this type of 'status inconsistency' may increase stress and psychological distress caused by uncertainty and conflicting role expectations (e.g., Gal et al. 2008). Germany's welfare system has often been described as one which reinforces social stratification along occupational and class lines, therefore, it could be argued that this influences societal norms and expectations regarding corresponding levels of education and household income. Continuing to apply Pfau-Effinger's (1998) framework of *gender order* and *gender culture*, the interconnectedness of institutional arrangements and societal values (in both causal directions) may contribute to increased mental health symptoms among status inconsistent women in Germany.

Building on the empirical results demonstrating a social gradient in health, as well as on the wealth of previous international research demonstrating IPV's impact on health, it was hypothesized that *all countries would show an impact of IPV exposure on health, beyond what could be attributed to social position* (H4b). The empirical results confirmed this hypothesis, both for self-assessed health ($H4b_1$) and mental health complaints ($H4b_2$). For the US, Germany, and Norway, IPV exposure increased the likelihood of poor self-assessed health and the number of mental health complaints reported. More specifically, in addition to the increased risk of poor health outcomes among women with lower social positions, women with IPV exposure had an even higher risk of poor health than women without IPV exposure. Cross-national research examining the health effects of IPV exposure (FRA 2014; Martinez et al. 2006; WHO 2005) provides little evidence to indicate that IPV's impact on physical or mental health varies dramatically across national contexts. In this sense, the present empirical findings fit with prior research, and they rather serve to emphasize the importance of recognizing the socioeconomic context in which IPV affects health, regardless of national context.

The final cross-national hypothesis was that *vulnerabilities to social position's impact on health among IPV survivors will be smallest in Norway and Germany, and greatest in the US* (H4c). Generally, this showed itself to be the case for self-assessed health ($H4c_1$), but the results did not provide evidence of significant vulnerability to social position's impact on mental health complaints among IPV survivors for any of the countries ($H4c_2$). To briefly summarize, household income's impact on self-assessed health varied according to IPV exposure for women in the US sample. In other words, severe IPV exposure presented itself as a serious risk for poor self-assessed health among women with low household incomes. Likewise, the empirical findings suggested that regardless of IPV exposure, higher levels of household income leveled out risk. Although women in the Germany and Norway samples also experienced similar levels of IPV exposure and social gradients in health as the US, IPV exposure did not magnify the social gradient in health in either of these countries.

I conjecture that this cross-national difference in vulnerability to poor self-assessed health among IPV survivors with limited household income may have to do with differences in policies related to access to health care, specifically the interrelated dimensions of affordability and entitlement to health care. Access to care has repeatedly been linked to health outcomes in the US (Hoffman and Paradise 2008; Wisdom et al. 2005). During the mid-1990s, health care coverage in the US was linked to employment status rather than being understood as a social right, which introduces a number of complications for the health of IPV survivors. Women in the US who are economically dependent on their abusive partners may rely on their partner's employment for health insurance. Especially for those women with chronic health issues related to the IPV, this has been shown to result in a vicious circle of poor health and abuse (Scott et al. 2002; Thomas et al. 2008). Likewise, ending a relationship may leave economically dependent women without economic resources of their own and either uninsured or relying on Medicaid (Brandwein 1999). Related to this, high health care costs in the US may prevent women from seeking the care they need. Although on the rise internationally, the US has the second highest per capita out-of-pocket costs among OECD countries (Rice et al. 2013). Among survivors of IPV in the US, financial concerns, as well as being uninsured or under-insured, are often named as barriers to care (Postmus et al. 2009).

Moreover, the uninsured tend to forgo preventative care altogether. One US study showed that among women living in a domestic violence shelter, only half reported having a community health clinic or primary care physician, and only about one-third had had a preventative check-up in the previous year (Wilson et al. 2007). Some of these women could not afford co-payments even at the community health clinics. Altogether, this suggests that difficulties in access to care in the US are part of the explanation for vulnerabilities to poor self-assessed health among low-income women with IPV exposure.

Although the principles behind the health care systems and their implementation differ between Germany and Norway, they do agree on the importance of universal entitlement to health care and protection against high out-of-pocket costs. The principle of equal access to services according to medical need regardless of social status or income is central to Norway's health policy, ensuring women's access to care without relying on a partner. While health care coverage is related to social insurance contributions via employment in Germany, and could potentially mean that some women are reliant on an abusive partner's employment for health insurance, there are mechanisms in place to make sure that women maintain their health insurance when establishing an independent household. For example, health insurance is also available in Germany for those with part-time employment, insurance contributions are relative to income earned, and the contributions for the unemployed and those receiving social assistance are covered by the state. Moreover, both countries have mechanisms in place (e.g., annual ceilings and/or cost-sharing exemptions) to ensure affordability of care and limit private out-of-pocket costs.

Despite these measures, it is important to mention that evidence of inequalities in access to health care still exist to some extent in both Germany and Norway. For example, in terms of availability of providers, patients in Norway are subject to much longer waiting times than in the US or Germany. Furthermore, both education and geographical accessibility have been found to impact specialist visits in Norway (Iversen and Kopperud 2003, 2005), and significantly more individuals in the lowest income quintile in Germany reported an unmet health need due to cost than those in the highest income quintile (Eurostat 2014). Even so, analyses of the same German national survey data used in this book found that the health care system is the top source of external help sought by IPV survivors (Müller and Schröttle 2004), and that personal and social resources did not have an impact on whether IPV survivors sought medical care (Brzank 2012). This would imply that IPV survivors in Germany are generally able to access the health care they need for their physical health complaints, which has also been supported by at least one qualitative study (Larsen et al. 2014).[3] Thus, despite these issues of access, I argue that the institutional arrangements in Germany and Norway related to affordability and entitlement provide the infrastructure necessary for IPV survivors to address their overall health issues, even in cases of limited resources.

[3]In comparison, however, women faced greater barriers when seeking mental health care.

As previously mentioned, it was predicted that IPV exposure would magnify the effect of the social gradient in mental health for the US, but to a lesser degree in Germany and Norway. However, the empirical evidence did not reveal a vulnerability to social position's impact on mental health complaints for IPV survivors in any of the countries. This is contrary to what was predicted given the substantial effect of IPV exposure on mental health (Dillon et al. 2013) and the tremendous gap in health insurance coverage for mental health services in the US (Rice et al. 2013). According to Rice et al. 2013, lack of health insurance coverage is linked to unmet mental health needs: only one-third of those with mental health issues in the US are being treated. Leaving mental health issues untreated due to lack of financial resources has consistently been found among IPV survivors in the US (Rodríguez et al. 2009; Wilson et al. 2007). Although Germany's mental health care services have been criticized as overly complex and fragmented (Salize et al. 2007) and mental health patients in Norway are frequently met with long waiting times (Ringard et al. 2013), access to care is universal with limited out-of-pocket costs. Although the present empirical results do not support the hypothesis that policies related to access to care affect the vulnerability to the social gradient in mental health for IPV survivors, this issue warrants further research and investigation.

9.3 Further Relevant Contextual Comparisons

The current section explores additional cross-national similarities and differences in the social and policy context which were not hypothesized due to the concentration on the welfare state, but were nonetheless sparked by the empirical analyses of IPV exposure and health outcomes across the three countries. To begin, the differences in national policies on violence against women merit discussion, as do the institutional arrangements affecting access to divorce, and those governing alimony and child support after partnership dissolution.

The *national policies on violence against women* and the surrounding context for each of the countries were briefly reviewed in Chap. 4 in order to provide a foundation for the case descriptions. A further comparison of these policies here is also worthwhile for understanding the similarities and differences in the empirical results of this book, as it provides a sense of victim-specific assistance beyond the general services provided by the welfare state. Violence against women as a topic deserving national attention came to the forefront in all three countries through feminist mobilization in civil society (Htun and Weldon 2012). While each country has developed extensive national policies combating violence against women and has been successful in positively influencing societal discourse on the topic, they have slightly different approaches to the issue which ultimately affect the types of resources available to IPV survivors. The US Violence Against Women Act places its emphasis on "coordinated community care" (i.e., among law enforcement, prosecutors, attorneys, and victim services) focusing on criminalization and prosecution of violence against women (Modi et al. 2014). While reforms for improved prosecution of violence against women were also key to Germany's National Action Plans (BMFSFJ 1999, 2007), so were prevention efforts, awareness raising, and cooperation between state and non-governmental organizations (Hagemann-White 2005). Norway's National Action Plans (Ministry of Health 2011; Ministry of Justice and Public Security 2012; Ministry of Justice and the Police 2004) however, offer the starkest contrast to the approaches of the previous two countries. The focus of the Norwegian plans is on changing societal attitudes and improving the capabilities of existing state institutions (i.e., the police, education, and support services) in preventing and coping with violence against women (Saur et al. 2011).

These different approaches are visible, for example, in the level of shelters available for women fleeing abusive relationships. Given that shelters are typically an option of last resort and predominantly serve women without the socioeconomic resources to pursue other options (Haj-Yahia and Cohen 2009; Jonassen and Skogøy 2010), shelter space is a reasonable indicator of the support available for IPV survivors. For instance, the number of shelter spaces available in Norway greatly exceeds the recommended minimum for a country of its size and shelters were primarily funded by government resources up until 2011. In Germany, however, the number of available spaces falls short of the recommended minimum with unregulated funding at the state level, and the US faces a shortage of available shelter spaces with usually only nominal government funding (NNEDV 2012; Stelmaszekn and Fisher 2012). In short, when comparing support specifically aimed at survivors of IPV, the safety net available in Norway appears to be a bit wider than that in either Germany or the US, and seems to go to greater lengths to change societal norms around violence. In light of the present empirical results indicating lesser vulnerabilities to health in Norway and Germany, it should be considered that Norwegian national policies on violence against women may also place women in Norway in a better position for dealing with IPV and its health consequences.

Implicit in the examination of intimate partner violence is the topic of partnership dissolution and it would be remiss not to mention the institutional arrangements surrounding it, although it is not directly related to the welfare state context in my hypotheses. Legislation can potentially make partnership dissolution in the case of married couples more or less burdensome and thereby affect *access to divorce*, which is relevant when considering how it relates to women's exposure to IPV. For example, it has been shown that changes in divorce laws between 1950 and 2003 in Europe were significantly related to divorce rates (González and Viitanen 2006), and likewise in the US, a significant positive effect has been found on divorce rates in those states with implementation of 'no-fault' divorce laws (Nakonezny et al. 1995). In both Germany and Norway, 'no-fault' divorces do not require justification for seeking divorce and are granted after a one-year waiting period in which the couple has established separate households (Martiny and Schwab 2002; Sverdrup 2002).[4] However, both countries allow the required

[4]In Germany, if one member of the couple contests the divorce, this waiting period can be extended to 3 years.

waiting period to be eliminated if violence in the household is documented. In the US, the laws governing divorce are legislated by the states rather than at the federal level. While nearly half of US states hold 'no-fault' divorce laws, the rest require proof of 'irreconcilable differences' before granting a divorce (Legal Information Institute 2014a). Whether a waiting period is required and its corresponding length also vary by state: over half of US states stipulate a waiting period before seeking divorce, ranging from 60 days in Kentucky to 3 years in Rhode Island, Utah, and Texas (American Bar Association 2013).

Comparatively, this suggests that access to divorce among IPV survivors would be easier in Germany and Norway, and more difficult in the US. However, the current empirical findings suggest that across the countries, laws governing divorce sufficiently allowed for partnership dissolution for partnered women who have been exposed to IPV. Specifically, IPV exposure from a current or former partner was significantly related to being unmarried or not partnered in all three countries, even after accounting for other predictive variables This implies that those with IPV exposure who were currently unmarried or not partnered had ended an abusive relationship within the past 5 years.

A further examination of the importance of cohabitation in each of the countries may partially explain why the differences in access to divorce do not appear to be related to partnership dissolution for the samples in these countries. For example, cohabitation is much more common in Norway than in the other two countries. The percentage of the population above age 20 currently cohabitating was 5.3 % in Germany, 5.5 % in the US, and 10.7 % in Norway (OECD 2013). Likewise, of those between ages 20 and 34, 13.6 % in Germany were cohabitating as opposed to 22.7 % in Norway.[5] Moreover, cohabitating couples in Norway are afforded nearly all rights of married couples (e.g., pensions, social security, and taxation) if they have a child in common or have lived together for at least 2 years, but without the duty to provide for one another financially (Lyngstad et al. 2010; Noack 2001). In Germany, however, marriage is protected by law, and in the early 2000s, cohabitating partners did not have the right to the health insurance of their partner, nor the right to alimony after separation (Ostner 2001). Laws in the US run this entire spectrum depending on the state, ranging from no rights at all to being treated equivalently to marriage (Bowman 2004). Thus, it may be that the combination of divorce laws and cohabitation laws even out the playing field across the countries regarding access to partnership dissolution and its relation to IPV exposure.

Household income was a contributing factor to IPV exposure for both the US and Germany, so in addition to family policy, laws related to *spousal maintenance* following partnership dissolution are worth exploring to assess whether they play a role in women's abilities to establish an independent household. Maintenance in both Norway and Germany is based on the idea that each individual is responsible for supporting themselves, and that the obligation to support one another ends with divorce (Martiny and Schwab 2002; Sverdrup 2002). However, in the case that one

[5]No comparable OECD data was available for the US for this indicator.

of the partners cannot support themselves after dissolution, they are entitled to maintenance payments from the other partner. In Norway, this is only the case "if the ability and opportunity of the spouse to ensure support have been reduced as a result of caring for children of the marriage or of the distribution of joint tasks during cohabitation" (Sverdrup 2002, p. 12). In practice, such maintenance payments are rather the exception than the rule. The duration of maintenance in Norway is limited to 3 years and generally the amount is one-third of the income of the ex-spouse if the claimant has no income of their own. In Germany, maintenance payments in the case that one partner cannot support themselves are based on the principle of *nacheheliche Solidarität*, or post-divorce solidarity of spouses, and similar to Norway, the concept of 'marriage-created need' (*ehebedingte Bedürftigkeit*) plays a role (Martiny and Schwab 2002, p. 23). In contrast to Norway, however, maintenance is not necessarily limited to a short period in Germany, but can also be claimed for much longer periods of time. Typically, the amount of maintenance in the early 2000s for an individual who has none of their own income was approximately three-sevenths of the income of the ex-spouse (Martiny and Schwab 2002).

In the US, however, there is "no accepted legal theory to explain why one spouse should have to continue financially supporting the other after their marriage has been legally terminated" (McCoy 2005, p. 514). Instead, the laws for spousal maintenance vary by state. Throughout the country, there are a variety of different types of spousal maintenance, including: permanent lifelong support, rehabilitative support until the claimant is able to establish an independent household of their own, and reimbursement support to cover the expenses one spouse bore during the marriage (e.g., education). While some states provide no guidelines whatsoever to aid the courts in determining the amount and duration of maintenance payments, others require the consideration of an extensive number of factors, such as: marital standard of living, marriage duration, contribution of each partner to the marriage, age, and physical and mental health (McCoy 2005). In states which require proof of fault for the divorce, marital misconduct can also be taken into account to determine the amount of payments. In sum, based on these similarities and differences across the three countries in spousal maintenance, no clear pattern emerges to explain the connection between household income and IPV exposure in the US and Germany but not in Norway.

Relatedly, I did not specifically hypothesize whether differences in laws governing *child support* after partnership dissolution may affect the social gradient in IPV exposure by influencing women's abilities to maintain an independent household. Children in the household can affect the decision to leave abusive relationships for a number of different reasons, particularly if women are economically dependent on their partner (Moxnes 1991; Stöckl et al. 2011).[6] Thus,

[6]Beyond the scope of this book, but still central in the literature, is the wish of many women to maintain an intact family for the benefit of the children and/or the wish for the children to maintain a relationship with their father (Meyer 2012; Stöckl et al. 2011). On the other side of the spectrum, concerns about the abusive father gaining custody of children after relationship dissolution are

access to financial support for children in the household after partnership dissolution may play a deciding factor in exiting an abusive relationship where children are involved. The present empirical data revealed that in the US sample, a greater number of children in the household was related to increased risk of minor and severe IPV exposure, while this was not the case for Germany or Norway. This finding reflects the pattern of institutional arrangements regarding child support in the three countries. In the US, court orders specifying the financial contributions of noncustodial parents toward children's basic living expenses are common during divorce proceedings (Legal Information Institute 2014b), however, there are often issues of compliance and a lack of enforcement (Peters et al. 1993). In cases of noncompliance, only some states allow the court to directly garnish the noncompliant parent's wages in order to ensure that the custodial parent receives the appropriate financial support (Legal Information Institute 2014b). In the case of an abusive relationship, research has found that noncompliance places a particular financial burden on women who have established independent households after leaving the relationship (Bell 2003; Pearson et al. 1999).

Meanwhile, noncustodial parents in Germany and Norway are required to pay child support according to their economic resources, with the size of the payments being highly regulated by law.[7] In cases of noncompliance in Norway, the state steps in and provides the custodial parent with a minimum standard of child support and is responsible for collecting the noncompliant parent's outstanding debts (Strand 2012). Similarly, in cases of non-compliance in Germany, single parents can apply for Advanced Child Maintenance (*Unterhaltvorschuss*), which allows for a legally fixed minimum payment to be made to the custodial parent for a period of up to 6 years as long as the children are under 12 years of age (Leitner et al. 2008; OECD 2003). In guaranteeing a minimum standard of child support after partnership dissolution—also in cases of noncompliant parents—the institutional arrangements in Germany and Norway remove some of the financial burden involved in establishing an independent household. Related to my empirical findings, this may potentially also improve women's abilities to exit abusive relationships so that having children in the household does not significantly impact women's IPV exposure. Thus, in considering differences in IPV exposure across the three countries, child support laws also deserve attention.

(Footnote 6 continued)

very real and may also influence decisions about relationship dissolution (Davies et al. 2009; Jaffe and Crooks 2004; Wuest et al. 2006).

[7]In the early 2000s in Norway, payments were based on a minimum fixed percentage of the noncustodial parent's income. In the meantime, however, child support payments have developed into a "standard budget calculation based on the actual cost associated with bringing up a child, developed by the National Institute for Consumer Research (*Statens institutt for forbruksforskning*). The costs are stratified according to the age of the child and shared proportionally between the parents according to income and personal agreements on visiting arrangements" (Strand 2012, p. 92). In Germany, the monthly payment is based on the children's age and the income of the noncustodial parent (Leitner et al. 2008).

9.4 Discussion

The main goal of this chapter was to examine the policy entry points where macro-level institutional arrangements may influence health inequities for survivors of IPV. Based on the conceptual framework, it was hypothesized that policies affecting women's *ability to establish independent households* would also influence their IPV exposure, and that policies affecting *access to health care* would influence vulnerabilities to social position's impact on health for IPV survivors. Comparing the US, Germany, and Norway has enabled a discussion of whether patterns in differential exposure and vulnerability vary across welfare state contexts, and whether institutional arrangements may contribute to health inequities for IPV survivors. Using a combination of the detailed descriptions of the policy contexts for each case in Chap. 4 and the empirical results in Chaps. 6, 7, and 8, the macro-level, cross-national hypotheses were examined and a number of policy effects were proposed.

Although it was expected across-the-board that social position would have a smaller impact in Norway than in Germany or the US, instead it seems that specific patterns in policies supporting women in establishing independent households reflect patterns of how social position impacts IPV exposure. Specifically, Norway's dual-earner family policy strategy may be related to why employment was associated with IPV exposure only in Norway and why household income did not affect IPV exposure there, although it did for the other two countries. As an institutional explanation, one might look specifically to Norway's transitional allowance and support for single parents to help balance work and family responsibilities—unique among the three cases—along with flexible work arrangements and subsidized childcare. This combination may positively influence women's decisions to exit an abusive relationship by ensuring a minimal standard of income while establishing an independent household. Meanwhile, the emphasis on employment activation in Norway may have alternatively left the minority of women who were not employed with fewer opportunities for establishing independent households and opened them up to specific vulnerabilities to IPV exposure.

Additionally, Germany's male breadwinner/female part-time carer strategy of family policy may account for why lower levels of household income predicted the highest levels of IPV exposure. Women who became single parents when establishing an independent household may not have fit the typical mold for benefits from the welfare state, and thus may instead have needed to rely on means-tested income assistance if they were not already tied into the labor market. Moreover, more traditional societal norms associated with this model of family policy may have contributed to minor levels of IPV exposure if male partners with traditional gendered ideologies felt threatened by their female partner's education levels. Finally, it seems that the overall lack of institutional supports in the US affected women's exposure to IPV by weakening their abilities to establish independent households without falling into poverty.

To a limited extent, policies ensuring access to health care appear to have been related to reduced social inequalities in health for IPV survivors. Specifically, the vulnerability to poor self-assessed health in the US among IPV survivors with limited household income may have been related to institutional arrangements affecting affordability and entitlement to health care. As opposed to Germany and Norway, health policies in the US do not ensure either one of these factors, leading to high out-of-pocket costs and leaving significant portions of the population without health insurance. In this context of institutional arrangements hindering access to health care, financial resources play a significant role in shaping perceived health for IPV survivors. On the other hand, the entitlement to health care and mechanisms which limit out-of-pocket costs in Germany and Norway appear to ensure access to care, even in cases of limited resources, and provide the social structure necessary for IPV survivors to address their health issues.

The comparative findings presented in this chapter make important contributions to a limited body of evidence linking institutional arrangements to IPV exposure and health outcomes. Although macro-level factors are often assumed to play a role, they are rarely systematically investigated (Whitaker 2014). Even so, it is important to acknowledge issues with the research design. The ability to statistically connect individual-level variables of social position, IPV exposure, and health outcomes to macro-level policies was limited by a lack of directly comparable cross-national survey data. Thus, assessment of the cross-national hypotheses was conducted using descriptive comparison of the empirical results of three diverse countries. While the countries were chosen to represent a wide spectrum of institutional arrangements, a broader set of countries may be necessary for further research. Finally, although other relevant cross-national differences in the social and policy contexts are acknowledged which may have also contributed to the outcomes, it is not possible to eliminate all competing explanations. Instead, the results presented in this chapter should be used to inform further research on the effect of the policy context on the health of women with IPV exposure.

In sum, these results fit with expectations of the broader role of policy in impacting women's health (Wisdom et al. 2005) and that political commitment to social provision more effectively addresses the needs of IPV survivors (Peter 2006). The implications these results have for welfare state policy to intervene in preventing health inequities for IPV survivors will be explored in the following chapter.

References

American Bar Association. (2013). Grounds for divorce and residency requirements. *Family Law Quarterly, 46*(4), 530–533.

Anderson, D. K., & Saunders, D. G. (2003). Leaving an abusive partner: An empirical review of predictors, the process of leaving, and psychological well-being. *Trauma, Violence, and Abuse, 4*(2), 163–191. doi:10.1177/1524838002250769

Andreß, H.-J., Borgloh, B., Brockel, M., Giesselmann, M., & Hummelsheim, D. (2006). The economic consequences of partnership dissolution: A comparative analysis of panel studies from Belgium, Germany, Great Britain, Italy, and Sweden. *European Sociological Review, 22*(5), 533–560. doi:10.1093/esr/jcl012

Atkinson, M. P., Greenstein, T. N., & Lang, M. M. (2005). For women, breadwinning can be dangerous: Gendered resource theory and wife abuse. *Journal of Marriage and Family, 67*(5), 1137–1148.

Beckfield, J., & Krieger, N. (2009). Epi + demos + cracy: Linking political systems and priorities to the magnitude of health inequities—Evidence, gaps, and a research agenda. *Epidemiologic Reviews, 31*(1), 152–77. doi:10.1093/epirev/mxp002

Bell, H. (2003). Cycles within cycles. *Violence Against Women, 9*(10), 1245–1262. doi:10.1177/1077801203255865

Bergqvist, K., Åberg Yngwe, M., & Lundberg, O. (2013). Understanding the role of welfare state characteristics for health and inequalities—An analytical review. *BMC Public Health, 13*(1), 1234–1253. doi:10.1186/1471-2458-13-1234

BMFSFJ. (1999). *Aktionsplan der Bundesregierung zur Bekämpfung von Gewalt gegen Frauen [Action plan of the federal government combating violence against women].* Berlin: Bundesministerium für Familie, Senioren, Frauen und Jugend.

BMFSFJ. (2007). *Aktionsplan II der Bundesregierung zur Bekämpfung von Gewalt gegen Frauen [Action plan II of the federal government combating violence against women].* Berlin: Bundesministerium für Familie, Senioren, Frauen und Jugend.

Bowman, C. G. (2004). Legal treatment of cohabitation in the United States. *Law and Policy, 26*(1), 119–151.

Brandwein, R. A. (1999). Family violence, women and welfare. In R. A. Brandwein (Ed.), *Battered women, children, and welfare reform: The ties that bind* (pp. 3–16). Thousand Oaks, CA: Sage Publications.

Brzank, P. (2012). *Wege aus der Partnergewalt. Frauen auf der Suche nach Hilfe [Escaping partner violence: Women seeking help].* Wiesbaden: Springer VS.

Budig, M. J., Misra, J., & Boeckmann, I. (2012). The motherhood penalty in cross-national perspective: The importance of work-family policies and cultural attitudes. *Social Politics: International Studies in Gender, State and Society, 19*(2), 163–193. doi:10.1093/sp/jxs006

Davies, L., Ford-Gilboe, M., & Hammerton, J. (2009). Gender inequality and patterns of abuse post leaving. *Journal of Family Violence, 24*(1), 27–39. doi:10.1007/s10896-008-9204-5

Deaton, A. (2002). Policy implications of the gradient of health and wealth. *Health Affairs, 21*(2), 13–30. doi:10.1377/hlthaff.21.2.13

Diderichsen, F., Evans, T., & Whitehead, M. (2001). The social basis of disparities in health. In T. Evans, M. Whitehead, F. Diderichsen, A. Bhuyia, & M. Wirth (Eds.), *Challenging inequities in health: From ethics to action* (pp. 12–23). New York, NY: Oxford University Press.

Dillon, G., Hussain, R., Loxton, D., & Rahman, S. (2013). Mental and physical health and intimate partner violence against women: A review of the literature. *International Journal of Family Medicine*, 1–15. doi:10.1155/2013/313909

Esping-Andersen, G. (1990). *The three worlds of welfare capitalism.* London: Polity.

European Union Agency for Fundamental Rights [FRA]. (2014). *Violence against women: An EU-wide survey.* Luxembourg. http://fra.europa.eu/sites/default/files/fra-2014-vaw-survey-main-results_en.pdf. Accessed November 01, 2014.

Eurostat. (2014). *Self reported unmet need for medical examination or treatment, by income quintile.* http://epp.eurostat.ec.europa.eu/portal/page/portal/statistics/search_database. Accessed October 31, 2014.

Gal, G., Kaplan, G., Gross, R., & Levav, I. (2008). Status inconsistency and common mental disorders in the Israel-based world mental health survey. *Social Psychiatry and Psychiatric Epidemiology, 43*(12), 999–1003. doi:10.1007/s00127-008-0393-2

González, L., & Viitanen, T. K. (2006). *The effect of divorce laws on divorce rates in Europe* (No. 2023). Bonn, Germany: Forschungsinstitut zur Zukunft der Arbeit.

Gornick, J. C., & Meyers, M. K. (2009). Institutions that support gender equality in parenthood and employment. In J. C. Gornick & M. K. Meyers (Eds.), *Gender equality: Transforming family divisions of labor* (pp. 3–64). London: Verso.

Gornick, J. C., Meyers, M. K., & Ross, K. E. (1998). Public policies and the employment of mothers: A cross-national study. *Social Science Quarterly, 79*, 35–54.

Hagemann-White, C. (2005). Surveying prevalence of violence against women in the context of the German National Action Plan. *Statistical Journal of the United Nations, 22*, 301–309.

Haj-Yahia, M. M., & Cohen, H. C. (2009). On the lived experience of battered women residing in shelters. *Journal of Family Violence, 24*(2), 95–109. doi:10.1007/s10896-008-9214-3

Hansen, H.-T., Jürgens, O., Strand, A. H. H., & Voges, W. (2006). Poverty among households with children: A comparative study of Norway and Germany. *International Journal of Social Welfare, 15*(4), 269–279. doi:10.1007/s10896-008-9214-3

Hobson, B. (1994). Solo mothers, social policy regimes and the logics of gender. In D. Sainsbury (Ed.), *Gendering welfare states* (pp. 170–187). London, Thousand Oaks, CA: Sage Publications.

Hoffman, C., & Paradise, J. (2008). Health insurance and access to health care in the United States. *Annals of the New York Academy of Sciences, 1136*, 149–160. doi:10.1196/annals.1425.007

Htun, M., & Weldon, S. L. (2012). The civic origins of progressive policy change: Combating violence against women in global perspective, 1975–2005. *American Political Science Review, 106*(03), 548–569. doi:10.1017/S0003055412000226

Iversen, T., & Kopperud, G. S. (2003). The impact of accessibility on the use of specialist health care in Norway. *Health Care Management Science, 6*(4), 249–261. doi:10.1023/A:1026233725045

Iversen, T., & Kopperud, G. S. (2005). Regulation versus practice—The impact of accessibility on the use of specialist health care in Norway. *Health Economics, 14*(12), 1231–1238.

Jaffe, P. G., & Crooks, C. V. (2004). Partner violence and child custody cases: A cross-national comparison of legal reforms and issues. *Violence Against Women, 10*(8), 917–934. doi:10.1177/1077801204266447

Jonassen, W., & Skogøy, E. (2010). *A home for us, a home for you.... A study of change in user population and use of shelters for battered women*. Oslo, Norway: NKVTS: Nasjonalt kunnskapssenter om vold og traumatisk stress.

Kjeldstad, R. (2000). Employment strategy policies and lone parenthood: The case of Norway. *Social Politics: International Studies in Gender, State and Society, 7*(3), 343–371. doi:10.1093/sp/7.3.343

Knudsen, K., & Waerness, K. (2001). National context, individual characteristics and attitudes on mothers' employment: A comparative analysis of Great Britain, Sweden and Norway. *Acta Sociologica, 44*(1), 67–79.

Korpi, W., Ferrarini, T., & Englund, S. (2013). Women's opportunities under different family policy constellations: Gender, class, and inequality tradeoffs in Western countries re-examined. *Social Politics: International Studies in Gender, State and Society, 20*(1), 1–40. doi:10.1093/sp/jxs028

Larsen, M., Krohn, J., Püschel, K., & Seifert, D. (2014). Experiences of health and health care among women exposed to intimate partner violence: Qualitative findings from Germany. *Health Care for Women International, 35*(4), 359–379. doi:10.1080/07399332.2012.738264

Legal Information Institute. (2014a). Divorce and separation: An overview. http://www.law.cornell.edu/wex/divorce. Accessed July 05, 2014.

Legal Information Institute. (2014b). Child support: An overview. http://www.law.cornell.edu/wex/child_support. Accessed July 05, 2014.

Leisering, L. (2001). Germany—Reform from within. In P. Alcock & G. Craig (Eds.), *International social policy: Welfare regimes in the developed world* (pp. 161–82). London: Palgrave.

Leitner, S., Ostner, I., & Schmitt, C. (2008). Family policies in Germany. In I. Ostner & C. Schmitt (Eds.), *Family policies in the context of family change: The Nordic countries in comparative perspective* (pp. 175–202). Wiesbaden: VS Verlag für Sozialwissenschaften. doi:10.1007/978-3-531-90895-3_9

Link, B. G., & Phelan, J. (1995). Social conditions as fundamental causes of disease. *Journal of Health and Social Behavior, 35*(Extra Issue), 80–94.

Lyngstad, T. H., Noack, T., & Tufte, P. A. (2010). Pooling of economic resources: A comparison of Norwegian married and cohabiting couples. *European Sociological Review, 27*(5), 624–635. doi:10.1093/esr/jcq028

Martinez, M., Schröttle, M., Condon, S., Springer-Kremser, M., Timmerman, G., Hagemann-White, C., et al. (2006). *State of European research on the prevalence of interpersonal violence and its impact on health and human rights*. Co-ordination Action on Human Rights Violations (CAHRV).

Martiny, D., & Schwab, D. (2002). Grounds for divorce and maintenance between former spouses: Germany. *Commission on European Family Law*. http://ceflonline.net/wp-content/uploads/Germany-Divorce.pdf. Accessed July 05, 2014.

McCoy, J. (2005). Spouse support disorder: An overview of problems in current alimony law. *Florida State University Law Review, 33*, 501–526.

Meyer, S. (2012). Why women stay: A theoretical examination of rational choice and moral reasoning in the context of intimate partner violence. *Australian and New Zealand Journal of Criminology, 45*(2), 179–193. doi:10.1177/0004865812443677

Ministry of Health. (2011). *The National Health and Care Plan 2011–2015* (No. 16, 2010–2011). Oslo, Norway.

Ministry of Justice and Public Security. (2012). *Action plan against domestic violence 2012*. Norway: Oslo.

Ministry of Justice and the Police. (2004). *Domestic violence action plan (2004–2007)*. Norway: Oslo.

Misra, J., Moller, S., & Budig, M. J. (2007). Work family policies and poverty for partnered and single women in Europe and North America. *Gender and Society, 21*(6), 804–827. doi:10.1177/0891243207308445

Modi, M. N., Palmer, S., & Armstrong, A. (2014). The role of Violence Against Women Act in addressing intimate partner violence: A public health issue. *Journal of Women's Health, 23*(3), 253–259. doi:10.1089/jwh.2013.4387

Moe, A. M., & Bell, M. P. (2004). Abject economics. *Violence Against Women, 10*(1), 29–55. doi:10.1177/1077801203256016

Moxnes, K. (1991). *Kjernesprengning i familien? Familieforandring ved samlivsbrudd og dannelse av nye samliv [Destroying the core of the family? Family change during breakups and the formation of new relationships]*. Oslo, Norway: Universitetsforlaget.

Müller, U., & Schröttle, M. (2004). *Lebensituation, Sicherheit und Gesundheit von Frauen in Deutschland: Eine repräsentative Untersuchung zu Gewalt gegen Frauen in Deutschland [Health, well-being and personal safety of women in Germany: A representative study of violence against women in Germany]*. Berlin: Bundesministerium für Familie, Senioren, Frauen und Jugend.

Nakonezny, P. A., Shull, R. D., & Rodgers, J. L. (1995). The effect of no-fault divorce law on the divorce rate across the 50 states and its relation to income, education, and religiosity. *Journal of Marriage and the Family, 57*(2), 477–488. doi:10.2307/353700

National Network to End Domestic Violence. (2012). *Domestic violence counts 2012: A 24-hour census of domestic violence shelters and services*. Washington, DC.

Noack, T. (2001). Cohabitation in Norway: An accepted and gradually more regulated way of living. *International Journal of Law, Policy and the Family, 15*(1), 102–117. doi:10.1093/lawfam/15.1.102

OECD. (2003). *Benefits and wages: Germany 2003*. http://www.oecd.org/social/soc/36215432.pdf. Accessed May 09, 2013.

OECD. (2013). Cohabitation rate and prevalence of other forms of partnership. *OECD family database*. http://www.oecd.org/els/soc/SF3_3_Cohabitation_rate_and_prevalence_of_other_forms_of_partnership_Jan2013.pdf. Accessed May 09, 2013.

Olafsdottir, S. (2007). Fundamental causes of health disparities: Stratification, the welfare state, and health in the United States and Iceland. *Journal of Health and Social Behavior, 48*(3), 239–253. doi:10.1177/002214650704800303

Orloff, A. (1996). Gender in the welfare state. *Annual Review of Sociology, 22*(1), 51–78. doi:10.1146/annurev.soc.22.1.51

Ostner, I. (2001). Cohabitation in Germany—Rules, reality and public discourses. *International Journal of Law, Policy and the Family, 15*(1), 88–101. doi:10.1093/lawfam/15.1.88

Pearson, J., Thoennes, N., & Griswold, E. A. (1999). Child support and domestic violence: The victims speak out. *Violence Against Women, 5*(4), 427–448. doi:10.1177/10778019922181293

Peter, T. (2006). Domestic violence in the United States and Sweden: A welfare state typology comparison within a power resources framework. *Women's Studies International Forum, 29*, 96–107. doi:10.1016/j.wsif.2005.10.001

Peters, H. E., Argys, L. M., Maccoby, E. E., & Mnookin, R. H. (1993). Enforcing divorce settlements: Evidence from child support compliance and award modifications. *Demography, 30*(4), 719–735. doi:10.2307/2061815

Pfau-Effinger, B. (1998). Gender cultures and the gender arrangement—A theoretical framework for cross-national gender research. *Innovation: The European Journal of Social Science Research, 11*(2), 147–166. doi:10.1080/13511610.1998.9968559

Pfau-Effinger, B. (2012). Women's employment in the institutional and cultural context. *International Journal of Sociology and Social Policy, 32*(9), 530–543. doi:10.1108/01443331211257634

Postmus, J. L., Severson, M., Berry, M., & Yoo, J. A. (2009). Women's experiences of violence and seeking help. *Violence Against Women, 15*, 852–868. doi:10.1177/1077801209334445

Ray, R., Gornick, J. C., & Schmitt, J. (2010). Who cares? Assessing generosity and gender equality in parental leave policy designs in 21 countries. *Journal of European Social Policy, 20*(3), 196–216. doi:10.1177/0958928710364434

Rice, T., Rosenau, P., Unruh, L. Y., & Barnes, A. J. (2013). United States of America: Health system review. *Health Systems in Transition, 15*(3), 1–431 (European Observatory on Health Systems and Policies).

Ringard, Å., Sagan, A., Saunes, I. S., & Lindahl, A. K. (2013). Norway: Health system review. *Health Systems in Transition, 15*(18), 1–162 (European Observatory on Health Systems and Policies).

Rodríguez, M., Valentine, J. M., Son, J. B., & Muhammad, M. (2009). Intimate partner violence and barriers to mental health care for ethnically diverse populations of women. *Trauma, Violence, and Abuse, 10*(4), 358–374. doi:10.1177/1524838009339756

Salize, H. J., Rössler, W., & Becker, T. (2007). Mental health care in Germany: Current state and trends. *European Archives of Psychiatry and Clinical Neuroscience, 257*(2), 92–103. doi:10.1007/s00406-006-0696-9

Saur, R., Hustad, A. E., & Heir, T. (2011). *Violence prevention in Norway: Activities and measures to prevent violence in close relationships*. Oslo, Norway: Norwegian Centre for Violence and Traumatic Stress Studies (NKVTS).

Scott, E. K., London, A. S., & Myers, N. A. (2002). Dangerous dependencies. *Gender and Society, 16*, 878–897. doi:10.1177/089124302237893

Skevik, A., & Hatland, A. (2008). Family policies in Norway. In I. Ostner & C. Schmitt (Eds.), *Family policies in the context of family change: The Nordic countries in comparative perspective* (pp. 89–107). Wiesbaden: VS Verlag für Sozialwissenschaften. doi:10.1007/978-3-531-90895-3_5

Stelmaszekn, B., & Fisher, H. (2012). *Country report 2012: Reality check on data collection and European services for women and children survivors of violence: A right for protection and support?*. Vienna, Austria: WAVE Network.

Stöckl, H., Heise, L., & Watts, C. (2011). Factors associated with violence by a current partner in a nationally representative sample of German women. *Sociology of Health and Illness, 33*(5), 694–709. doi:10.1111/j.1467-9566.2011.01319.x

Strand, A. H. H. (2012). *The welfare state matters: On the economic consequences of partnership dissolution in Norway and Britain*. University of Bergen. Retrieved from https://bora.uib.no/bitstream/handle/1956/6174/Dr.thesis_AnneHegeHendenStrand.pdf?sequence=1. Accessed April 11, 2014.

Sverdrup, T. (2002). Grounds for divorce and maintenance between former spouses: Norway. *Commission on European Family Law*. http://ceflonline.net/wp-content/uploads/Norway-Divorce.pdf. Accessed April 11, 2014.

Swanberg, J., & Logan, T. (2007). Intimate partner violence, employment and the workplace: An interdisciplinary perspective. *Journal of Interpersonal Violence, 22*(3), 263–267. doi:10.1177/0886260506295379

Syltevik, L. J. (1999). Endret velferdspolitikk for alenemødre—Fra relasjonelt til individualisert alenemoderskap [Changing welfare policies for lone mothers—From relational to individualistic lone motherhood]. *Tidsskrift for velferdsforskning, 2*, 85–101.

Thomas, K. A., Joshi, M., Wittenberg, E., & McCloskey, L. A. (2008). Intersections of harm and health: A qualitative study of intimate partner violence in women's lives. *Violence Against Women, 14*, 1252–1273. doi:10.1177/1077801208324529

van Damme, M., Kalmijn, M., & Uunk, W. (2009). The employment of separated women in Europe: Individual and institutional determinants. *European Sociological Review, 25*(2), 183–197. doi:10.1093/esr/jcn042

Whitaker, M. P. (2014). Linking community protective factors to intimate partner violence perpetration. *Violence Against Women, 20*(11), 1338–1359.

WHO. (2005). *WHO multi-country study on women's health and domestic violence against women: Initial results on prevalence, health outcomes and women's responses*. Geneva.

Wilson, K. S., Silberberg, M. R., Brown, A. J., & Yaggy, S. D. (2007). Health needs and barriers to healthcare of women who have experienced intimate partner violence. *Journal of Women's Health, 16*, 1485–1498. doi:10.1089/jwh.2007.0385

Wisdom, J. P., Berlin, M., & Lapidus, J. A. (2005). Relating health policy to women's health outcomes. *Social Science and Medicine, 61*, 1776–1784. doi:10.1016/j.socscimed.2005.03.030

Wuest, J., Ford-Gilboe, M., Merritt-Gray, M., & Lemire, S. (2006). Using grounded theory to generate a theoretical understanding of the effects of child custody policy on women's health promotion in the context of intimate partner violence. *Health Care for Women International, 27*(6), 490–512. doi:10.1080/07399330600770221

Chapter 10
Conclusion

Abstract This book sets out to address the issue of health inequities experienced by IPV survivors and identify areas where social policy may be able to intervene. This involved investigating at the individual level: to what extent social position impacts IPV exposure; and to what extent women with IPV exposure are more vulnerable to social position's impact on health. Whether the poorer health outcomes of IPV survivors are structurally produced through social policy was also examined. In particular, whether social position's impact on IPV exposure is reflective of family policies supporting women in establishing independent households and whether the vulnerabilities to social position's impact on health among IPV survivors are reflective of national health policies affecting access to care. This final chapter begins with a discussion of the main findings related to each of the research questions and their theoretical implications. This is followed by a brief look at the general limitations, as well as some suggestions for future research. Based on the conceptual framework, implications for welfare policy are also discussed, before closing with some final thoughts regarding the health inequities of IPV survivors.

This book sets out to address the issue of health inequities experienced by IPV survivors and identifies areas where social policy may be able to intervene. This involved investigating at the individual level: to what extent social position impacts IPV exposure (RQ1); and to what extent women with IPV exposure are more vulnerable to social position's impact on health (RQ2). Whether the poorer health outcomes of IPV survivors are structurally produced through social policy was also examined. In particular, whether social position's impact on IPV exposure is reflective of family policies supporting women in establishing independent households (RQ3) and whether the vulnerabilities to social position's impact on health among IPV survivors are reflective of national health policies affecting access to care (RQ4). Specifically, social position was measured using indicators of household income, education, and employment, while health was measured using indicators of self-assessed health and mental health complaints. To assess IPV exposure, measures of physical and sexual abuse from a current or former partner were combined, and a measurement of severity via injury from abuse was created. In answering these questions, this research makes several important contributions to

© Springer International Publishing Switzerland 2016

M.M. Larsen, *Health Inequities Related to Intimate Partner Violence Against Women*, Social Disparities in Health and Health Care,
DOI 10.1007/978-3-319-29565-7_10

the literature on IPV exposure, health inequities, and social policy. First, it reveals context-specific nuances in the intersections between social position and IPV exposure and their impact on health, which has often been neglected in the research from a gendered and feminist perspective. Second, it does this using nationally representative data covering a broader spectrum of socioeconomic, IPV, and health outcomes than is often available in community-based studies. Third, and perhaps most importantly, this research applies a cross-national comparative approach in order to assess the role of institutional welfare arrangements in the health inequities of IPV survivors, which has been missing in the literature until now.

This final chapter begins with a discussion of the main findings related to each of the research questions and their theoretical implications. This is followed by a brief look at the general limitations, as well as some suggestions for future research. Based on the conceptual framework, implications for welfare policy are also discussed, before closing with some final thoughts regarding the health inequities of IPV survivors.

10.1 Discussion of Findings

Throughout this work a conceptual framework was applied arguing that differential exposure to IPV and differential vulnerability to poor health are two primary mechanisms driving health inequities for survivors of IPV. The hypotheses related to *differential exposure to IPV* were informed by two different bodies of theory. At the individual level, it was assumed that women's socioeconomic resources impact their ability to exercise agency so that limited resources increase their dependence on male partners, making it difficult to exit relationships, and therefore, potentially increases their risk of IPV. Thus, at the individual level, it was expected that household income, education, and employment shape women's abilities to exit (potentially) abusive relationships. At the macro-level, Hobson's (1990) and Orloff's (1993) theories of defamilization and women's economic dependencies related to the welfare state served as the foundation. Based on their theories, it was assumed that institutional arrangements affecting *women's abilities to establish independent households* was the policy entry point shaping women's decisions about exiting abusive relationships, thereby also shaping their IPV exposure. In particular, family policies were considered regarding parental leave, childcare provision and the organization of the school day, family and child allowances, flexible working time arrangements, and taxation systems.

Furthermore, to inform the hypotheses related to *differential vulnerability to poor health*, theoretical literature on both health care access and health inequalities was referenced. In particular, Penchansky and Thomas' (1981) 'affordability' and 'availability' aspects of access to care were applied. These have to do with the financial costs of health care in relation to the patients' ability and readiness to pay for care, as well whether the supply of health care providers is sufficient for meeting the health care needs of the population. Moreover, when looking at issues of equity,

Table 10.1 Overview of final results

	Hypotheses[a]	Predictors	Outcomes		
			IPV	SAH	Mental health
Chapter 7: Differential exposure to IPV	1a	Household income	/	–	–
	1b	Education	/	–	–
	1c	Employment	/	–	–
Chapter 8: Differential vulnerability to poor health	$2a_1$, $2a_4$	Household income	–	✓	✓
	$2a_2$, $2a_5$	Education	–	✓	/
	$2a_3$, $2a_6$	Employment	–	✓	x
	2b	IPV exposure	–	✓	✓
	$2c_1$, $2c_4$	Household income*IPV exposure	–	/	x
	$2c_2$, $2c_5$	Education*IPV exposure	–	x	x
	$2c_3$, $2c_6$	Employment*IPV exposure	–	x	x
Chapter 9: Comparing the policy context	3	Social gradient in IPV/country	/	–	–
	4a	Social gradient in health/country	–	✓	/
	4b	IPV's impact on health/country	–	✓	✓
	4c	Social position*IPV/country	–	✓	x

✓ confirmed, x not confirmed, / mixed results, – not applicable
[a]Hypotheses simplified for presentation purposes

Whitehead's (2000) concept of equal 'entitlement' to health care was also used, which argues for equal access to care according to need. Thus, at the individual level, it was assumed that social position shapes women's access to health care and thereby their health outcomes. Moreover, it was expected that IPV exposure has an additional influence on health, beyond what can be explained by social position, and that IPV exposure magnifies social position's impact on health. At the macro-level, it was assumed that institutional arrangements enabling *access to health care* would be the policy entry point improving the health outcomes of IPV survivors in lower social positions. Specifically, health policies were considered addressing entitlement to health care, affordability of care, and availability of providers. Table 10.1 provides a brief overview of the results presented in this book. For each hypothesis, it is specified whether the results confirmed the assumptions for the corresponding outcomes.[1]

[1]For detailed descriptions of the hypotheses, please refer to Chaps. 7, 8, and 9.

10.1.1 Findings on Differential Exposure to IPV

A key finding of the research was that higher levels of social position were generally related to lower IPV exposure in the US, Germany, and Norway. Interestingly, the results also demonstrated distinctive patterns across the countries, meaning that not all social position indicators were equally important for all countries. Given the extensiveness of Norway's dual-earner family policies, as compared to the US's market-oriented policies, and Germany's family policies which presupposed a male breadwinner/female (part-time) carer norm, it was hypothesized that social position's impact on IPV exposure would be generally smaller in Norway, and greater in the US and Germany. However, the empirical evidence suggests that the policy link is less straightforward, but is still reflective of national differences in family policy arrangements.

For instance, higher levels of household income predicted lower levels of exposure for the US and Germany. In the US, it was argued that the lack of institutional supports for women's dual roles as earners and carers, today as well as in the mid-1990s, makes it more difficult to maintain economic independence through labor market participation, thereby increasing the risk of IPV exposure associated with lower household incomes either during or after a relationship. Within the context of male breadwinner/female part-time carer arrangements found in Germany, particularly in the early 2000s, women who became single parents did not fit the typical mold for benefits from the welfare state and faced greater risk of poverty after dissolution of a partnership (Hansen et al. 2006; Strand 2012). This may have negatively influenced women's decisions to exit abusive relationships, thereby contributing to the association between IPV exposure and lower household income either during or after a relationship. Moreover, it is noteworthy that household income did not prove to be empirically related to IPV exposure in Norway. This reflects to some degree the institutional supports available for women to offset financial losses due to relationship dissolution, both today and in the early 2000s, such as family and cash-for-care allowances, as well as the transitional allowance for newly single parents.

Meanwhile, being employed was the strongest predictor of decreased risk of IPV exposure for the Norwegian sample, but it did not play a role in either the US or Germany. Norwegian family policy emphasizes employment as the best strategy to improve living standards and simultaneously discourages long gaps between employment for both men and women. This is accomplished using daylong childcare available after the age of one, subsidized activities for school-age children to fill the gap between the end of the school day and the end of the work day, flexible working arrangements for parents, and the continuing education available to single parents to help them improve their employment chances. Thus, employment offers women greater opportunities for establishing independent households. Notably, the present findings also suggest that the minority of women who are not employed may be neglected within Norway's institutional arrangements, and may not have the resources necessary to exit abusive relationships.

Another important observation was that education was related to IPV exposure in all three countries. For the US and Norway, increased education was related to lower IPV exposure, while in Germany, increased education was related to increased risk of minor IPV (i.e., IPV without injury). Women in the US and Norwegian samples with fewer years of education, especially those with less than a high school education, had an increased risk of severe IPV exposure. Regardless of household income, a lack of education may increase women's economic dependence on a partner and make it more difficult to exit an abusive relationship. However, the traditional *gender culture* interacting with Germany's family policies may affect minor IPV exposure when male partners with traditional gendered ideologies feel threatened by female partners' education levels.

Taken together, these results stress the importance of considering women's socioeconomic resources within the context of IPV, implying that increased resources generally serve as a protection against IPV exposure by enabling women to exit abusive relationships. Even more, policies which support women's economic independence and their abilities to establish independent households appear to also have an influence on the social gradient in IPV exposure. Additionally, in line with previous research (Budig et al. 2012), the results demonstrate the need to also consider the interaction between policy and the gender culture. While the importance of macro-level factors for IPV exposure has been theorized (e.g., Heise 1998), there have been only a limited number of attempts to link these together (e.g., Kaya and Cook 2010; Whitaker 2014). In this sense, the research presented in this book bridges the divide between gendered welfare state literature and the literature on the risk factors related to IPV. That the impact of social position on IPV exposure can be so nuanced depending on the specific national policy context is a meaningful contribution to the literature, implying that policy can indeed affect IPV exposure.

10.1.2 Findings on Differential Vulnerability to Poor Health

Related to vulnerability to poor health, there were a number of noteworthy findings presented in this book. First, the results demonstrated a social gradient in health for the US, Germany, and Norway. Specifically, not being employed, as well as lower levels of household income and education, was related to increased odds of poor self-assessed health for all three countries. Additionally, lower household income predicted more mental health complaints in both the US and Norway, as did fewer years of education in the US. In Germany, however, the greatest levels of mental health complaints were reported among those with high household income but low levels of education, and those with high levels of education but low household income.

Second, the empirical results also demonstrated that IPV exposure within the past five years negatively contributed to health outcomes beyond what was attributable to social position. Specifically, in the US and Germany, severe IPV exposure (i.e., IPV exposure with injury) nearly doubled the odds of poor self-assessed health. In Norway, those with either minor or severe IPV exposure had odds of poor self-assessed health that were more than twice as high as for women without exposure. Moreover, the incident rate for mental health complaints was also nearly twice as high for those in Germany and Norway with severe IPV exposure. Meanwhile, in the US, both minor and severe IPV exposures lead to higher incident rates of mental health complaints. Given that lower social positions co-occurred with IPV exposure in all three countries, this empirical evidence provided support for further examining whether social position and IPV exposure produce susceptibilities to one another.

Regarding IPV exposure's moderating effect on the relationship between social position and health, the empirical evidence indicated that social position's impact on health increased with IPV exposure for the US data. Specifically, the effect of household income on poor self-assessed health was strongest for those with severe IPV exposure. Women in the US at the lowest household income levels with severe IPV exposure were the most vulnerable to poor self-assessed health, being more than twice as likely as women with a history of minor or no IPV exposure to report poor self-assessed health. Conversely, at higher levels of household income, there was very little difference in the probabilities of poor self-assessed health based on women's IPV exposure. These findings imply two things for the US sample. First, the lack of financial resources represented a serious risk for poor self-assessed health among women with severe IPV exposure. Second, the risk of poor self-assessed health levels out as household income increases, regardless of IPV exposure. However, such an effect was not found for mental health complaints in the US, or for either health outcome in Germany or Norway.

In Chap. 9, it was argued that this cross-national difference in vulnerability to poor self-assessed health among IPV survivors with limited household income may have to do with cross-national differences in policies related to entitlement and affordability of health care. Up until recently, health care coverage was not considered an entitlement in the US. Instead, it has been primarily attained via employment status, meaning that women who were economically dependent on their abusive partners may also have relied on their partner for health insurance. Likewise, ending a relationship may have left economically dependent women without employment or only part-time employment and either uninsured or reliant upon Medicaid. Related to this, high health care costs in the US, especially for the uninsured, may have prevented women with lower household income with severe IPV exposure from seeking the care they needed.[2] In contrast, the principle of equal entitlement to care according to medical need is incorporated throughout Norway's health policy, ensuring women's access to care without relying on a partner. While health care coverage is related to social insurance contributions via employment in Germany, in the early 2000s as well as today, there are mechanisms in place that

[2]It is acknowledged, of course, that in addition to financial costs there are a great number of barriers preventing IPV survivors from accessing the health care they need in the US (e.g., fear of judgment, issues of confidentiality, and conflicts with transportation or scheduling). However, given the prevalence of barriers associated with cost (Postmus et al. 2009; Wilson et al. 2007), this is the primary focus of the research presented in this book.

help make sure that women maintain their health insurance when establishing an independent household (e.g., insurance for part-time employment and the unemployed, contributions relative to income). Moreover, both countries continue to have annual ceilings and/or cost-sharing exemptions to ensure affordability of care and limit private out-of-pocket costs. Altogether, this suggests that lack of entitlement and minimal regulation of health care costs in the US may partially explain the empirical evidence found for vulnerabilities to poor self-assessed health among low-income women with severe IPV exposure. On the flip side, this suggests that universal entitlement to care, as well as measures ensuring the affordability of health care, has a protective effect against the double burden of low social position and IPV exposure.

However, no evidence of differential vulnerabilities according to education or employment was found for any of the three countries. It has been previously shown that income, education, and employment are not interchangeable measures of social position (Geyer et al. 2006). Thus, it is conceivable that lower levels of education and unemployment alone are not sufficient for creating the same vulnerabilities to poor health for IPV survivors as those created by limited financial resources, especially in contexts without universal entitlement to health care and without mechanisms controlling out-of-pocket costs. In this particular type of health policy context—where health insurance is not guaranteed even for the employed, and where costs are high for both the insured and the uninsured—access to financial resources appears to be the deciding factor for IPV survivors' overall health.

A surprising observation was that no evidence of differential vulnerability to poor mental health among IPV survivors was found for any of the three countries. Comparison of cross-national differences in health policy hints at vulnerabilities, so questions remain as to why this was not evident for mental health outcomes. As described in Sect. 9.2, this is quite contrary to what might be expected given the substantial effect of IPV exposure on mental health and the tremendous gap in health insurance coverage for mental health services in the US as opposed to Germany and Norway. In Sect. 8.3 the possibility was discussed that the mental health variable was not sensitive enough to detect significant interactions. Thus, it is essential that further theorizing and investigation into the generation of vulnerabilities to poor mental health for IPV survivors be done.

In summary, the evidence presented supports the conceptual framework proposed for the generation of health inequities for IPV survivors. The empirical evidence confirms the negative health consequences of IPV exposure for three countries diverse in both their approach to violence against women and to health. Moreover, although it has been argued theoretically, up until now there has been only minimal empirical research suggesting that limited income and IPV exposure magnify their impact on health. The present research helps fill this gap by establishing the vulnerabilities created by household income and IPV exposure in the US, and acknowledging that it may overpower any possible vulnerabilities related to education or employment in the US context. Importantly, the findings presented in this book trace the link between policy and health inequities for IPV survivors from a cross-national perspective, addressing a critical gap in the literature and opening up a discussion of where social policy can intervene to reduce these inequities.

10.2 Critical Issues

Like all research, the research detailed in this book was subject to limitations. Those issues specific to the analyses were described in detail at the end of Chaps. 7, 8, and 9. Therefore, the current section will focus on more general issues.

First, it bears repeating that causal claims could not be made based on the use of cross-sectional data. Although unobserved heterogeneity in the data was reduced as much as possible, it remains a possibility that it has biased the effects of the variables of interest. Therefore, in practice, empirical associations between the variables were reported, which were then used to test hypotheses grounded in a conceptual framework assuming causality.

Second, this research was based on data from three different national prevalence surveys on violence against women: the US's *National Violence Against Women Survey*, the *Health, Well-Being, and Safety of Women in Germany Survey*, and Norway's *Survey of Everyday Safety*. These data sets were not designed to be directly comparable and have methodological differences which require consideration in their comparison. Thus, it remains a possibility that some of the cross-national differences observed in the analyses may have been due to slight differences in measurement and operationalization of the key variables of interest. Moreover, cultural differences in replying to sensitive questions regarding health and experiences of violence cannot be ruled out. These are issues facing a great number of attempts at comparing data on violence against women. Even so, cross-national comparison is vital to understanding the risk factors for IPV exposure and it consequences. Therefore, to minimize the impact of this critical issue, a structured approach recommended for comparing national data sets on violence against women and health was applied (Schröttle et al. 2006). This involved harmonization of the three data sets, including comprehensive documentation of (1) the similarities and differences across surveys in sampling, methodology, and data collection; (2) the exact definitions of violence, health, reference groups, and age groups to be analyzed; and (3) consideration of methodological influences on the outcomes in the data. These exhaustive efforts should increase confidence in the patterns found in the empirical evidence.

Finally, the use of somewhat older data sets was necessitated by the fact that nationally representative data on violence against women and health are not typically collected on a frequent or ongoing basis.[3] For example, the most recent

[3]A recent exception to this is the US's National Intimate Partner and Sexual Violence Survey which began in 2010 as an annual survey conducted by the CDC, NIJ, and Department of Defense

available data for the US were collected in 1995–1996, while the most recent data for Germany were collected in 2003, and in 2003–2004 for Norway. Therefore, the present cross-national comparison of policy contexts only considered institutional arrangements corresponding to the period of data collection of the respective surveys. It goes without saying, however, that welfare policy is not static. Since these surveys were conducted, a number of important reforms have taken place in the US and Germany, with more minor reforms in Norway.

Perhaps most notable in the IPV literature is the US's 'welfare reform' which went into effect in 1997, placing a 5-year lifetime maximum on assistance for low-income families and requiring beneficiaries to be employed within two years, regardless of the age of children and the affordability of childcare (Christopher 2004; Kamerman and Kahn 2001; Olsen 2007). A major point of contention is that this reform increased women's dependencies on partners and that it was particularly dangerous for women in abusive relationships, despite the exceptions made for women in abusive relationships (Brandwein 1999; Green and Brownell 2007; Scott et al. 2002). In light of these reforms, one might expect to find that lower household income continues to be related to more IPV exposure, perhaps to an even greater degree than what was presented in this book. Even more recently, the US health care reform of 2010 requires all Americans to purchase health insurance, expands Medicaid coverage for the low-income, disallows discrimination on the private health insurance market based on gender or health history, and seeks to bring health care costs under control (Rice et al. 2013). The degree to which this reform is successful remains to be seen, but access to health care in the US will likely improve. One could therefore speculate that the interaction between household income and IPV would have a somewhat decreased effect on health today than it did in the present analyses from the mid-1990s.

Germany's health care system also underwent reform in the past decade, resulting in some shifting of costs to patients in the form of co-payments for physician's visits and prescription medications. It is argued that this may limit access for low-income populations (Gerlinger 2010). Even so, it is unlikely that such reforms would substantially change the results presented in this book. In the meantime, there has also been a push toward 'sustainable family policy' (*nachhaltige Familienpolitik*) in Germany, which has included expansion of childcare places for younger children and the introduction of an income replacement benefit during parental leave (*Elterngeld*) (Leitner 2011; Ray 2008). Thus, the assumption of Germany as strictly a male breadwinner/female part-time carer model needs to be reexamined (Ostner 2010). In this case, one might expect to find employment playing a slightly larger role for IPV exposure today in Germany as compared to the early 2000s.

(Footnote 3 continued)

(Black et al. 2011). However, the data were not publically available when analysis for this book began.

Finally, even further expansion of family policy has also occurred in Norway, with the establishment in 2009 of the legal right to childcare, with 97 % of children aged three to five and 80 % of children aged one to two attending childcare (Eydal and Rostgaard 2011). Thus, it could be speculated that the role of employment for IPV exposure for Norway might be even larger today than what was presented in this book. Despite these changes in the policy landscapes, however, the lessons drawn from this research remain valid from a broader standpoint. These results illustrate the links between social position, IPV exposure, and health within specific policy contexts and offer important insights into how policy is intertwined with women's lives. The conclusions regarding which policies are most protective against IPV exposure and poor health outcomes offer crucial lessons for continued improvement of policy, which are relevant across many different policy contexts.

10.3 Suggestions for Further Research

These results give rise to several suggestions for future research. First, ongoing research could expand upon this work using a broader spectrum of welfare states. The US, Germany, and Norway were selected as cases based on their differences in policies affecting social stratification, women's abilities to establish independent households, and access to health care. These three countries are often considered prototypes of liberal, conservative, and social democratic welfare states, respectively, but welfare states falling into the same categories can still differ significantly in their family and health policies (Kasza 2002). This opens two potential lines of research: further testing the hypotheses using other similar welfare states (e.g., Australia, France, Denmark, respectively) to examine whether similar patterns emerge; and/or dissimilar welfare states (e.g., Southern or Central and Eastern European welfare states) to discover what other types of patterns may emerge from the data (Szikra and Szelewa 2010). This would be helpful for determining whether the results for the US, Germany, and Norway hold up to further testing. Of course, this would be dependent upon nationally representative data on violence and health that is also available to researchers for secondary analysis.

Relatedly, access to cross-nationally comparable data on health and violence against women would improve the specificity of conclusions drawn regarding social policy's effects on health inequities. This type of data would allow the appropriate policy indicators (e.g., number of fully paid weeks of maternity leave, private out-of-pocket payments in percent of total health expenditure) to be linked to individual outcomes using multi-level statistical modeling. It would also allow for the comparison of a greater number of countries at one time. This would extend the spectrum of social policies under consideration and potentially reveal more detailed patterns in the relationships between social position, IPV exposure, health, and social policy. An example of such data is the 2012 cross-national survey on health and violence against women conducted by the EU Agency for Fundamental Rights (2014) among 42,000 women in all 28 member states of the EU. To its advantage, the data are based on a standardized questionnaire and data collection procedures. Released to the public in late 2015, it could drastically improve upon the methodological restrictions present in this book's research, although cultural differences across countries would still need to be considered. Such data would also extend the present analysis by allowing a more current examination of policy entry points in the generation of health inequities for IPV survivors, reflective of the latest reforms in family and health policy.

As mentioned previously, the lack of significant findings for vulnerabilities to poor mental health requires continued investigation. Although the differences in policy contexts would indicate vulnerabilities for IPV survivors to poor mental health according to social position, this was not found in the data. Perhaps finer measures of mental health or IPV exposure would reveal such vulnerabilities. Alternatively, it is also possible that the conceptual framework for mental health outcomes does not hold up with IPV as a moderator and must therefore be reconsidered.

The connection between increased education and increased risk of minor IPV in Germany also deserves further research. Although it was speculated that a potential imbalance in resources between partners may be threatening for male partners holding traditional gender ideologies, this was not tested directly. Using a sample of women in current partnerships and sociodemographic information for their partners, it would be worthwhile to assess whether women with higher levels of education than their partners are indeed at risk of greater risk of IPV. Additionally, the interaction between household income and education in its effect on mental health in Germany is worthy of further investigation. Qualitative research may be useful for exploring in greater detail why women in Germany living with household incomes inconsistent with their education reported a higher number of mental health complaints than women with more consistent income and education.

Finally, given the limitations present in the national data analyzed, this book operated under mostly heteronormative assumptions regarding IPV. In essence, socioeconomic resources were understood to play a role in IPV exposure and health outcomes, but assumed this was also influenced by a patriarchal structure steeped in hegemonic masculinity.[4] However, a growing body of literature demonstrates that IPV also occurs in homosexual relationships, seemingly with similar rates (Freedberg 2006) and patterns (Renzetti 1992), and with similar influences of individual-level factors (Jeffries and Ball 2008). Yet, it is clear that conclusions based on research of men's violence against women cannot simply be carried over to homosexual relationships. Instead, further research is needed to understand the specific intersections of gender, sexuality, and power involved in abusive relationships among lesbian, gay, bisexual, and transgender individuals. Moreover, it is necessary to consider the macro-level social dynamics that may additionally play a role in exiting abusive relationships (e.g., homophobia, limited services available

[4]Hegemonic masculinity is a sociological understanding of the social norms men need to adhere to in order to be legitimized as men (Connell 1995).

for homosexual survivors of IPV) (Oliffe et al. 2014; St Pierre and Senn 2010). These may be crucial for improved understanding of the generation of health inequities for IPV survivors.

10.4 Policy Implications

The discovery of policy intervention points preventing the generation of health inequities for IPV survivors was one of the main drivers of the present research. The results point toward the intertwining of social policy with the health outcomes for women who have been exposed to violence by a partner. In addition to the implications for family policy in addressing differential exposure to IPV, there are also implications for policies related to social stratification and those affecting the impact of social position on health.

To begin, the results imply that IPV exposure can and should be addressed in a broad range of policy. While national action plans and criminal justice initiatives addressing violence against women are vital, they should go hand-in-hand with social policy ensuring that women have access to the socioeconomic resources necessary to exit violent relationships (Hahn and Postmus 2014). Broader structural approaches which address women's abilities to establish independent households are vital for reducing women's exposure to IPV (Davies et al. 2009; Purvin 2007). For policy contexts with institutional arrangements assuming women should balance work and caregiving responsibilities with help from the market, it is crucial to note that those with limited socioeconomic resources may instead find themselves in situations of economic dependency. Policies which strengthen women's ties to the labor market and decrease economic dependence on partners are necessary for increasing women's opportunities for preventing or ending abusive relationships. Such intervention could be in the form of paid parental leave, subsidized childcare, and flexible working arrangements. Moreover, policy makers should also aim at preventing poverty during the transition period after relationship dissolution. One particular example is Norway's transitional support for single parents, providing income, education, and employment assistance while single parents with small children get back on their feet. By increasing women's abilities to establish autonomous households, social policy can play a vital role for women exiting abusive relationships. Without these types of broader social policy support, criminal justice efforts toward curbing IPV will be for naught for women with limited socioeconomic resources.

These implications also apply to policy contexts which assume a primary breadwinner and part-time caregiver in the household. While these contexts provide a great deal of support for families, it is also necessary to broaden support to allow for the possibility of having both partners be full-time earners. This includes income replacement during parental leave, increasing childcare availability for children under the age of three, and extending childcare and school hours so that they do not conflict with a typical work schedule. This increases women's economic independence and gives them the voice to be able to exit relationships.

Additionally, policy contexts with an emphasis on employment activation and the encouragement of dual-earner families should also be aware of the vulnerabilities to IPV exposure existing for women who are not employed. Without employment, these women need special attention to enable them to establish an autonomous household and to recover from the consequences of IPV, which may have prevented their employment. Transitional assistance for single parents may also need to allow for extra support for those exiting abusive relationships without employment.

In developing a health system response to IPV, the most frequent approaches are improved recognition of IPV by physicians and health professionals through training, and consistent screening for IPV in health care settings (Brzank and Blättner 2010; McCaw and Kotz 2009; Plichta 2004). This is vital for "helping to identify abuse early, providing victims with the necessary treatment, and referring women to appropriate care. Health services must be places where women feel safe, are treated with respect, are not stigmatized, and where they can receive quality, informed support" (WHO 2005, p. vi). While these approaches are critical for addressing the health consequences of IPV, the present results suggest that they may be irrelevant if women's access to care is limited because they are not entitled to coverage or if costs are unaffordable. Particularly in a policy context without entitlement to health care and with minimal regulation of costs, the combination of low household income and IPV exposure magnifies the risk of poor physical health. Thus, it is not enough to screen for IPV in health care settings. Health policy makers should also ensure that women have entitlement to health care without dependence on a partner. Likewise, policy should include mechanisms which control the out-of-pocket costs of care so that women with IPV exposure can afford the health care they require. Especially in times of reform and economic difficulty for welfare states, these implications are also valuable lessons for health policy contexts which already have such systems in practice. In seeking to reform health policies and systems, the importance of ensuring access to care should not be forgotten for its ability to address health inequities for survivors of IPV.

10.5 Final Reflections

In this work, policy interventions were identified that address the special needs of IPV survivors in order to reduce their inequities in health. Importantly, empirical analysis was integrated with analysis of the policy context in order to capture the complexities of women's lives. Because the living conditions of IPV survivors are intricately connected to the setup of social policy, they are particularly sensitive to policy changes and their experiences are an important gauge of the effects of policy. Focusing specifically on a vulnerable group and the particular social policies likely to affect them directly highlights, perhaps more effectively than a one-size-fits-all strategy, where policy can intervene to stop the production of health inequities. In doing so, this book has illustrated how deeply entrenched IPV is in the social structure and that the most effective response is one that is interwoven into wider policies addressing the needs of all women.

> Until the issue of domestic violence is addressed as a social problem with universal provisions, this type of violence will continue to reach epidemic proportions—no matter how much work is done to combat such abuse (Peter 2006, p. 100).

References

Black, M. C., Basile, K. C., Breiding, M. J., Smith, S. G., Walters, M. L., Merrick, M. T., Stevens, M. R. (2011). *The National Intimate Partner and Sexual Violence Survey (NISVS): 2010 summary report*. Atlanta, GA: CDC

Brandwein, R. A. (1999). Family violence, women and welfare. In R. A. Brandwein (Ed.), *Battered women, children, and welfare reform: The ties that bind* (pp. 3–16). Thousand Oaks, CA: Sage Publications.

Brzank, P., & Blättner, B. (2010). Screening nach Gewalt gegen Frauen durch den Partner [Screening for violence against women by a partner]. *Bundesgesundheitsblatt - Gesundheitsforschung - Gesundheitsschutz, 53*(2), 221–232. doi:10.1007/s00103-009-1018-y

Budig, M. J., Misra, J., & Boeckmann, I. (2012). The motherhood penalty in cross-national perspective: The importance of work-family policies and cultural attitudes. *Social Politics: International Studies in Gender, State and Society, 19*(2), 163–193. doi:10.1093/sp/jxs006

Christopher, K. (2004). Welfare as we [don't] know it: A review and feminist critique of welfare reform research in the United States. *Feminist Economics, 10*(2), 143–171. doi:10.1080/1354570042000217757

Connell, R. W. (1995). *Masculinities*. Berkeley: University of California Press.

Davies, L., Ford-Gilboe, M., & Hammerton, J. (2009). Gender inequality and patterns of abuse post leaving. *Journal of Family Violence, 24*(1), 27–39. doi:10.1007/s10896-008-9204-5

European Union Agency for Fundamental Rights [FRA]. (2014). *Violence against women: An EU-wide survey*. Luxembourg. http://fra.europa.eu/sites/default/files/fra-2014-vaw-survey-main-results_en.pdf. Accessed November 1, 2014.

Eydal, G. B., & Rostgaard, T. (2011). Gender equality revisited—Changes in Nordic childcare policies in the 2000s. *Social Policy and Administration, 45*(2), 161–179. doi:10.1111/j.1467-9515.2010.00762.x

Freedberg, P. (2006). Health care barriers and same-sex intimate partner violence: A review of the literature. *Journal of Forensic Nursing, 2*(1), 15–24.

Gerlinger, T. (2010). Health care reform in Germany. *German Policy Studies, 6*(1), 107–142.

Geyer, S., Hemström, O., Peter, R., & Vågerö, D. (2006). Education, income, and occupational class cannot be used interchangeably in social epidemiology. Empirical evidence against a common practice. *Journal of Epidemiology and Community Health, 60*(9), 804–810. doi:10.1136/jech.2005.041319

Green, D. L., & Brownell, P. (2007). Poverty, women, welfare, work, and domestic violence. In *Battered women and their families: Intervention strategies and treatment programs* (3rd ed., pp. 423–450). New York, NY: Springer Publishing.

Hahn, S. A., & Postmus, J. L. (2014). Economic empowerment of impoverished IPV survivors: A review of best practice literature and implications for policy. *Trauma, Violence, and Abuse, 15* (2), 79–93. doi:10.1177/1524838013511541

Hansen, H.-T., Jürgens, O., Strand, A. H. H., & Voges, W. (2006). Poverty among households with children: A comparative study of Norway and Germany. *International Journal of Social Welfare, 15*(4), 269–279. doi:10.1111/j.1468-2397.2006.00469.x
Heise, L. (1998). Violence against women: An integrated, ecological framework. *Violence Against Women, 4*(3), 262–290.
Hobson, B. (1990). No exit, no voice: Women's economic dependency and the welfare state. *Acta Sociologica, 33*(3), 235–250. doi:10.1177/000169939003300305
Jeffries, S., & Ball, M. J. (2008). Male same-sex intimate partner violence: A descriptive review and call for further research. *Murdoch e-Law Review, 15*(1), 134–179.
Kamerman, S. B., & Kahn, A. J. (2001). Child and family policies in the United States at the opening of the twenty-first century. *Social Policy and Administration, 35*(1), 69–84. doi:10.1111/1467-9515.00220
Kasza, G. J. (2002). The illusion of welfare "regimes". *Journal of Social Policy, 31*(02), 271–287. doi:10.1017/S0047279401006584
Kaya, Y., & Cook, K. J. (2010). A cross-national analysis of physical intimate partner violence against women. *International Journal of Comparative Sociology, 51*(6), 423–444. doi:10.1177/0020715210386155
Leitner, S. (2011). Germany outpaces Austria in childcare policy: The historical contingencies of "conservative" childcare policy. *Journal of European Social Policy, 20*(5), 456–467. doi:10.1177/0958928710380482
McCaw, B., & Kotz, K. (2009). Developing a health system response to intimate partner violence. In C. Mitchell & D. Anglin (Eds.), *Intimate partner violence: A health-based perspective* (pp. 419–428). New York, NY: Oxford University Press.
Oliffe, J. L., Han, C., Maria, E. S., Lohan, M., Howard, T., Stewart, D. E., et al. (2014). Gay men and intimate partner violence: A gender analysis. *Sociology of Health and Illness, 36*(4), 564–579. doi:10.1111/1467-9566.12099
Olsen, G. M. (2007). Toward global welfare state convergence? Family policy and health care in Sweden, Canada and the United States. *Journal of Sociology and Social Welfare, 34*(2), 143–164.
Orloff, A. (1993). Gender and the social rights of citizenship: The comparative analysis of gender relations and welfare states. *American Sociological Review, 58*(3), 303–328.
Ostner, I. (2010). Farewell to the family as we know it: Family policy change in Germany. *German Policy Studies, 6*(1), 211–244.
Penchansky, R., & Thomas, J. W. (1981). The concept of access: Definition and relationship to consumer satisfaction. *Medical Care, 19*, 127–140.
Peter, T. (2006). Domestic violence in the United States and Sweden: A welfare state typology comparison within a power resources framework. *Women's Studies International Forum, 29*, 96–107. doi:10.1016/j.wsif.2005.10.001
Plichta, S. B. (2004). Intimate partner violence and physical health consequences: Policy and practice implications. *Journal of Interpersonal Violence, 19*(11), 1296–1323. doi:10.1177/0886260504269685
Postmus, J. L., Severson, M., Berry, M., & Yoo, J. A. (2009). Women's experiences of violence and seeking help. *Violence Against Women, 15*, 852–868. doi: 10.1177/1077801209334445
Purvin, D. M. (2007). At the crossroads and in the crosshairs: Social welfare policy and low-income women's vulnerability to domestic violence. *Social Problems, 54*(2), 188–210. doi:10.1525/sp.2007.54.2.188
Ray, R. (2008). *A detailed look at parental leave policies in 21 OECD countries*. Washington, DC: Center for Economic and Policy Research.
Renzetti, C. (1992). *Violent betrayal: Partner abuse in lesbian relationships*. Thousand Oaks, CA: Sage Publications.

Rice, T., Rosenau, P., Unruh, L. Y., & Barnes, A. J. (2013). United States of America: Health system review. *Health Systems in Transition, 15*(3), 1–431. European Observatory on Health Systems and Policies.

Schröttle, M., Martinez, M., Condon, S., Jaspard, M., Piispa, M., & Westerstrand, J., et al. (2006). *Comparative reanalysis of prevalence of violence against women and health impact data in Europe—Obstacles and possible solutions. Testing a comparative approach on selected studies.* http://www.cahrv.uni-osnabrueck.de/reddot/D_20_Comparative_reanalysis_of_prevalence_of_violence_pub.pdf. Accessed April 14, 2010.

Scott, E. K., London, A. S., & Myers, N. A. (2002). Dangerous dependencies. *Gender and Society, 16*, 878–897. doi:10.1177/089124302237893

St Pierre, M., & Senn, C. Y. (2010). External barriers to help-seeking encountered by Canadian gay and lesbian victims of intimate partner abuse: An application of the barriers model. *Violence and Victims, 25*(4), 536–552. doi:10.1891/0886-6708.25.4.536

Strand, A. H. H. (2012). *The welfare state matters: On the economic consequences of partnership dissolution in Norway and Britain.* Bergen: University of Bergen. https://bora.uib.no/bitstream/handle/1956/6174/Dr.thesis_Anne Hege Henden Strand.pdf?sequence=1. Accessed April 11, 2014.

Szikra, D., & Szelewa, D. (2010). Do Central and Eastern European countries fit the "Western" picture? The example of family policies in Hungary and Poland. In C. Klenner & S. Leiber (Eds.), *Welfare states and gender inequality in Central and Eastern Europe* (pp. 81–116). Brussels: ETUI.

Whitaker, M. P. (2014). Linking community protective factors to intimate partner violence perpetration. *Violence Against Women, 20*(11), 1338–1359. doi:10.1177/1077801214552854

Whitehead, M. (2000). *The concepts and principles of equity and health.* Copenhagen: WHO Regional Office for Europe.

WHO. (2005). *WHO multi-country study on women's health and domestic violence against women: Initial results on prevalence, health outcomes and women's responses.* Geneva: WHO.

Wilson, K. S., Silberberg, M. R., Brown, A. J., & Yaggy, S. D. (2007). Health needs and barriers to healthcare of women who have experienced intimate partner violence. *Journal of Women's Health, 16*, 1485–1498. doi: 10.1089/jwh.2007.0385

CPSIA information can be obtained
at www.ICGtesting.com
Printed in the USA
LVOW02*2228050516
486884LV00001B/48/P

9 783319 295633